Lecture Notes in Artificial Intelligence 1504

Subseries of Lecture Notes in Computer Science
Edited by J. G. Carbonell and J. Siekmann

Lecture Notes in Computer Science

Edited by G. Goos, J. Hartmanis and J. van Leeuwen

T0223088

Springer
Berlin
Heidelberg
New York
Barcelona
Budapest
Hong Kong
London
Milan
Paris
Singapore
Tokyo

Otthein Herzog   Andreas Günter (Eds.)

KI-98: Advances in Artificial Intelligence

22nd Annual German Conference
on Artificial Intelligence
Bremen, Germany, September 15-17, 1998
Proceedings

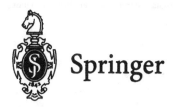

Springer

Series Editors

Jaime G. Carbonell, Carnegie Mellon University, Pittsburgh, PA, USA
Jörg Siekmann, University of Saarland, Saarbrücken, Germany

Volume Editors

Otthein Herzog
Andreas Günter
Universität Bremen, Technologie-Zentrum Informatik
Universitätsallee 22, D-28359 Bremen, Germany
E-mail: herzog@informatik.uni-bremen.de
         guenter@tzi.de

Cataloging-in-Publication Data applied for

Die Deutsche Bibliothek - CIP-Einheitsaufnahme

Advances in artificial intelligence : proceedings / KI-98, 22th
Annual German Conference on Artificial Intelligence, Bremen,
Germany, September 15 - 17, 1998. Otthein Herzog ; Andreas Günter
(ed.). - Berlin ; Heidelberg ; New York ; Barcelona ; Budapest ; Hong
Kong ; London ; Milan ; Paris ; Singapore ; Tokyo : Springer, 1998
  (Lecture notes in computer science ; Vol. 1504 : Lecture notes in
  artificial intelligence)
  ISBN 3-540-65080-6

CR Subject Classification (1991): I.2, J.3

ISBN 3-540-65080-6 Springer-Verlag Berlin Heidelberg New York

© Springer-Verlag Berlin Heidelberg 1998
Printed in Germany

Typesetting: Camera ready by author
SPIN 10638986   06/3142 – 5 4 3 2 1 0   Printed on acid-free paper

Preface

A central aspect of the annual conferences on Artificial Intelligence of the AI chapter of the "Gesellschaft für Informatik" is the presentation of research results. Apart from all contributions chosen by the program committee, the present volume additionally contains full papers of four of the six invited talks as well as a compilation of to-date German AI projects, thus presenting a comprehensive survey of AI research in Germany.

The 22nd Annual Conference on Artificial Intelligence (KI-98) took place in September 1998 at the University of Bremen and featured predominantly technical papers, six invited talks, 16 workshops with numerous contributions, four application-oriented user panels, a technical exhibition, and a poster session.

With its emphasis on "Methods of Artificial Intelligence in Medicine and Environmental Protection" it was our aim at this conference to illustrate a trend which as such is not new but still developing: as "conventional" methods are not powerful enough, many applications are frequently only made possible by artificial intelligence methods. This fact still constitutes a great opportunity and challenge for the application of these methods.

The focus of this conference was further broadened by the combination with the

- 12th International Symposium "Computer Science for Environmental Protection" - Umwelt-Informatik '98
- and the 43rd Annual Conference of the "Deutsche Gesellschaft für Medizinische Informatik, Biometrie und Epidemiology e.V.".

The overlapping of the different conferences with joint workshops, a joint technical exhibition, and invited talks demonstrated as well the synergistic potential of this conference week.

The Best-Paper-Award donated by the Springer publishing company was awarded by the program committee to the authors:

Dirk Hähnel, Wolfram Burgard, and Gerhard Lakemeyer
for their contribution
"GOLEX - Bridging the Gap betweet Logic (GOLOG) and a Real Robot".

We would like to thank the program committee, the referees, and all those who put considerable effort into the preparation of this conference.

Bremen, July 1998

Otthein Herzog
Andreas Günter

22nd Annual German Conference on Artificial Intelligence (KI-98)

Conference Chairs

Andreas Günter, Bremen   Otthein Herzog, Bremen

Program Committee Chair

Otthein Herzog, Bremen

Program Committee Members

Hans-Jürgen Appelrath, Oldenburg
Wolfgang Bibel, Darmstadt
Siegfried Bocionek, Erlangen
Hans-Jürgen Bürckert, Saarbrücken
Hans-Dieter Burkhard, Berlin
Armin B. Cremers, Bonn
Wolfgang Dilger, Chemnitz
Norbert E. Fuchs, Zürich
Ulrich Furbach, Koblenz
Günter Görz, Erlangen
Eberhard Greiser, Bremen
Andreas Günter, Bremen
Hans-Dietrich Haasis, Bremen
Werner Horn, Wien

Kai von Luck, Hamburg
Katharina Morik, Dortmund
Bernhard Nebel, Freiburg
Bernd Neumann, Hamburg
Heinrich Niemann, Erlangen
Frank Puppe, Würzburg
Michael M. Richter, Kaiserlautern
Claus Rollinger, Osnabrück
Erik Sandewall, Linköping
Kurt Sundermeyer, Berlin
Robert Trappl, Wien
Wolfgang Wahlster, Saarbrücken
Thomas Wetter, Heidelberg

Workshop Chair

Hans-Dieter Burkhard, Berlin

Exhibition Chairs

Christoph Klauck, Hamburg   Ubbo Visser, Bremen

Directory of German AI Research Projects

Steffen Hölldobler, Dresden   Enno Sandner, Dresden

List of Additional Referees

Baumgartner, Peter
Beetz, Michael
Dellen, Barbara
Dix, Jürgen
Fox, Dieter
Gast, Helmar
Giesl, Jürgen
Goldmann, Sigrid
Hatzack, Wolfgang
Haustein, Stefan
Holzbaur, Christian
Hoos, Holger
Ittner, Andreas
Joachims, Thorsten
Kamp, Vera
Khalil, Hesham
Klinkenberg, Ralf
Kramer, Stefan
Lenski, Wolfgang
Möller, Ralf
Müller, Martin
Ronthaler, Marc
Sauer, Jürgen
Schulz, Dirk
Seipel, Dietmar
Sperschneider, Volker
Stolzenburg, Frieder
Strohmaier, Antje
Stützle, Thomas
Volk, Martin
Vollrath, Ivo
Wilke, Wolfgang
Wirth, Claus-Peter
Zeidler, Jens

Table of Contents

Invited Papers

Technical Papers - Section 1

Technical Papers - Section 2

Technical Papers - Section 3

Technical Papers - Section 4

Technical Papers - Section 5

Part II

Information Processing and Knowledge Generation in the Nervous System

Ernst Pöppel
Universität München

Abstract

In a classical psychological view data are gathered by the sensory systems and then processed sequentially in distinct neuronal structures. This bottom-up analysis is hierarchically organized, and somewhere on the way of this analysis data are turned into information (like in the sense organs), and information is turned into knowledge (like somewhere in cortical structures). Sometimes, "information" and "knowledge" are used, however, interchangeably. Although this is a classical view, it is still with us, often present as an implicit hypothesis. In a modern view, bottom-up and top-down analyses are intertwined. It might be useful to emphasize with the term "information processing" the bottom-up component and with the term "knowledge generation" the top-down component not forgetting of course their respective dependence.

The distinction between the two aspects of analysis can for instance be demonstrated in the temporal analysis of information and organization of knowledge. Different transduction times in the visual and auditory modality or within the visual modality for surfaces with different flux, and the spatial distribution of neuronal activities which are basic to integrated mental activity result in a logistical problem: How does the brain structure the chaos of undefined (and undefinable) temporal availability of information that is basic to any percept or the programming of any precise movement?

It is suggested that the brain creates endogenously atemporal system states within which incoming information is treated as co-temporal. According to the model a system state is implemented by relaxation-type neuronal oscillations, each period representing one such system state. Experimental evidence suggests that the duration of these system states or elementary processing units is approximately 30 to 40 msec. Support comes from studies on temporal order threshold, choice reaction time, latency of eye movements, stereopsis, midlatency response of the auditory evoked potential or the execution of simple movements.

On a theoretical level, it is suggested that the integrated information within such system states is the neuronal basis of "primordial events". The sequence of such events is temporally integrated up to approximately 2 to 3 seconds. This temporal integration process is pre-semantic and it defines a "working platform" for mental activity. Experimental evidence for such a universal integration process comes from studies on temporal reproduction, short term memory, spontaneous segmentation of speech, the duration of intentional acts, sensorimotor synchronization or the endogenous modulation of the mismatch negativity as studied with the MEG.

Because of its omnipresence in different domains of the mental repertory, this integration process can be used to define each singular "state of being conscious" (STOBCON). Experimental evidence shows that the content within such STOBCONs is strongly modulated in a top-down way. What can be referred to as "knowledge" represented within such STOBCONs according to this model is up-dated in regular intervals by external information. The brain is "asking" autonomously in intervals of approximately 3 seconds "what is new in the world?" and by doing so re-generating its knowledge basis.

Data Mining with Graphical Models

Rudolf Kruse and Christian Borgelt

Dept. of Knowledge Processing and Language Engineering
Otto-von-Guericke-University of Magdeburg
Universitätsplatz 2, D-39106 Magdeburg, Germany
e-mail: {kruse,borgelt}@iws.cs.uni-magdeburg.de

Abstract. The explosion of data stored in commercial or administrational databases calls for intelligent techniques to discover the patterns hidden in them and thus to exploit all available information. Therefore a new line of research has recently been established, which became known under the names "Data Mining" and "Knowledge Discovery in Databases". In this paper we study a popular technique from its arsenal of methods to do dependency analysis, namely learning inference networks (also called "graphical models") from data. We review the already well-known probabilistic networks and provide an introduction to the recently developed and closely related possibilistic networks.

1 Introduction

Due to the advances in hardware and software technology, large databases (product databases, customer databases, etc.) are nowadays maintained in almost every company and scientific or administrational institution. But often the data is only recorded; evaluation is restricted to simple retrieval and aggregation operations that can be carried out e.g. by SQL queries. It is clear that such operations cannot discover broader structures or general patterns that are present in the data. This, obviously, is a waste of information, since knowing such patterns can give a company a decisive competitive edge. Therefore from recent research a new area called "Data Mining" has emerged, which aims at finding "knowledge nuggets" that are hidden in huge volumes of data. It is the operational core of a process called "Knowledge Discovery in Databases", which (in addition to data mining) comprises data selection, data preprocessing, data transformation, visualization, and result evaluation and documentation [9].

Data mining itself can be characterized best by a set of tasks like classification, clustering (segmentation), prediction, etc. In this paper we focus on dependency analysis, i.e. the task to find dependencies between the attributes that are used to describe a domain of interest. A popular method for this task is the automatic induction of *inference networks*, also called *graphical models* [36, 20], from a set of sample cases.

Graphical models are best known in their probabilistic form, i.e. as Bayesian networks [26] or Markov networks [22]. Efficient implementations of inference systems based on them include HUGIN [1] and PATHFINDER [16]. They are learned from data by searching for the most appropriate decomposition of the multivariate probability distribution induced by a given dataset [6, 17].

Unfortunately probabilistic graphical models suffer from severe difficulties to deal with imprecise, i.e. set-valued, information in the database to learn from. However, the incorporation of imprecise information is more and more recognized as being indispensable for industrial practice. Therefore graphical models are studied also with respect to other uncertainty calculi, either based on a generalization of the modeling technique to so-called valuation-based networks [30, 31], implemented e.g. in PULCINELLA [28], or based on a specific derivation of possibilistic networks, implemented e.g. in POSSINFER [13, 21]. Recently learning possibilistic networks from data has also been studied [12, 14, 2, 3].

2   Notation and Presuppositions

Notation. Let $V = \{A^{(1)}, \ldots, A^{(m)}\}$ be a finite set of attributes $A^{(k)}$, which are used to describe the section of the world under consideration. We assume the domains $\mathrm{dom}(A^{(k)}) = \{a_1^{(k)}, \ldots, a_{n_k}^{(k)}\}$ of these attributes to be finite sets of categorical values (i.e. we confine to the important case of *discrete graphical models*.) With these presuppositions the reasoning space in which all inferences take place is the joint domain $\Omega = \mathrm{dom}(A^{(1)}) \times \cdots \times \mathrm{dom}(A^{(m)})$, which is sometimes called the *universe of discourse*. Each possible state of the world is described by a tuple $\omega = (a_{i_1}^{(1)}, \ldots, a_{i_m}^{(m)})$ containing the values which the attributes in V assume for this state. For simplicity (and because states with identical describing tuples cannot be distinguished) we identify each $\omega \in \Omega$ with a possible state of the world.

Several times we need to refer to subspaces of Ω and projections of tuples ω to these subspaces. A subspace $\Omega_W \subseteq \Omega$ is the joint domain of a subset $W \subseteq V$ of attributes, i.e. $\Omega_W = \times_{A \in W} \mathrm{dom}(A)$. A projection of a tuple $\omega \in \Omega$ to this subspace is a tuple $\mathrm{proj}_W^V(\omega) = \omega_W \in \Omega_W$, which contains only the values of the attributes in W.

Presuppositions. Graphical models are concerned with drawing inferences from observations. For a situation in which we are about to draw inferences, we assume that the considered section of the world is in a specific state, whose description $\omega_0 \in \Omega$ we do not know or do not know completely. The inferences to be drawn aim at identifying this state, i.e. at determining the values in ω_0.

To be able to carry out such inferences, *generic knowledge* about dependencies between the values of different attributes must be available. This knowledge is represented as a distribution $\mathcal{D}$ on Ω, which assigns to each tuple $\omega \in \Omega$ a value d_ω, which expresses the probability or (degree of) possibility of the combination of values present in ω. Depending on the values d_ω can have and the interpretation of these values we distinguish between probability and possibility distributions (details are given below). Generic knowledge may be obtained from experts, textbooks, databases etc. Since we are concerned with "data mining", we focus on learning generic knowledge from data.

In addition to generic knowledge we need knowledge to start the inferences from — also called *evidential knowledge* —, which consists in restrictions on the possible values of some of the attributes. This knowledge could be obtained e.g. from observations made about the current state ω_0. From the evidential knowledge about the values of some attributes we infer, using the generic knowledge, restrictions about the values of other attributes, thus narrowing the set of states that have to be considered possible or likely for ω_0.

It is obvious that storing the generic knowledge directly, i.e. the distribution $\mathcal{D}$, would make reasoning very simple, since then we only have to select all $\omega \in \Omega$ compatible with the given evidential knowledge and to combine the corresponding values d_ω appropriately. But, unfortunately, if there are more than only very few attributes, the number of values d_ω to be stored in this case would exceed any reasonable limit. Hence other ways of representing the generic knowledge have to be found. One of them is to use a graphical model, which we discuss in the next section.

3 Graphical Models

In graphical modeling a directed or undirected (hyper)graph is used to represent the generic knowledge about the domain in which the inferences take place. Each vertex corresponds to an attribute, each edge to a dependence between attributes. The edges are the paths along which knowledge about the values of one attribute can be transferred to other attributes, i.e. along which inferences can be drawn. This is understandable, since no information can be transferred from an attribute to another, which is independent of the first.

But even if attributes are dependent, they are sometimes unconnected in a graphical model. The idea underlying this is that an inference need not be direct. If the dependence between two attributes is captured completely by the consecutive dependences on a path connecting the two attributes via other attributes, a direct connection is not necessary. All inferences from one of the attributes to the other can then be carried out along this path.

Conditional independence. Such situations can be characterized by the notion of *conditional independence* [7, 26]. If two attributes get independent, if certain other attributes are fixed, their dependence is not genuine, but only mediated through other attributes. Therefore they need not be connected directly in the graph. Thus the topology of the graph is used to represent an independence model, i.e. a set of conditional independence statements, of the domain under consideration [26].

Of course, not just any notion of conditional independence will do, since, as stated above, the aim is to replace an inference along a direct connection between attributes by an indirect inference. In order to allow such a replacement, the used notion of conditional independence has to satisfy certain axioms, which are known as the *semi-graphoid axioms* [7, 25]. If we denote the independence of a set of attributes X from a set of attributes Y given a set of attributes Z as $X \perp\!\!\!\perp Y \mid Z$, they can be written as

symmetry:	$(X \perp\!\!\!\perp Y \mid Z) \Longleftrightarrow (Y \perp\!\!\!\perp X \mid Z)$
decomposition:	$(W \cup X \perp\!\!\!\perp Y \mid Z) \Longleftrightarrow (W \perp\!\!\!\perp Y \mid Z) \wedge (X \perp\!\!\!\perp Y \mid Z)$
weak union:	$(W \cup X \perp\!\!\!\perp Y \mid Z) \Longleftrightarrow (X \perp\!\!\!\perp Y \mid Z \cup W)$
contraction:	$(W \perp\!\!\!\perp Y \mid Z) \wedge (X \perp\!\!\!\perp Y \mid Z \cup W) \Longleftrightarrow (W \cup X \perp\!\!\!\perp Y \mid Z)$

The *symmetry* axiom states that in any state of knowledge Z, if Y tells us nothing new about X, then X tells us nothing new about Y. The *decomposition* axiom asserts that if two combined items of information are judged irrelevant to X, then each separate item is irrelevant as well. The *weak union* axiom states that learning irrelevant information W cannot help the irrelevant information Y become relevant to X. The *contraction* axiom states that if we judge W irrelevant to X after learning some irrelevant information Y, then W must have been irrelevant before we learned Y. Together the weak union and contraction properties mean that irrelevant information should not alter the relevance of other propositions in the system; what was relevant remains relevant, and what was irrelevant remains irrelevant [26]. It is plausible that any reasonable notion of conditional independence should satisfy these axioms.

Independence graphs. Given an appropriate notion of conditional independence an *independence graph* can be defined. In such a graph the *conditional independence* of two attribute sets given a third is expressed by *separation* of the corresponding node sets by the nodes corresponding to the third set.

What is to be understood by "separation" depends on whether the graph is directed or undirected. If it is undirected, separation is defined as follows: If X, Y, and Z are three disjoint subsets of nodes, then Z separates X from Y, iff after removing the nodes in Z and their associated edges from the graph there is no path, i.e. no sequence of consecutive edges, from a node in X to a node in Y. Or, in other words, Z separates X from Y, iff all paths from a node in X to a node in Y contain a node in Z.

For directed graphs, which have to be acyclic, the so-called *d-separation criterion* is used [26]: If X, Y, and Z are three disjoint subsets of nodes, then Z is said to *d-separate* X from Y, iff there is no path, i.e. no sequence of consecutive edges (of any directionality), from a node in X to a node in Y along which the following two conditions hold:

1. every node with converging edges either is in Z or has a descendant in Z,

2. every other node is not in Z.

With these notions we can define the *Markov properties* of graphs [36]:

pairwise: Attributes, whose nodes are non-adjacent in the graph, are independent conditional on all remaining attributes.

local: Conditional on the attributes corresponding to the adjacent nodes, an attribute is independent of all remaining attributes.

global: Any two subsets of attributes, whose corresponding node sets are separated by a third node set, are independent conditionally only on the attributes corresponding to the nodes in the third set.

Note that the local Markov property is contained in the global, and the pairwise Markov property in the local.

Since the pairwise Markov property refers to the independence of only two attributes, it would be most natural (at least for undirected graphs) to use it to define an independence graph: If two attributes are dependent given all other attributes, there is an edge between their corresponding nodes, otherwise there is no edge [36]. But, unfortunately, the three types of Markov properties are not equivalent in general, and it is obvious that we need the *global* Markov property for inferences from multiple observations. However, the above definition can be used, if — in addition to the semi-graphoid axioms — the following axiom holds:

intersection: $(W \perp\!\!\!\perp Y \mid Z \cup X) \wedge (X \perp\!\!\!\perp Y \mid Z \cup W) \Longleftrightarrow (W \cup X \perp\!\!\!\perp Y \mid Z)$

The semi-graphoid axioms together with this one are called the *graphoid axioms* [7, 25]. If they hold for a given notion of conditional independence, an independence graph can be defined via the pairwise Markov condition, since the intersection axiom allows us to infer the global Markov property from the pairwise. If the intersection axiom does not hold, the global Markov property has to be used to define an independence graph.

It is obvious that an independence graph for a given domain is easy to find. For example, the complete undirected graph, i.e. the graph in which every node is connected directly to every other, always is an independence graph. But a complete graph would not reduce the amount of data to be stored (see below). Therefore, in graphical modeling, we have to add the condition that the independence graph has to be *sparse* or even *minimal*, i.e. should contain as few edges as possible.

Note that directed acyclic graphs and undirected graphs represent conditional independence relations in fundamentally different ways. In particular, there are undirected graphs that represent a conditional independence that cannot be represented by a single directed acyclic graph, and vice versa.

The quantitative part of a graphical model. The independence graph is also called the *qualitative* part of a graphical model, since it specifies which attributes are dependent and which are independent, but not the details of the dependences. How the latter information, which is called the *quantitative* part of a graphical model, is described, depends again on the type of the graph. In a directed acyclic graph, it is represented as a set of conditional distributions: one for each attribute conditional on all of its parents in the graph. If an attribute does not have any parents, its associated distribution simplifies to an unconditional distribution.

For an undirected graph, the quantitative part is represented as a set of marginal distributions: one for each maximal clique of the independence graph, where a maximal clique is a fully connected subgraph that is not contained in another fully connected subgraph. Because of this representation an undirected *hyper*graph is often used instead of a normal undirected graph. The nodes of each maximal clique of the normal graph are then connected by one *hyper*edge in the hypergraph. Unfortunately, this approach suffers from the fact that the resulting hypergraph can have cycles. This causes problems, because during an inference process the same information can travel along more than one path and thus may be used several times to update the knowledge about an attribute. If the inference mechanism is not idempotent, i.e. if a second incorporation of already included information changes the result, this can invalidate the conclusions drawn.

In order to avoid these problems, the discussion is usually restricted to *triangulated* undirected graphs, i.e. to graphs in which each cycle of length four or larger contains a *chord*, where a chord is an edge between two non-consecutive nodes in the cycle. It can be shown that the maximal clique hypergraph of a triangulated undirected graph is always a *hypertree*, i.e. does not contain any cycles. In addition, this type of graphs is important, because it can be shown that a triangulated undirected graph is isomorphic to a directed acyclic graph. Thus, with the restriction to triangulated graphs, the difference between directed and undirected graphs vanishes.

It is worth noting that especially the representation using undirected graphs suggests to view graphical modeling as a decomposition method: The (global) distribution $\mathcal{D}$ is decomposed into a set of (local) distributions $\{\mathcal{D}_{X_1}, \ldots, \mathcal{D}_{X_n}\}$ on subspaces, which are the cross-products of the domains of the attributes in a maximal clique. Because of this decomposition, global reasoning, i.e. drawing inferences using $\mathcal{D}$, can be replaced by local reasoning, which involves only the distributions $\mathcal{D}_{X_k}$.

Reasoning in graphical models. The reasoning process, which we describe here exemplary for an undirected graph, basically is this: Information obtained e.g. by observations about the values of an attribute is extended to the distributions on all hyperedges containing the attribute and then projected to the intersections of these hyperedges with other hyperedges. From there it is extended and projected again etc. until the information is distributed to all attributes.

A general local propagation algorithm for hypertrees has been developed for so-called *valuation-based systems* [30]. The axiomatic framework of a valuation-based system [32] can represent various uncertainty calculi such as probability theory, Dempster-Shafer theory, and possibility theory.

Learning graphical models from data. When we consider learning graphical models from data, problems arise from the fact that various kinds of prior information can be available, expert knowledge as well as a database of sample cases, both of which should be considered in a unified framework. However, since our focus is on "data mining", we restrict ourselves to a purely data-oriented approach, i.e. we assume only a database of observations to be given.

Since constructive methods are rarely available, data oriented learning methods nearly always consist of two parts: a search method and an evaluation measure. The evaluation measure estimates the quality of a given (hyper)graph and the search method governs which (hyper)graphs are inspected. Often the search is guided by the value of the evaluation measure, since it is usually the goal to maximize (or to minimize) its value. Commonly used search methods include optimum weight spanning tree construction [5] (for undirected graphs) and greedy parent selection [6] (for directed graphs). Evaluation measures depend on the underlying uncertainty calculus and are considered below.

4 Probabilistic Graphical Models

In purely probabilistic approaches quantitative knowledge about the dependencies between the attributes in V is described by a probability distribution P on Ω. $P(\omega) = p \in [0, 1]$ means that the combination of attribute values in ω has the probability p. A conditional probability distribution is defined in the usual way, i.e. as

$$P(\omega_X \mid \omega_Y) = \frac{P(\omega_{X \cup Y})}{P(\omega_Y)}.$$

Conditional independence is defined in accordance with the usual notion of stochastic independence as follows: Let X, Y, and Z be three disjoint subsets of attributes in V. X is called *conditionally independent* of Y given Z w.r.t. P, abbreviated $X \perp\!\!\!\perp_P Y \mid Z$, iff

$$\forall \omega \in \Omega : \quad P(\omega_{X \cup Y} \mid \omega_Z) = P(\omega_X \mid \omega_Z) \cdot P(\omega_Y \mid \omega_Z)$$

whenever $P(\omega_Z) > 0$.

Bayesian networks. The most popular kind of probabilistic graphical models in artificial intelligence is the *Bayesian network*, also called *belief network* [26]. A Bayesian network consists of a directed acyclic graph and a set of conditional probability distributions $P(\omega_A \mid \omega_{\mathrm{parents}(A)})$, $A \in V$, where parents(A) is the set of attributes corresponding to the parents of the attribute A in the graph.

A Bayesian network describes a decomposition of a joint probability distribution P on Ω into a set of conditional probability distributions: A strictly positive probability distribution P on Ω *factorizes* w.r.t. a directed acyclic graph, if

$$\forall \omega \in \Omega : \quad P(\omega) = \prod_{A \in V} P(\omega_A \mid \omega_{\mathrm{parents}(A)}).$$

In this case P satisfies the *global Markov property* (cf. section 3). It follows, that a Bayesian network can be seen as a graphical representation of a Markov chain.

Since a Bayesian network is a directed graph, it is well-suited to represent direct causal dependencies between variables. In many cases this is quite natural for knowledge representation, e.g. in expert systems designed for diagnostic reasoning (abductive inference) in medical applications.

Markov networks. An alternative type of probabilistic graphical models uses undirected graphs and is called a *Markov network* [22]. Similar to a Bayesian network it describes a decomposition of the joint probability distribution P on Ω, but it uses a *potential representation*: A strictly positive probability distribution P on Ω *factorizes* w.r.t. an undirected graph, if

$$\forall X \in \mathrm{cliques}(G) : \exists \phi_X : \forall \omega \in \Omega : \quad P(\omega) = \prod_{X \in \mathrm{cliques}(G)} \phi_X(\omega_X),$$

where cliques(G) is the set of all maximal cliques, each of which is represented by the set of attributes whose corresponding nodes are contained in it. The ϕ_X are strictly positive functions defined on Ω_X, $X \subseteq V$.

Learning probabilistic networks from data. When learning probabilistic networks from data, we have to distinguish between quantitative and qualitative network induction.

Quantitative network induction for a given network structure consists in estimating the joint probability distribution P, where P is selected from a family of parameterized probability distributions. A lot of approaches have been developed in this field, using methods such as maximum likelihood, maximum penalized likelihood, or fully Bayesian approaches, which involve different computational techniques of probabilistic inference such as the expectation maximization (EM) algorithm, Gibbs sampling, Laplace approximation, and Monte Carlo methods. For an overview, see e.g. [34].

Qualitative network induction consists in learning a network structure from a database of sample cases. In principle one could use the factorization property of a probabilistic network to evaluate its quality by comparing for each $\omega \in \Omega$ the probability computed from the network with the relative frequency found in the database to learn from. But this approach is usually much too costly. Other methods include the extensive testing of conditional independences (CI tests) [35] and a Bayesian approach [6]. Unfortunately, CI tests tend to be unreliable unless the volume of data is enormous, and with an increasing number of vertices they soon become computationally intractable. Bayesian learning requires debatable prior assumptions (for example, default uniform priors on distributions, uniform priors on the possible graphs) and also tends to be inefficient unless greedy search methods are used. Nevertheless, several network induction algorithms have successfully been applied. The oldest example is an algorithm to decompose a multi-variate probability distribution into a tree of two-dimensional distributions [5]. It uses mutual information as the evaluation measure and optimum weight spanning tree construction as the search method. Another example is the $K2$ algorithm [6], which uses a greedy parent search and a Bayesian evaluation measure. Its drawback, which consists in the fact that it needs a topological order of the attributes, can be overcome by a hybrid algorithm [33], which combines CI tests (to find a topological order) and $K2$ (to construct the Bayesian network with respect to this topological order). Several evaluation measures, which can be used with optimum weight spanning tree construction and greedy parent search as well as other search methods, are surveyed in [2, 3].

5 Possibilistic Graphical Models

Possibility distributions. A *possibility distribution* π on a universe of discourse Ω is a mapping from Ω into the unit interval, i.e. $\pi : \Omega \rightarrow [0, 1]$ [38, 8]. From an intuitive point of view, $\pi(\omega)$ quantifies the degree of possibility that $\omega = \omega_0$ is true, where ω_0 is the actual state of the world (cf. section 2): $\pi(\omega) = 0$ means that $\omega = \omega_0$ is impossible, $\pi(\omega) = 1$ means that $\omega = \omega_0$ is possible without any restrictions, and $\pi(\omega) \in (0, 1)$ means that $\omega = \omega_0$ is possible only with restrictions, i.e. that there is evidence that supports $\omega = \omega_0$ as well as evidence that contradicts $\omega = \omega_0$.

Several suggestions have been made for semantics of a *theory of possibility* as a framework for reasoning with uncertain and imprecise data. The interpretation of a degree of possibility we prefer is based on the context model [11, 21]. In this model possibility distributions are seen as *information-compressed* representations of (not necessarily nested) random sets and a degree of possibility as the one-point coverage of a random set [23].

To be more precise: Let ω_0 be the actual, but unknown state of a domain of interest, which is contained in a set Ω of possible states. Let $(C, 2^C, P)$, $C = \{c_1, c_2, \ldots, c_m\}$, be a finite probability space and $\gamma : C \to 2^\Omega$ a set-valued mapping. C is seen as a set of contexts that have to be distinguished for a set-valued specification of ω_0. The contexts are supposed to describe different physical and observation-related frame conditions. $P(\{c\})$ is the (subjective) probability of the (occurrence or selection of the) context c.

A set $\gamma(c)$ is assumed to be the *most specific correct set-valued specification* of ω_0, which is implied by the frame conditions that characterize the context c. By "most specific set-valued specification" we mean that $\omega_0 \in \gamma(c)$ is guaranteed to be true for $\gamma(c)$, but is not guaranteed for any proper subset of $\gamma(c)$. The resulting *random set* $\Gamma = (\gamma, P)$ is an imperfect (i.e. imprecise *and* uncertain) specification of ω_0. Let π_Γ denote the *one-point coverage of Γ* (the *possibility distribution induced by Γ*), which is defined as

$$\pi_\Gamma : \Omega \to [0, 1], \quad \pi_\Gamma(\omega) = P(\{c \in C \mid \omega \in \gamma(c)\}).$$

In a complete model the contexts in C must be specified in detail to make the relationships between all contexts c_j and their corresponding specifications $\gamma(c_j)$ explicit. But if the contexts are unknown or ignored, then $\pi_\Gamma(\omega)$ is the total mass of all contexts c that provide a specification $\gamma(c)$ in which ω_0 is contained, and this quantifies the *possibility of truth* of the statement "$\omega = \omega_0$" [11, 13].

That in this interpretation a possibility distribution represents uncertain *and* imprecise knowledge can be understood best by comparing it to a probability distribution and to a relation. A probability distribution covers *uncertain*, but *precise* knowledge. This becomes obvious, if one notices that a possibility distribution in the interpretation described above reduces to a probability distribution, if $\forall c_j \in C : |\gamma(c_j)| = 1$, i.e. if for all contexts the specification of ω_0 is precise. On the other hand, a relation represents *imprecise*, but *certain* knowledge about dependencies between attributes. Thus, not surprisingly, a relation can also be seen as a special case of a possibility distribution, namely if there is only one context. Hence the context-dependent specifications are responsible for the imprecision, the contexts for the uncertainty in the imperfect knowledge expressed by a possibility distribution.

Possibilistic networks. Although well-known for a couple of years [18], a unique concept of possibilistic independence has not been fixed yet. In our opinion, the problem is that possibility theory is a calculus for uncertain *and* imprecise reasoning, the first of which is related to probability theory, the latter to relational theory (see above). But these two theories employ different notions of independence, namely stochastic independence and lossless join decomposability.

Stochastic independence is an *uncertainty-based* type of independence, whereas lossless join decomposability is an *imprecision-based* type of independence. Since possibility theory addresses both kinds of imperfect knowledge, notions of possibilistic independence can be uncertainty-based or imprecision-based.

W.r.t. this consideration two definitions of possibilistic independence have been justified [4], namely uncertainty-based possibilistic independence, which is derived from *Dempster's rule of conditioning* [29] adapted to possibility measures, and imprecision-based possibilistic independence, which coincides with the well-known concept of *possibilistic non-interactivity* [8]. The latter can be seen as a generalization of lossless join decomposability to the possibilistic setting, since it treats each α-cut of a possibility distribution like a relation.

Because of its consistency with the *extension principle* [37], we confine to possibilistic non-interactivity. As a concept of possibilistic independence it can be defined as follows: Let X, Y, and Z be three disjoint subsets of variables in V. Then X is called *conditionally independent* of Y given Z w.r.t. π, abbreviated $X \perp\!\!\!\perp_\pi Y \mid Z$, iff

$$\forall \omega \in \Omega : \quad \pi(\omega_{X \cup Y} \mid \omega_Z) = \min\{\pi(\omega_X \mid \omega_Z), \pi(\omega_Y \mid \omega_Z)\}$$

whenever $\pi(\omega_Z) > 0$, where $\pi(\cdot \mid \cdot)$ is a non-normalized conditional possibility distribution, i.e.

$$\pi(\omega_X \mid \omega_Z) = \max\{\pi(\omega') \mid \omega' \in \Omega \wedge \operatorname{proj}_X^V(\omega) = \omega_X \wedge \operatorname{proj}_Z^V(\omega) = \omega_Z\}.$$

Both mentioned types of possibilistic independence satisfy the *semi-graphoid axioms* (see section 3). Possibilistic independence based on Dempster's rule in addition satisfies the intersection axiom and thus can be used within the framework of the valuation-based systems already mentioned above [30]. However, the intersection axiom is related to uncertainty-based independence. Relational independence does not satisfy this axiom, and therefore it cannot be satisfied by possibilistic non-interactivity as a more general type of imprecision-based independence.

Similar to probabilistic networks, a possibilistic network can be seen as a decomposition of a multi-variate possibility distribution. The factorization formulae can be derived from the corresponding probabilistic factorization formulae (for Markov networks) by replacing the product by the minimum.

Learning possibilistic networks from data. Just as for probabilistic networks, it is possible in principle to estimate the quality of a given possibilistic network by exploiting its factorization property. For each $\omega \in \Omega$ the degree of possibility computed from the network is compared to the degree of possibility derived from the database to learn from. But again this approach can be costly.

Contrary to probabilistic networks, the induction of possibilistic networks from data has been studied much less extensively. A first result, which consists in an algorithm that is closely related to the $K2$ algorithm for the induction of Bayesian networks, was presented in [12]. Instead of the Bayesian evaluation measure used in $K2$, it relies on a measure derived from the *nonspecificity* of a possibility distribution. Roughly speaking, the notion of nonspecificity plays the same role in possibility theory that the notion of *entropy* plays in probability theory. Based on the connection of the imprecision part of a possibility distribution to relations, the nonspecificity of a possibility distribution can also be seen as a generalization of *Hartley information* [15] to the possibilistic setting.

In [14] a rigid foundation of a learning algorithm for possibilistic networks is given. It starts from a comparison of the nonspecificity of a given multi-variate possibility distribution to the distribution represented by a possibilistic network, thus measuring the loss of specificity, if the multi-variate possibility distribution is represented by the network. In order to arrive at an efficient algorithm, an approximation for this loss of specificity is derived, which can be computed locally on the hyperedges of the network. As the search method a generalization of the optimum weight spanning tree algorithm to hypergraphs is used. Several other heuristic local evaluation measures, which can be used with different search methods, are presented in [2, 3].

It should be emphasized, that, as already discussed above, an essential advantage of possibilistic networks over probabilistic ones is their ability to deal with imprecision, i.e. multi-valued, information. When learning possibilistic networks from data, this leads to the convenient situation that missing values in an observation or a set of values for an attribute, all of which have to be considered possible, do not pose any problems.

6 Application

Although a good theory may be the most practical thing to have, all theory must hold its own in a test against reality. As a test case we chose the Danish Jersey cattle blood group determination problem [27], for which a Bayesian network designed by domain experts (cf. figure 1) and a database of 500 real world sample cases exists (an extract of this database is shown in table 1). The problem with this database is that it contains a pretty large number of unknown values — only a little over half of the tuples are complete (This can already be guessed from the extract shown in table 1: the stars denote missing values).

As already indicated above, missing values can make it difficult to learn a Bayesian network, since an unknown value can be seen as representing imprecise information: It states that all values contained in the domain of the corresponding attribute are possible. Nevertheless it is still feasible to learn a Bayesian network — similar to the expert designed one — from the database in this case, since the dependencies are rather strong and thus the remaining small number of tuples is still sufficient to recover the underlying structure. However, learning a possibilistic network from the same dataset is much easier, since possibility theory was especially designed to handle imprecise information. Hence no discarding or special treatment of tuples is necessary. An evaluation of the learned network showed that it was of comparable quality. Thus we can conclude that learning possibilistic networks from data is an important alternative to the established probabilistic methods.

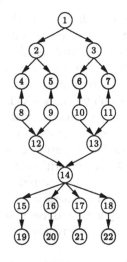

1 – parental error
2 – dam correct?
3 – sire correct?
4 – stated dam ph.gr. 1
5 – stated dam ph.gr. 2
6 – stated sire ph.gr. 1
7 – stated sire ph.gr. 2
8 – true dam ph.gr. 1
9 – true dam ph.gr. 2
10 – true sire ph.gr. 1
11 – true sire ph.gr. 2

12 – offspring ph.gr. 1
13 – offspring ph.gr. 2
14 – offspring genotype
15 – factor 40
16 – factor 41
17 – factor 42
18 – factor 43
19 – lysis 40
20 – lysis 41
21 – lysis 42
22 – lysis 43

The grey nodes correspond to observable attributes.
Node 1 can be removed to simplify constructing the
clique tree for propagation.

Fig. 1. Domain expert designed network for the Danish Jersey cattle blood type determination example

n	y	y	f1	v2	f1	v2	f1	v2	f1	v2	v2	v2	v2v2	n	y	n	y	0	6	0	6
n	y	y	f1	v2	**	**	f1	v2	**	**	**	**	f1v2	y	y	n	y	7	6	0	7
n	y	y	f1	v2	f1	f1	f1	v2	f1	f1	f1	f1	f1f1	y	y	n	n	7	7	0	0
n	y	y	f1	v2	f1	f1	f1	v2	f1	f1	f1	f1	f1f1	y	y	n	n	7	7	0	0
n	y	y	f1	v2	f1	v1	f1	v2	f1	v1	v2	f1	f1v2	y	y	n	y	7	7	0	7
n	y	y	f1	f1	**	**	f1	f1	**	**	f1	f1	f1f1	y	y	n	n	6	6	0	0
n	y	y	f1	v1	**	**	f1	v1	**	**	v1	v2	v1v2	n	y	y	y	0	5	4	5
n	y	y	f1	v2	f1	v1	f1	v2	f1	v1	f1	v1	f1v1	y	y	y	y	7	7	6	7

Table 1. An extract from the Danish Jersey cattle blood group determination database.

7 Conclusions

In this paper we reviewed, although briefly, the ideas underlying probabilistic networks and provided an equally brief introduction to possibilistic networks. The main advantage of the latter is that they can handle directly imprecise, i.e. set-valued, information. This is especially useful, if an inference network is to be learned from data and the database to learn from contains a considerable amount of missing values. Whereas in order to learn a probabilistic network these tuples have to be discarded or treated in some complicated manner, possibilistic network learning can easily take them into account and can thus, without problem, make use of all available information. These considerations proved to be well-founded in an application on a real-world database.

References

1. S.K. Andersen, K.G. Olesen, F.V. Jensen, F. and Jensen. HUGIN — a shell for building Bayesian belief universes for expert systems. *Proc. 11th International Joint Conference on Artificial Intelligence*, pp. 1080–1085, 1989

2. C. Borgelt and R. Kruse. Evaluation measures for learning probabilistic and possibilistic networks. *Proc. 6th IEEE Int. Conf. on Fuzzy Systems*, pp. 669–676, Barcelona, Spain, 1997

3. C. Borgelt and R. Kruse. Some Experimental Results on Learning Probabilistic and Possibilistic Networks with Different Evaluation Measures. *Proc. 1st Int. J. Conf. on Qualitative and Quantitative Practical Reasoning, ECSQARU-FAPR'97*, 71–85, Bad Honnef, Germany, 1997

4. L.M. de Campos, J. Gebhardt, and R. Kruse. *Syntactic and semantic approaches to possibilistic independence*. Technical report, University of Granada, Spain, and University of Braunschweig, Germany, 1995

5. C.K. Chow and C.N. Liu. Approximating discrete probability distributions with dependence trees. *IEEE Trans. on Information Theory* 14(3) 462–467, 1968

6. G. Cooper and E. Herskovits. A Bayesian method for the induction of probabilistic networks from data. *Machine Learning* 9:309–347, 1992

7. A. Dawid. Conditional independence in statistical theory. *SIAM Journal on Computing* 41:1–31, 1979

8. D. Dubois and H. Prade. *Possibility Theory*. Plenum Press, New York, NY, 1988

9. U.M. Fayyad, G. Piatetsky-Shapiro, P. Smyth, and R. Uthurusamy, eds. *Advances in Knowledge Discovery and Data Mining*. AAAI Press / MIT Press, Cambridge, MA, 1996

10. J. Gebhardt and R. Kruse. A new approach to semantic aspects of possibilistic reasoning. In: M. Clarke, R. Kruse, and S. Moral, eds. *Symbolic and Quantitative Approaches to Reasoning and Uncertainty* (Lecture Notes in Computer Science 747), pp. 151–160, Springer, Berlin, Germany, 1993

11. J. Gebhardt and R. Kruse. The context model — an integrating view of vagueness and uncertainty. *Int. Journal of Approximate Reasoning* 9:283–314, 1993

12. J. Gebhardt and R. Kruse. Learning possibilistic networks from data. *Proc. 5th Int. Workshop on Artificial Intelligence and Statistics*, pp. 233–244, Fort Lauderdale, FL, 1995

13. J. Gebhardt and R. Kruse. POSSINFER — A software tool for possibilistic inference. In: D. Dubois, H. Prade, and R. Yager, eds. *Fuzzy Set Methods in Information Engineering: A Guided Tour of Applications*, pp. 407–418, Wiley, New York, NY, 1996

14. J. Gebhardt and R. Kruse. Tightest hypertree decompositions of multivariate possibility distributions. *Proc. Int. Conf. on Information Processing and Management of Uncertainty in Knowledge-based Systems (IPMU'96)*, pp. 923–927, Granada, Spain, 1996

15. R.V.L. Hartley. Transmission of information. *The Bell Systems Technical Journal* 7:535–563, 1928

16. D. Heckerman. *Probabilistic Similarity Networks*. MIT Press, Cambridge, MA, 1991

17. D. Heckerman, D. Geiger, and D.M. Chickering. Learning Bayesian Networks: The Combination of Knowledge and Statistical Data. *Machine Learning* 20:197–243, Kluwer, Dordrecht, Netherlands, 1995

18. E. Hisdal. Conditional possibilities, independence, and noninteraction. *Fuzzy Sets and Systems* 1:283–297, 1978

19. F.V. Jensen and J. Liang. drHUGIN — a system for value of information in Bayesian networks. *Proc. 5th Int. Conf. on Information Processing and Management of Uncertainty in knowledge-based Systems*, 1994

20. R. Kruse, E. Schwecke, and J. Heinsohn. *Uncertainty and Vagueness in Knowledge-based Systems: Numerical Methods.* Series: Artificial Intelligence, Springer, Berlin, Germany, 1991

21. R. Kruse, J. Gebhardt, and F. Klawonn. *Foundations of Fuzzy Systems.* Wiley, Chichester, England, 1994 Translation of the book: *Fuzzy Systeme (Series: Leitfäden und Monographien der Informatik).* Teubner, Stuttgart, Germany, 1994

22. S.L. Lauritzen and D.J. Spiegelhalter. Local computations with probabilities on graphical structures and their application to expert systems. *Journal of the Royal Stat. Soc., Series B* 2(50):157–224, 1988

23. H.T. Nguyen. Using Random Sets. *Information Science* 34:265–274, 1984

24. J. Pearl. Fusion, propagation, and structuring in belief networks. *Artificial Intelligence* 29:241–288, 1986

25. J. Pearl and A. Paz. Graphoids: a graph based logic for reasoning about relevance relations. In: B.D. Boulay et. al, eds. *Advances in Artificial Intelligence 2*, pp. 357–363 North Holland, Amsterdam, Netherlands, 1987

26. J. Pearl. *Probabilistic Reasoning in Intelligent Systems: Networks of Plausible Inference (2nd edition).* Morgan Kaufmann, San Mateo, CA, 1992

27. L.K. Rasmussen. *Blood Group Determination of Danish Jersey Cattle in the F-blood Group System.* Dina Research Report no. 8, 1992

28. A. Saffiotti and E. Umkehrer. PULCINELLA: a general tool for propagating uncertainty in valuation networks. *Proc. 7th Conf. on Uncertainty in Artificial Intelligence*, pp. 323–331, Morgan Kaufmann, San Mateo, CA, 1991

29. G. Shafer. *A Mathematical Theory of Evidence.* Princeton University Press, Princeton, NJ, 1976

30. G. Shafer and P.P. Shenoy. *Local computations in hypertrees*, Working paper 201. School of Business, University of Kansas, Lawrence, KS, 1988

31. P.P. Shenoy. *Conditional independence in valuation-based systems*, Working Paper 236, School of Business, University of Kansas, Lawrence, KS, 1991

32. P.P. Shenoy. Valuation-based systems: a framework for managing uncertainty in expert systems. In: L.A. Zadeh and J. Kacprzyk, eds. *Fuzzy Logic for the Management of Uncertainty*, pp. 83–104, Wiley, New York, NY, 1992

33. M. Singh and M. Valtorta. An algorithm for the construction of Bayesian network structures from data. *Proc. 9th Conf. on Uncertainty in Artificial Intelligence* Washington, pp. 259–265, 1993

34. D. Spiegelhalter, A. Dawid, S. Lauritzen, and R. Cowell. Bayesian analysis in expert systems. *Statistical Science* 8(3):219–283, 1993

35. T.S. Verma and J. Pearl. An algorithm for deciding if a set of observed independencies has a causal explanation. *Proc. 8th Conf. on Uncertainty in Artificial Intelligence* pp. 323–330, 1992

36. J. Whittaker. *Graphical Models in Applied Multivariate Statistics.* Wiley, Chichester, England, 1990

37. L.A. Zadeh. The concept of a linguistic variable and its application to approximate reasoning. *Information Sciences* 9:43–80, 1975

38. L.A. Zadeh. Fuzzy sets as a basis for a theory of possibility. *Fuzzy Sets and Systems* 1:3–28, 1978

Artificial Intelligence for Nature - Why Knowledge Representation and Problem Solving Should Play a Key Role in Environmental Decision Support

Peter Struss

Department of Computer Science, Technical University of Munich, Orleansstr. 34,
D-81667 Munich, Germany, email: struss@in.tum.de,
and OCC'M SoftwareGmbH, Gleissentalstr. 22, D-82041 Deisenhofen, Germany

Abstract. Decision Support Systems for the environment have to incorporate and exploit knowledge about the phenomena and the interdependencies in the affected natural systems, i.e. a model. Using an ongoing project on mangrove forest management as an example, we discuss different tasks and requirements and propose to use methods and techniques developed in research on modeling and model-based systems in Artificial Intelligence for computer support to solving the problems.

1   Introduction

Every day, we can witness how effectively modern technology influences and changes the world and our lives. The most outstanding effects, indeed, are destructive. By "destructive", we mean that human activities destroy the existing balance of complex natural systems - irreversibly, at a large and even global scale. Or is it not "impressive" that it took only a few decades to eliminate the stability of self-organizing systems that have existed and developed over thousands and millions of years: rivers, rain forests, even oceans and the atmosphere, interrelationships of species?

Despite this "success", humans will not be able to destroy the system of life on earth itself. It will survive human impact as it survived the impact of a meteor 60 million years ago, move to a different balance, develop new species, and eliminate others (perhaps including the human species). However, the impact of human activities has started to change and threaten the living conditions and even the lives of the originators of the disturbances.

In general, no person intended these effects. The original goals are usually constructive, positive: generating energy, producing food and timber, improving health, depositing garbage... To use an example we will return to later, the purpose of dams of the Cauvery River in South India is to avoid flooding and/or to generate electricity. The fact that the dams change the downstream transportation of sediments, which results in changed patterns of sediment deposits in the river delta, causing slopes to turn into troughs, which capture stagnant tidal water with the effect of increased salinity through evaporation, up to a point where it causes the dying of mangroves, hence, reduced shelter against cyclones, etc. - far from the dam - these are "side-effects".

The term "side-effect" is part of an ideology: it seems to categorize interdependencies between natural phenomena, but, actually, it characterizes human intentions and/or ignorance. Nature does not distinguish between primary and secondary effects. Some of them are the target of human activities, the others are "side-effects" because they are undesired and, often, unanticipated or unknown to us. We do not understand the "environment" well enough. "Environment" - this is an even more ideological term: environment of what? The environment of human society and activity. It's the world, after all! An incredibly complex gigantic system - reduced to an "environment", the mere backdrop for our activities, or, even worse, to a set of "resources", subject to human exploitation (Fig. 1a). Let us "manage" "resources", but in a "sustainable" manner!

This is not a discussion about terminology. It is this ridiculous worm's-eye view of the anthropocentric ideology that prevents us from solving our "environmental problems" because it prevents us from *understanding* their causes. What is required is a deeper analysis of the interactions among individuals and populations of living organisms and between them and their physical conditions, including the embedding of human activities into this system (Fig. 1b). This view, certainly alien to politics and economy, has gained influence in research and created scientific progress. We need to develop *models* of the natural systems we are interacting with that reflect their complex interdependencies.

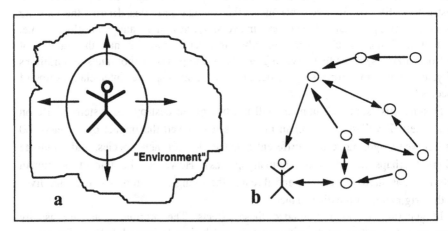

Fig. 1. 1a The anthropocentric view   1b A "natural" view

2   The Role of Information Technology

This insight is a great achievement. However, it is only the starting point of the difficulties. It only poses the question. Finding the answers is the hard part. Why? Just because the systems we are looking at are so complex, incorporate so many participating substances and organisms, contain so many interactions, actual ones as well as potential and hidden ones. We are simply overwhelmed by the complexity when we try to model them, by the amount and structure of data when we try to identify behavioral patterns and to exploit them for explanation of existing phenomena or prediction of future ones, by unforeseen responses of the systems when we attempt to influence them according to our intentions. We know only bits and pieces. And even when we believe to have understood some fundamental mechanisms in one system, they almost certainly have to be revised when we try to apply them to a similar system, because some hidden preconditions are not satisfied, or new phenomena cancel out the expected effects.

Now, there exists also a technology that has been developed to cope with large amounts of data and complex information, to prevent them from overwhelming us. Computers and information technology have provided effective tools that can support research and decision making on "environmental problems". They enabled substantial results in acquiring information and in the analysis and prediction of the behavior of natural systems and their response to human impact. In particular, they help to

- acquire data, e.g. through remote sensing and image processing,
- store and retrieve data, e.g. in data bases and geographical information systems,
- transfer data, e.g. via the internet,
- process data, e.g. in statistical analysis and in simulating numerical models of ecosystems.

Although these computer systems are often extremely useful and even prerequisites for improving our understanding and decision making, they do not directly address these tasks that we have identified to be crucial. They provide and process *data*, rather than knowledge, and, in fact, using them *requires* substantial *knowledge*:

- A basic understanding is already necessary to determine what kind of data should be acquired or retrieved to provide insight.
- If we have a model as an input to a simulation system, the most difficult part of the work has already been done.
- And having obtained data, by means of sensing, retrieval, or simulation, they are of no use without an interpretation based on prior knowledge. Knowledge is what turns data into information.

Currently, all these knowledge-intensive tasks have to be carried out solely by human experts, mainly researchers, and computer support for them is almost non-existent. In a sense, the improved facilities for acquiring and generating data even creates problems rather than solving them: huge amounts of data are buried on tapes and data bases, and many of them will never be excavated because interpreting them and drawing conclusions is by orders of magnitude more time-consuming than creating and storing them.

But is it really feasible to build computer systems that support such knowledge-intensive tasks? Does this not imply that they must be able to capture and manipulate at least a substantial part of the knowledge that their users need to solve problems? Yes, it does. Artificial Intelligence pursues the goal of providing theoretical foundations, methods, and systems for such capabilities. They have proven to be of use in other application domains, and, in particular, in modeling other kinds of physical systems, namely technical systems, artifacts, and solving problems related to them, such as configuration and diagnosis. We will discuss what can carry over to establish solutions to the problems discussed here.

To become more specific, we will use a particular project we are involved in to extract typical tasks, problems, and requirements from it.

3   Tasks and Requirements

We started a collaboration with the M.S. Swaminathan Research Foundation (MSSRF) and the Indian Institute of Technology (IIT) Madras. MSSRF is conducting research on the causes of degradation of mangrove forests in the coastal wetlands of South India. As in other regions of the world, this degradation has reached a stage that represents a serious threat to function of the mangrove forests as a shelter against cyclones, a habitat for various species, and a source of timber and food for the local population. While MSSRF can investigate the interdependencies in this ecosystem and the factors influencing its development and, based on these results, develop strategies for the restoration and management of the mangrove forests, ultimately decisions and actions have to be taken locally, by forest departments and the authorities of the local self-administration.

As the local conditions and relevant factors (in terms of geomorphology, hydrology, climate, species, exploitation etc.) vary considerably, it is impossible to produce general management plans that can be applied to all sites without further investigation, modification and specialization. On the other hand, MSSRF's experts are not available for continuous consultation at the various mangrove areas. In response to this situation, our collaboration aims at capturing their growing expertise in a knowledge-based system which can then support local investigations, problem solving, and decision making at the various sites in reflection of their specificity. Certainly, a geographic information system is a useful tool which can store the specific data of each site. But it is fairly obvious that it cannot provide the solution to the ambitious goals. Pure retrieval of existing data, although important to the work of the experts, offers very limited help to the kind of users involved in the management of the mangrove areas. On the one hand, they would have to know what to inquire, and, on the other hand, for most of the problems, one cannot expect the solution to have been produce in advance and stored in the data base. Rather, it has to be constructed by reasoning about facts from the data base under the guidance of principled knowledge about the domain and task. For the non-experts, at least part of this knowledge and the appropriate reasoning mechanisms have to be provided by the knowledge-based system.

We informally discuss some of the problem solving tasks and their requirements. In section 4, we will revisit them and propose how to formalize them in order to provide a basis for automated reasoning systems.

Situation Assessment (What's Going on?)

Given a set of observations (measurements, descriptions of geomorphological or biological features, results of visual inspection, etc.) and general domain knowledge, determine the relevant phenomena and processes which cannot be or have not been observed directly. We might distinguish two different kinds of this tasks, although they frequently have to be solved together:

- *System Identification* which again has two aspects. One is *structure* identification, i.e. determining the (types of) constituents of the system and their interactions. Second, *parameter* identification, i.e. determining constants that characterize the particular instances of such constituents. The starting point is a description of the entities that are directly observable (the topography, present species, etc.) and measurable quantities (salinity of the water, current, etc.). The goal is to establish a behavior model of the target system. Obviously, this is a reasoning task which requires scientific knowledge and expertise, since it is about recognizing the processes that are caused by the visible configuration of entities, but happen behind them, often difficult or impossible to observe (e.g. deposit of sediments, chemical processes, etc.). Computer support to this task should satisfy a number of requirements. First, knowledge that has been gained in modeling similar systems and through generalization should be *re-used* directly where appropriate. Thus, we want to avoid having to build a model of each mangrove area from scratch. Second, the input to such a modeling system should be entered in a way that is natural to the user who may be a domain expert or a local semi-expert and whom we cannot force to use some mathematical formalism or computer language. Third, many of the available observations are inherently qualitative in nature, such as "trough-shaped area" or "increased degradation", but, nevertheless, carry crucial information that has to be taken into account. .
- *State Identification* interprets observation in order to infer internal states or tendencies in the system *at a particular time*. Obviously, this is based on, or combined with, system identification.

Both tasks can occur as "diagnostic" tasks if the given observations do not match the expectations or a given model.

Diagnosis (What's Going Wrong?)

This step tries to identify the causes of deviations of a system from what we consider normal or healthy. For instance, the threatening degradation of mangroves is a particular area of the Pichavaram forest mentioned earlier would require tracing the cause-effect chain sketched earlier back to the Cauvery dam. This is an example of

- *Identification of Ultimate Causes*, whereas
- *Identification of Controllable Causes* focuses on determining hooks for curing the symptoms in case we are not able or willing to remove the ultimate causes or if this does not suffice to also remove the undesirable effects. Since it is not easy to remove or open the dam, increasing the drainage rate of the water in the troughs is an options for reducing the salinity (whereas influencing the evaporation rate is not).

For diagnosis, the system needs, besides the objective description of the system under analysis, an appropriate representation of the desired states of evolution of the system. Note that this diagnostic reasoning may involve more than hypothesizing abnormal parameters or state values, but may involve the revision or extension of the original model in order to include the origins of the disturbances and all their effects. Again, the computer tool has to address the requirements stated above, in this task even more, since it should be part of the continuous use of the local authorities.

Therapy (What Can be Done?)

Given descriptions of a disturbed system (including the causes for the disturbance as discussed above) and of our goals, determine actions suited to re-establish a state that complies with our goals. In the simplest case, such actions are designed to shift a single quantity in the proper direction, e.g. increasing the flow from the trough to the sea by digging canals (which is what is actually being done). In general, the task can require planning a sequence of actions over time achieving a number of different sub-goals ("First, take steps to decrease salinity, then introduce species X to change the soil, finally, re-introduce species Y"). In addition to representing the ecosystem itself and the goals of management or conservation, computer support to this task needs to incorporate knowledge about the potential interventions, and, more specifically, this has to be done in a way that enables the analysis of their impact on the ecosystem.

Prediction (What's Going to Happen?)

Given a system model and some, potentially incomplete, description of its state (the identified actual one or a hypothesized one), anticipate the possible evolution of the system in the future. The purpose can be to check whether the actual state may lead to a critical one, or to explore the consequences of some action (of exploitation or therapy) before it is actually taken. Although this may sound like ordinary numerical simulation, one has to keep in mind that the initial conditions as well as the parameters may be specified only partially (e.g. qualitatively) and lead to ambiguous predictions. This is particularly true for the evaluation of potential actions which we cannot or would not want to describe numerically. Initially, we may be only interested in determining whether a certain class of measures could move the system in a proper or tolerable direction: "What will happen if a crab farm is established in this bay?", "What is the consequence of digging a canal from the trough-shaped areas to the sea?". Second, also the output, the predicted behavior, has to be stated in terms of concepts that are familiar to the user, rather than tables of numbers.

Explanation (Why Does It Happen?)

Describe the ecosystem and its response to disturbances and interventions in a way that is comprehensible to the user. Suppose the computer system had hypothesized the reduction of sediment deposit as a potential cause of mangrove degradation (a rather difficult task), then we would like it to deliver a "causal chain" of the kind presented in section 1. This is a crucial feature, because it enables the critical assessment of the performance of the system particularly for validation of the knowledge base. Furthermore, it is essential to the educational purpose of the system with regard to the local decision makers.

Discovery (What Can Possibly Happen, and under which Conditions?)

Given the existing theory about a domain (such as mangrove ecosystems), a description of a specific system (mangrove forest), and system observations that contradict the general theory or cannot be explained by it, propose revisions and extensions to the theory in order to account for the observations. This aims at supporting the research process itself and is certainly one of the most challenging tasks.

The easiest step is the mere detection of the contradiction. The following one would be to localize the elements of the theory that contribute to the contradiction (again, a "diagnostic" task!) and hence, are candidates for a revision. Beyond this, hypotheses for certain revisions of these elements or, more difficult, for undiscovered interactions could be generated. In order to decide which of these potential revisions is appropriate, helpful observations or experiments should be proposed. All this may sound too futuristic. However, we will see what is required to provide such tools, and there exist not only theories, but also implemented tools.

4   Artificial Intelligence Approaches to Modeling and Model-based Problem Solving

In our initial discussion, we emphasized in general terms the importance of explicitly representing general knowledge about the ecosystems under analysis in computer programs (as opposed to rules and algorithms special to particular goals and tasks). The examples in the previous section were meant to illustrate the crucial role of modeling and model-based reasoning.

Although traditional numerical modeling and simulation can and has to perform part of the work (e.g. in prediction when exact data are both available and necessary), the requirements discussed show that they cannot provide a solution to the central problems. For representation and presentation (in particular explanation) of existing and generated knowledge, conceptualization is essential.

- The system needs to maintain *a mapping to the phenomena in the physical world* as they are perceived by the user both for the model and the results obtained from it. In numerical modeling, this mapping has to exist in the heads of the experts when creating the model and when interpreting the generated data. But is lost in the mathematical model and in the simulation system. Differential equations and tables with numbers do not explain anything, and particularly for the non-expert users, they are not appropriate for conveying knowledge and information. This is why a weather report is presented (and, in fact, generated!) in terms of conceptual entities, such as low pressure systems, moving cold fronts, etc.
- Second, in our domain, much of the data, information, and knowledge can only be stated and should be communicated in *qualitative* terms. This is why qualitative and symbolic reasoning methods developed in Artificial Intelligence need to be exploited [Forbus 84], [Struss 97].

Both statements hold, especially, for spatial and temporal aspects that require an appropriate level of abstraction.

- The desired *re-use* of model elements also requires a structuring of the models in accordance with *conceptual entities* of basic phenomena and processes that occur in various systems in the domain.

This is why computer-supported conceptual modeling is needed [Heller-Struss 97]. We will outline some theories, methods, and techniques that have been developed in the Artificial Intelligence area of knowledge representation and reasoning and that offer means for tackling the tasks and requirements, without claiming to be comprehensive or to present ultimate solutions. Some of the aspects are discussed with more technical detail in another contribution to this volume [Heller-Struss 98] and in [Struss-Heller 98].

Process Modeling

Like to most other Artificial Intelligence approaches to modeling, compositionality is fundamental to process-oriented modeling [Forbus 84], [Struss-Heller 98]: the behavior model of a specific system is derived through aggregation of re-usable model fragments that represent elementary processes in the domain. Model composition follows *structure-to-function reasoning*. This means, a description of the configuration of objects that constitute the system entails a set of relevant interacting behavior model fragments which are additionally controlled by certain conditions on the quantities involved.

Knowledge connected to each (generic) process comprises the following elements:

- The *conditions* under which the process is included in the model. This is stated in terms of structural preconditions, i.e. certain objects and relations between them, and constraints on parameters and variables involved in the process. For instance, an evaporation process requires a water body in touch with the air and a humidity of less than 100%.
- A set of *relations* among quantities local to the process. According to the nature of knowledge in the domain, they can represent relationships in a qualitative way, e.g. as monotonic dependencies. In the evaporation example, the evaporation rate may be stated to grow monotonically with the water temperature.
- A set of *influences* that capture the contributions of such a process to changes in the system. This concept reflects a requirement that arises from the compositional modeling scheme: we need to describe the effects local to a model element; but without knowing which other model elements will affect the same quantity, no definite constraint can be established for the influenced quantity. For instance, the evaporation rate influences the amount of the (liquid) water body negatively. But this may, nevertheless, grow due to other processes, such as precipitation. Influences can be positive or negative and act on a variable or its derivative. Roughly, an influence is a statement about the partial derivative of the influenced variable w.r.t to the influencing one.

Somewhat simplified, we can formalize the concept of a process in logic by stating that the process conditions imply certain constraints (i.e. mathematical relations), influences, and, potentially, other structural properties (since a process may generate new objects and relations):

$$\text{STRUCTURE-CONDITIONS}_i \wedge \text{QUANTITY-SPEC}_i$$
$$\Rightarrow \text{CONSTRAINTS}_i \wedge \text{INFLUENCES}_i \wedge \text{STRUCTURE}'_i . \quad (1)$$

We can now categorize the contents of the knowledge base for our enterprise:

- The *domain theory* which represents the general knowledge about a particular type of ecosystem. Its core is the set of descriptions of generic processes as introduced above (a "library"). It has to be comprehensive in the sense that it contains all model elements required to model special ecological system of the respective type (of, course, it will never be complete).
- A *system structure* description which specifies the objects that constitute a particular system and their relations (e.g. spatial ones).
- *Quantity specifications* complete the specification of the ecosystem by determining parameters of objects involved. Secondly, they can represent observations about a particular *state* of this system.

We will now discuss how the various tasks can be formalized and implemented. It turns out that already the model composition step addresses some of the issues raised in section 3.

Situation Assessment, Step One: Model Composition

The idea underlying the process descriptions confines the input of a user to a "superficial" system description in terms of constellations of objects, their parameters, and observations about a particular state of the system. What the user does not have to enter or even know is what the relevant behavior models are. They are created automatically by the domain theory from the user input by applying process descriptions of the kind (1):

$$\text{DOMAIN-THEORY} \cup \text{STRUCTURE-DESCRIPTION} \cup \text{PARAM-SPEC}$$
$$\vdash \text{CONSTRAINTS} \cup \text{INFLUENCES.} \tag{2}$$

At this point, for each variable, all existing influences on it have to be combined to form a constraint. The problem lies in "*all* influences". If the initial structure description missed some facts or was based on certain assumptions, then (2) may fail to generate all relevant influences. Speaking in logical terms, in order to turn influences into a constraint, the system has to make "closed-world assumptions" (CWA) meaning that there exist no additional objects or relations that might generate another influence on a variable, y:

$$\text{INFLUENCES}(y) \wedge \text{CWA}_y \vdash \text{INFL-CONSTRAINT}(y). \tag{3}$$

Based on observations, the generated behavior model (a constraint network), can then complete the state description (as well as the parameter specification):

$$\text{CONSTRAINTS} \cup \text{QUANTITY-SPEC} \vdash \text{QUANTITY-SPEC}'.$$

Due to the lack of space, we an only mention that there are some non-trivial problems to solve because of the cyclic dependencies of behavior models (which can generate objects and derive quantity values) and process conditions on objects and quantities (which lead to behavior models) and refer to [Struss-Heller 98].

We also point out that (1), (2), and (3) enable the knowledge-based system to record which elements of the structure description, the quantity specification, the domain theory, and even the closed-world assumption lead to the existence of a particular constraint and, thus, to certain computed values. This is important, if some of these inputs are hypothetical or invalid in a given situation (e.g. due to disturbances in the system) and may have to be revised.

Model Revision - A Fundamental Task and Method

It turns out that several of the tasks of section 3 can be regarded and also implemented as a process of revising a given model. For instance, in situation assessment, we may start with a model of the normal state, but the given observations may contradict this model and force us to retract some normality assumptions to gain a picture of the actual situation.

Formally, the general revision process starts with a model that is inconsistent with the observations or some goals (both represented as sets of quantity specifications):

$$\text{MODEL}_0 \cup \text{OBSorGOALS} \vdash \perp. \tag{4}$$

Its result is a modified model (or several candidates) that removes the inconsistency with the observations (for situation assessment) or with the goals (for diagnosis and therapy):

$$\text{MODEL}_1 \cup \text{OBSorGOALS} \nvdash \perp. \tag{4'}$$

A stronger requirement would be that the revised model entails the observations (i.e. "explains" them) or the goals (i.e. accomplishes them):

$$\text{MODEL}_1 \vdash \text{OBSorGOALS} . \tag{4''}$$

Such a revision process is the core of model-based diagnosis systems that have been developed for technical systems and which currently enter industrial applications [Hamscher-Console-de Kleer 92], [Dressler-Struss 96]. Their techniques also form the basis for solutions in our domain. The key to a focused proposal of model revisions is the following: the inconsistencies occur as conflicting values for variables derived from observations and the constraints of the behavior model. Techniques that record the dependencies of the constraints and values on specific elements of MODEL_0 identify candidates for a revision. Guidance is usually given by some minimality criterion (w.r.t. sets, number, or probability of revisions).

Usually, there is not a unique proposed revision. Since the model-based system can explore the consequences of different hypotheses and, hence, their distinctions, it is able to propose measurements or tests that help to narrow down the set of candidates.

It is easy to see how these techniques can localize wrong assumptions about

Diagnosis

Here, the task is to identify the origins of contradictions between given goals and the description of the system and its state as it has been derived from situation assessment. We make parts of this description revisable, not because they may be wrong, but in order to find modifications of the model that remove the conflict with the goals,

$$\text{MODEL}_1 \cup \text{GOALS} \ \vdash\!\!\!\!/\ \perp ,$$

hence, could have caused the conflict, and provide a starting point for therapy:

$$\text{MODEL}_{rev} = \text{STRUCTURE}_{rev} \cup \text{PAR-SPEC}_{rev} \cup \text{VAR-SPEC}_{rev} \cup \text{CWAs},$$

Therapy

Therapy starts from a (not necessarily unique) result of the diagnostic step and has to identify actions that may implement the changes to the system proposed by this result:

$$\text{MODEL}_0 \cup \text{ACTIONS} \cup \text{GOALS'} \ \vdash\!\!\!\!/\ \perp .$$

This means the model knowledge base has to include actions. One way to achieve this is to represent the effects of an action as a process and the action itself as its (only) precondition. Thus, the revision process has to revise the closed-world assumption for variables that need to be influenced and then search for appropriate influences in the subset of the domain theory that represents potential actions.

Note that during therapy, the goal may be different from the ultimate ones, because it is in general impossible to satisfy them immediately. If the actual value of some variable is below what is specified by the goal, then an intermediate goal may be to increase the value, i.e. influence its derivative positively.

As stated above, the overall treatment may involve a real planning task which could exploit the model revision scheme presented here for generating steps of the plan and checking its compliance with the goals. Also, some goals may have to be violated temporarily, and by turning some goals into revisable options, the revision process can identify (minimal) sets of goals to be abandoned.

Prediction

This is simply the "model in action" over time, i.e. simulation:

$$\text{MODEL}(t=0) \ \vdash \ \text{MODEL}(t=t_1) \ .$$

But besides the computation of variable values over time (qualitative or numerical), a conceptual view of the evolution is derived in terms of activity of processes, creation and elimination of objects etc. This is important for the next task.

Explanation

This task now really benefits from the conceptual layer: rather than answering questions, such as "What happens?" or "Why does it happen?" by spitting out tables or plots of numerical values, it can present how certain processes were created, what their effects were, etc. Even questions why certain effects did *not* happen could be answered, based on the analysis of unsatisfied process conditions or influence combination.

Discovery

For all the previous tasks, the domain theory was not considered for revision. If we include elements of it (hypothetical processes or parts thereof) in the revisable part of the model, the general diagnostic technique could propose such elements for further inspection or modification. Finding missing processes could be supported by hypothesizing additional influences on variables that cannot be accounted for by existing process descriptions. Again, for alternative repairs of the theory, the system would be able to propose discriminating observations or experiments.

Of course, the ultimate driving force is the researcher. But a model-based system as his apprentice is a challenging perspective.

5   Conclusions

In this paper, we argued that
- solving our "environmental problems" requires to gain more insight in the complex interactions in ecosystems of which human activities are only a small part, i.e. *develop and use better models* of such systems,
- computer systems should be designed and implemented that support this task and, hence, have to support *conceptual modeling and problem solving* based on such models,
- theories, methods, and techniques developed in Artificial Intelligence research on knowledge representation and reasoning and, in particular, *qualitative modeling and model-based systems* are a promising starting point to pursue this goal.

This is why, although the goals are rather ambitious, there can be accomplishments, even in the short term. This is not the claim that we believe to have solved all fundamental problems. On the contrary, a lot of research and development of tools needs to be done. And we did not even touch some important research subjects, such as qualitative spatial and temporal reasoning. But there exists a strong basis in terms of theory, methods, *and implemented tools* and systems for tackling the tasks mentioned above in real applications.

What is required to progress? It is almost certain that wrong computer tools will be developed as long as the researchers in ecology do not pick up the offered solutions and spell out their requirements and Artificial Intelligence researchers do not expose their methods to these challenges. What is needed right now is closer collaboration between the domain experts and Artificial Intelligence researchers on developing principled solutions to specific problems.

Acknowledgments

Many thanks to the members of the MQM group at the Technical University of Munich for discussions and collaboration, and also to our project partners at the municipal department of water and sewage in Porto Alegre, Brazil, and the M.S. Swaminathan Research Foundation in Chennai, India, for supporting our work with their knowledge about the domain.

References

[Dressler-Struss 96] Dressler, O., Struss, P.: The Consistency-based Approach to Automated Diagnosis of Devices. In: Brewka, G. (ed.), Principles of Knowledge Representation, CSLI Publications, Stanford, ISBN 1-57586-057-0, pp. 267-311.

[Forbus 84] Forbus, K.: Qualitative Process Theory, in: Artificial Intelligence 24(1-3).

[Hamscher-Console-de Kleer 92] Hamscher, W., Console, L., de Kleer, J. (eds.): Readings in Model-based Diagnosis, Morgan Kaufmann Publishers, San Mateo.

[Heller-Struss 97] Heller, U., Struss, P.: Conceptual Modeling in the Environmental Domain. In: 15th IMACS World Congress on Scientific Computation, Modeling and Applied Mathematics, Berlin, August 1997, Vol. 6, pp. 147-152.

[Heller-Struss 98] Heller, U., Struss, P.: Diagnosis and Therapy Recognition for Ecosystems - Usage of Model-based Diagnosis Techniques. In: 12th International Symposium "Computer Science for Environmental Protection" (UI-98), Bremen, 1998, Metropolis Verlag, Marburg.

[Struss 97] Struss, P.: Model-based and qualitative reasoning: An introduction. In: Annals of Mathematics and Artificial Intelligence 19 (1997) III-IV, Baltzer Science Publishers.

[Struss-Heller 98] Struss, P., Heller, U.: Process-oriented Modeling and Diagnosis - Revising and Extending the Theory of Diagnosis from First Principles. In: Working Notes of the 9th International Workshop on Principles of Diagnosis (DX-98), Cape Cod.

The Infinite Variety of Logics

John F. Sowa

Abstract. Every knowledge representation language is a thinly disguised version of logic, often with a specialized ontology built into the notation. The number of possible notations for pure logic and the number of ontologies that could be combined with them are infinite. No single notation can ever be ideal for all possible applications, and new ones will always be found that can help to simplify various kinds of problems. Fortunately, the great diversity of logics can all be related to one another through a relatively small number of fundamental principles. This paper presents some examples that illustrate the advantages of different representations and the methods of mapping one to another.

1 Logical Trees, Graphs, and Algebra

In 1879, Gottlob Frege developed a tree notation he called the *Begriffsschrift*, which was the first complete version of first-order logic, but not even his students continued to use it. In his autobiography, Rudolf Carnap (1963) discussed his memories of Frege's lectures of 1913, which had an audience of three: Carnap, another student, and a retired army major who studied mathematics as a hobby. In 1919, Carnap studied Russell and Whitehead's *Principia Mathematica* and adopted its notation as "much more convenient."

The notation of the *Principia* is based on the algebraic notation developed independently by Charles Sanders Peirce (1883, 1885). Frege's compatriot Ernst Schröder was aware of the *Begriffsschrift*, but he didn't like the notation. Instead, he adopted Peirce's notation for his three-volume *Vorlesungen über die Algebra der Logik*. Later, the Italian mathematician Giuseppe Peano adopted the notation from Schröder, but he changed the symbols, since he wanted to mix mathematical and logical symbols in the same formulas. Peano began the practice of turning letters upside-down or backward to represent the logical symbols. As an illustration, Figure 1 represents the sentence *A cat is on a mat* in Frege's original *Begriffsschrift*, Peirce's algebraic notation, and Peano's version with the symbols $\land$ instead of $\bullet$ and $\exists$ instead of Σ. The fourth line shows Peirce's improvement of 1896: his *existential graphs* (EGs), which he continued to develop during the last eighteen years of his life.

In the last line of Figure 1, the bar between *cat* and *on* is called a *line of identity*; it represents an existential quantifier ($\exists x$). The other line of identity between *on* and *mat* represents the quantifier ($\exists y$). The words *cat* and *mat* represent the predicates $\mathrm{cat}(x)$ and $\mathrm{mat}(y)$, and *on* represents the predicate $\mathrm{on}(x, y)$.

Frege (1879): $\begin{array}{l}\text{on}(x,y)\\\text{mat}(y)\\\text{cat}(x)\end{array}$

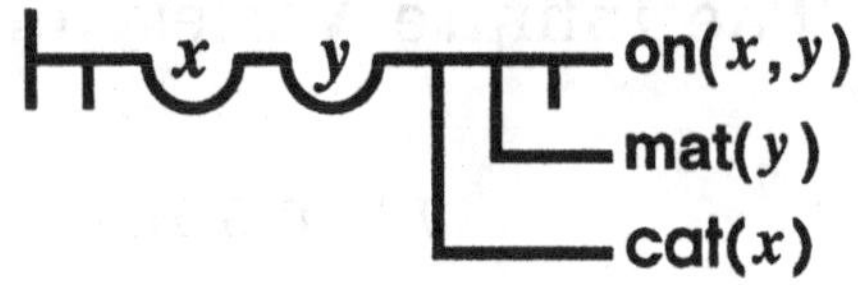

Peirce (1883): $\Sigma_x \Sigma_y (\text{cat}_x \cdot \text{mat}_y \cdot \text{on}_{xy})$

Peano (1895): $\exists x \exists y (\text{cat}(x) \wedge \text{mat}(y) \wedge \text{on}(x,y))$

Peirce (1896): cat —— on —— mat

Fig. 1. Four notations for representing "A cat is on a mat."

Therefore, Peirce's graph maps directly to his algebraic notation. Frege's tree, however, represents a more roundabout paraphrase:

$$\sim (\forall x)(\forall y)(cat(x) \supset (mat(y) \supset \sim on(x,y))).$$

This formula corresponds to the sentence *It is false that for all x and all y, if x is a cat then if y is a mat then x is not on y.* Even graphics cannot make such a cumbersome expression readable.

Peirce experimented with graph notations for logic as early as 1882, but his early graphs could not express the scope of quantifiers and negations. His invention of 1896 was the ultimate in simplicity: an oval enclosure for showing context, which also served to delimit scope. When marked with appropriate qualifiers, it could represent negation, modality, and other operators, such as knowledge, belief, desire, and purpose. As an example, Figure 2 shows an existential graph for the sentence *If there is a cat, then it is on a mat.*

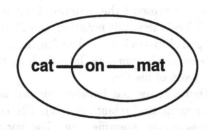

Fig. 2. Existential graph for "If there is a cat, then it is on a mat."

The default qualifier for each oval in Figure 2 is negation. Together, the two ovals represent implication, since $\sim (p \wedge \sim q)$ is equivalent to $(p \supset q)$. When overlaid on the graph at the bottom of Figure 2, the ovals express an if-then sentence. The line of identity for the cat has the scope of both ovals, but the line of identity for the mat is limited to just the inner oval. Therefore, Figure 3 may be translated to the following formula in predicate calculus:

$$\sim (\exists x)(cat(x) \wedge \sim (\exists y)(mat(y) \wedge on(x,y))).$$

By the operations of logic, this formula could be transformed to the following formula with the implication operator $\supset$:

$$(\forall x)(cat(x) \supset (\exists y)(mat(y) \wedge on(x,y))).$$

This formula illustrates a peculiar feature of the $\supset$ symbol: existential quantifiers in the antecedent must be moved to the front of the formula and be converted to universal quantifiers. That peculiarity has been a nuisance for linguists who have been trying to develop notations for representing the logical forms in natural language.

To simplify the mapping from language to logic, Hans Kamp (1981) invented *discourse representation structures* (DRS). The two primary operators in DRS are conjunction and the existential quantifier, and the implication operator has scoping rules that allow existential quantifiers in the antecedent to be preserved. Figure 3 shows the EG and DRS representations for the sentence *If a farmer owns a donkey, then he beats it*. The two notations are isomorphic: inside the contexts (ovals for EG or boxes for DRS), the implicit operators are conjunction and the existential quantifier; they have identical scoping rules for implication (a nest of two ovals for EG or two boxes connected by an arrow for DRS); and isomorphic mechanisms for cross references (lines of identity for EG or variables for DRS).

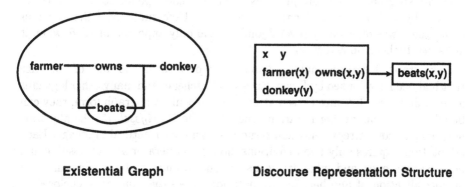

Existential Graph   Discourse Representation Structure

Fig. 3. EG and DRS for "If a farmer owns a donkey, then he beats it."

Peirce and Kamp both had a strong interest in representing contexts and the context-dependent references called *indexicals*. Peirce, in fact, coined the term *indexical,* and his interest in contexts led him to choose an oval enclosure for representing them. Although Peirce had not anticipated Kamp's rules for resolving indexical referents, Kamp's DRS rules can be applied directly to Peirce's EGs.

2 Rules of Inference

Besides readability, another important feature of a logical notation is computability, especially in support of the rules of inference. One reason why the *Begriffsschrift* is unreadable is that Frege chose to represent only those operators that were directly associated with his rules of inference: implication, negation, and the universal quantifier. Other operators like conjunction, disjunction, and the existential quantifier could only be represented by clumsy paraphrases. For the algebraic notation, Peirce followed Boole in patterning disjunction after addition, conjunction after multiplication, and implication after the less-than-or-equal operator (since the truth value of the antecedent is always less than or equal to the truth value of the consequent). Peirce defined the existential quantifier Σ as an infinite disjunction and the universal quantifier Π as an infinite conjunction. For the *Principia,* Russell adapted Frege's rules to the algebraic notation to create the most inefficient proof procedure that has ever been widely taught (but never widely learned). Better proof procedures for the algebraic notation were only invented many years later: *natural deduction* by Gerhard Gentzen (1935), *semantic tableaux* by Evert Beth (1955), and *resolution* by Alan Robinson (1965).

In 1897, a year after he invented existential graphs, Peirce discovered elegant rules of inference for them that are a generalization and simplification of Gentzen's rules of natural deduction. Peirce himself further generalized the rules to graph versions of modal logic and higher-order logic. It turns out that Peirce's rules are so general that any proof by resolution corresponds to the reverse of a proof by Peirce's form of natural deduction. Unfortunately, Peirce's paper about them was rejected by several journals and only appeared in 1906, when it attracted little or no attention.

The graph structures enabled Peirce to see patterns in the rules of inference that had been overlooked by Frege, Russell, Whitehead, and many other logicians for over 30 years. But once those patterns are recognized in graph form, they can be adapted to many other notations, including the *Begriffsschrift,* the algebraic notation, discourse representation structures, and even natural language. Each adaptation requires only two definitions: how each operator affects positive and negative contexts; and what it means for one formula to be a generalization or specialization of another. In any notation, a *positive context* is enclosed in an even number of negations, including a context with no negations at all; and a *negative context* is enclosed in an odd number of negations. The count of negations includes the number of explicit $\sim$ operators, but it also includes the implicit negations inside the definitions of the other logical operators. Each of them affects the *negation depth* of its operands:

- *Negation.* A negation $\sim$ increases the negation depth by one. For any expression of the form $\sim p$, the negation depth of the operand p is one greater than the negation depth of the containing context.
- *Conjunction.* A conjunction $\wedge$ has no effect on the number of negations. For an expression $p \wedge q$, the negation depth of both p and q is the same as the negation depth of the containing context.
- *Disjunction.* Since $p \vee q$ is defined as $\sim ((\sim p) \wedge (\sim q))$, a disjunction $\vee$ increases the negation depth of both p and q by two.
- *Implication.* Since $p \supset q$ is defined as $\sim (p \wedge \sim q))$, an implication $\supset$ increases the negation depth of p by one and the negation depth of q by two.
- *Existential.* The existential quantifier $\exists$ has no effect on the number of negations. For an expression $(\exists x)p$, the negation depth of p is the same as the negation depth of the containing context.
- *Universal.* Since the universal quantifier $(\forall x)p$ is defined as $\sim (\exists x) \sim p$, it increases the negation depth of p by two.

Existence and conjunction have no effect on the depth of nesting. Logically, philosophically, and computationally, they are the two simplest operators. Negation adds one to reverse the sign of a context: positive to negative or negative to positive. Implication reverses only the sign of its antecedent. Disjunction and the universal quantifier, which increase the depth by two, do not change the sign, but they introduce more computational complexity than $\exists$ and $\wedge$.

In natural deduction, either Peirce's or Gentzen's version, there is only one axiom: the blank statement, which is always true. In graph logic, the blank is represented by an empty sheet of paper or by a context with nothing in it. In the algebraic notation, however, blanks are not considered part of a formula; therefore, the blank must be represented by a place holder, such as the letter T for *truth*. The blank or T is the most general of all statements: all other statements, either graphs or formulas, can be derived by adding symbols that specialize the blank in one way or another. Peirce's rules are based on the principle that generalization in a positive context or specialization in a negative context preserves truth. The first step is to define specialization and generalization for the simplest of all logics, the existential-conjunctive (EC) subset of FOL, which uses only the operators $\wedge$ and $\exists$:

- *Specialization.* In EC logic, any statement may be specialized by adding more conjuncts to it. Any existential quantifier of the form $(\exists x)$ may be specialized by replacing all occurrences of x with some constant c.
- *Generalization.* Any formula in EC logic may be generalized by erasing one or more conjuncts (or equivalently replacing them by the place holder T). Any constant c may be generalized by replacing all occurrences of c with some variable such as x that does not occur in the formula and placing the quantifier $(\exists x)$ in front of the formula.

For EC logic, these definitions imply that q is more general than p if q is provable from p: $p \vdash q$. For any version of logic, provability is adopted as the definition of generalization. Since $p \vdash p$, every statement p is both a generalization and a specialization of itself.

Peirce's rules. After generalization and specialization have been defined for the EC subset, they can be recursively extended to any more complex formula by applying Peirce's five rules, which define the provability operator $\vdash$:

1. *Erasure.* In a positive context, any subgraph or subformula p may be erased. More generally, p may be replaced by any generalization q where $p \vdash q$. Since $p \vdash T$, erasure is the special case of replacing p with the blank.
2. *Insertion.* In a negative context, any subgraph or subformula p may be inserted. More generally, any statement q may be replaced by any specialization p where $p \vdash q$. Since $p \vdash T$, insertion is the special case of replacing the blank with p.
3. *Iteration.* If a subgraph or subformula p occurs in a context C, another copy of p may be written in the same context C or in any context nested in C.
4. *Deiteration.* Any subgraph or subformula p that could have been derived by iteration may be erased; i.e. any statement p may be erased if a copy of p occurs in the same context or any containing context.
5. *Double negation.* Two negations $\sim\sim$ with nothing between them may be erased or inserted around any subgraph or subformula.

These are sound and complete rules of inference for propositional logic. For existential graphs, they support full first-order logic with equality when they are applied to lines of identity. For the algebraic notation, they can be generalized to deal with variables, but the notation introduces more special cases that must be considered.

Proof in existential graphs To show how Peirce's rules can be applied to multiple notations, consider the following formula, which Leibniz called the *Praeclarum Theorema* (splendid theorem):

$$((p \supset r) \wedge (q \supset s)) \supset ((p \wedge q) \supset (r \wedge s)).$$

In the *Principia Mathematica*, this formula was one of the most difficult ones to be proved in Chapter 3. It required a total of 43 steps starting from five nonobvious axioms (one of which was redundant, but the proof of its redundancy was not discovered by the authors or any of their readers for 16 years). Figure 4 shows that the EG proof takes only 7 steps starting from an empty sheet; each step is numbered with the rule that is applied.

The EG at the end of the proof has four pairs of ovals, each pair corresponding to one of the $\supset$ symbols in the algebraic form. It would be possible to simplify the final graph by erasing a double negation, but then the exact correspondence with the algebraic notation would be lost. However, the resulting simplification is interesting in itself, since it corresponds to the negation of the collection of clauses used as the starting point in a proof by resolution:

$$p, q, \sim p \vee r, \sim q \vee s, \sim r \vee \sim s.$$

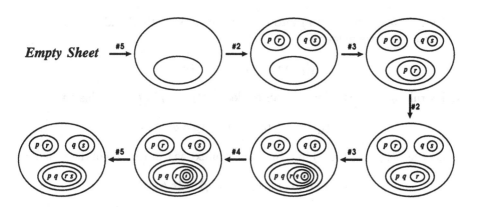

Fig. 4. Proof of the Praeclarum Theorema

From these clauses, resolution will derive the contradiction $\sim T$, which is the negation of the empty sheet at the start of Peirce's proof. But in terms of Peirce's rules, resolution can be proved as a derived rule of inference. Therefore, any proof by resolution can be converted to a proof by Peirce's rules just by drawing a negation around every step of the proof and reversing the order.

Proof in the algebraic notation. Although Peirce's rules apply to any notation for logic, some adjustment is needed to accommodate differences in syntax. In existential graphs, conceptual graphs, and discourse representation structures, a set of conjuncts may be written without intervening $\wedge$ symbols. In predicate calculus, however, another rule is needed to handle the extra *wedge* symbols.

- *Blanks.* The symbol T with the accompanying conjunction $\wedge$ may be inserted or deleted anywhere in a sequence of conjunctions.

This rule is implied by the other rules and the fact that p is equivalent to $p \wedge T$. In graph notations, in which the $\wedge$ symbol is implicit, this rule is unnecessary.

For each step in the proof of Figure 4, exactly the same rule can be applied to the algebraic formulas, although the linear notation makes the depth of nesting more obscure:

1. By rule #5, start by drawing two negative contexts around the blank or T: $\sim (T \wedge \sim T)$. Writing this formula as an implication,

$$T \supset T.$$

2. By rule #2, the first T may be replaced with any specialization. In particular, it may be replaced with the entire left side of the formula to be proved:

$$((p \supset r) \wedge (q \supset s)) \supset T.$$

3. By rule #3, copy $(p \supset r)$ into the same context with T and erase the now unneeded place holder T:

$$((p \supset r) \wedge (q \supset s)) \supset (p \supset r).$$

4. By rule #2, insert q into the antecedent of $(p \supset r)$ in the conclusion:

$$((p \supset r) \wedge (q \supset s)) \supset ((p \wedge q) \supset r).$$

5. By rule #3, copy $(q \supset s)$ into the same context as r at the end of the formula:

$$((p \supset r) \wedge (q \supset s)) \supset ((p \wedge q) \supset (r \wedge (q \supset s))).$$

6. By rule #4, erase the last copy of q and replace it with the blank or T:

$$((p \supset r) \wedge (q \supset s)) \supset ((p \wedge q) \supset (r \wedge (T \supset s))).$$

7. Finally, $(T \supset s)$ is equivalent to the double negation $\sim(\sim(s))$; therefore, by rule #5,

$$((p \supset r) \wedge (q \supset s)) \supset ((p \wedge q) \supset (r \wedge s)).$$

This example shows why no one but Peirce ever discovered these rules: although they can be applied to the algebraic notation, the linear form makes it difficult to see how the contexts are nested inside one another. In the EG form of Figure 4, the nesting is obvious. The graph notation is so perspicuous that Peirce discovered in one year what the best logicians in the world did not discover for another thirty years.

Comparison with Gentzen's proofs. Proofs by Peirce's rules are about the same length as proofs by Gentzen's rules, and both are much shorter than the proofs in the *Principia*. Peirce, however, discovered his rules thirteen years before the *Principia*, and the British journal *Mind* is one that refused to publish them. The major difference between Peirce's style of proofs and Gentzen's style is that every step in one of Peirce's proofs is a well-formed formula or graph. The first two steps in Figure 4 show why there is no need for Gentzen's book-keeping in making and discharging assumptions: step one introduces a dummy implication of the form $T \supset T$; then by replacing the first T with the antecedent of the theorem to be proved, the second step corresponds to a Gentzen-style assumption. The assumption never needs to be discharged by introducing the $\supset$ implies. symbol because that symbol was already introduced at step one.

A remarkable property of Peirce's rules, which permits the technique of starting with $T \supset T$, is that the rules depend only on the sign of the context, not its depth of nesting. Therefore, any proof that can be carried out on a blank sheet of paper can be " cut out" and " pasted" into any positive context nested at any depth. The formal statement of this property is called the *cut-and-paste theorem*:

- Theorem: If a statement q can be derived from a statement p by Peirce's rules of inference in the outermost context (nesting level 0), and if a copy of

p occurs in any positively nested context C, then the proof of q from p can be replicated by equivalent steps inside the context C.

Proof: Let the proof of q from P at level 0 be some sequence of statements $s_1, \ldots, s_n$, where the first step $p = s_1$ and the last step $q = s_n$. Since Peirce's rules depend only on the sign of a context, not its depth, every inference from s_i to s_{i+1} that is permissible on a blank sheet must also be permissible in C. Therefore, a copy of the sequence of graphs from $p = s_1$ to $q = s_n$ can be replicated inside C.

Other useful metatheorems can be derived from the cut-and-paste theorem as corollaries. The deduction theorem, for example, says that $p \vdash q$ implies $p \supset q$. It can be proved just by inserting p. in the antecedent of $T \supset T$, deriving q in the consequent, and erasing any intermediate results that may be left. In Gentzen's system, the deduction theorem is an assumption; in Peirce's system, it is a corollary.

3 Representing Music

Although logic is the most precise and the most fundamental of all declarative languages, it is by no means the only one. New notations, both graphic and linear, are constantly being invented in every field of science, engineering, business, and art. Musical notation, for example, has a history as long as logic. The mathematical relationships between the notes and scales were discovered by Pythagoras and his followers in ancient Greece. The modern notation with notes, staves, and clefs was developed by medieval monks working next door to the ones who were busily copying the textbooks on logic. Yet musical notation and other specialized notations are not competitors, but supplements to logic. Each of them represents a subset of logic with a built-in ontology tailored to a particular domain of interest.

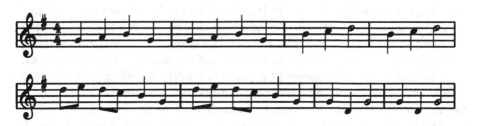

Fig. 5. A sample melody to be represented in logic

As an example, Figure 5 shows a sample melody, called " Frère Jacques" in French or " Brother John" in English. At the beginning of the first line, the *key signature* indicates one sharp for the key of G; the *time signature* 4/4 indicates 4 beats per *measure* with the quarter note having a duration of one time unit.

The vertical bars divide the melody in 8 measures, with a total of 32 notes. The vertical position of each note on the staff indicates a *tone*, designated by a letter from A through G (the letter may be qualified by a sharp or flat sign or by a number that indicates the octave). The shape of the note indicates duration: one time unit or *beat* for a quarter note; two units for a half note; or half a unit for an eighth note. The horizontal position of each note indicates that it is sounded after the one on the left and before the one on the right. These features, which represent the elements of an ontology for music, can be translated to logic supplemented with three predicates:

$tone(x, t)$	Note x has tone t.
$dur(x, d)$	Note x has the duration d.
$next(x, y)$	The next note after x is y.

To represent all 32 notes in the melody, the corresponding formula in predicate logic would require 32 variables, each with an existential quantifier. For each note, there would be three predicates to indicate its tone, duration, and successor. Following are the beginning and ending lines of the formula that represents the information in Figure 5:

$$(\exists x_1)(\exists x_2)(\exists x_3) \ldots (\exists x_{32})$$
$$(tone(x_1, G) \land dur(x_1, 1) \land next(x_1, x_2) \land$$
$$tone(x_2, A) \land dur(x_2, 1) \land next(x_2, x_3) \land$$
$$tone(x_3, B) \land dur(x_3, 1) \land next(x_3, x_4)$$
$$\land \ldots \land tone(x_{32}, G) \land dur(x_{32}, 2)).$$

The complete formula would start with 32 existential quantifiers and continue with 32 lines of predicates. The last line is shorter than the others because the last note does not have a successor.

Any musician would prefer to read music in the familiar notation of Figure 5 than in the translation to predicate calculus. But a translation to logic is a step toward implementing a program for analyzing the music or synthesizing it digitally. Logic is an *ontologically neutral* notation that can be adapted to any subject by adding one or more domain-dependent predicates. The full musical notation has many more features than those shown in Figure 5. Loudness, for example, is usually represented by abbreviations like **mf** for *mezzoforte* (medium loud). That feature could be represented by a predicate $mf(t_1, t_2)$, which indicates that a mezzoforte passage extends from time t_1 to t_2. But loudness is a continuously varying feature that is only roughly approximated by an abbreviation **mf** or predicate $mf(t_1, t_2)$. Subtle gradations in volume, timing, and phrasing make all the difference between a performance by Jascha Heifetz and the kid next door practicing the violin. Neither the musical score nor the logical formula represents those differences; each captures or omits exactly the same information.

Existential-Conjunctive Logic. Another observation about the translation gets to the essence of what logic can contribute: the only logical operators used in the formula are the existential quantifier $\exists$ and the conjunction $\land$. As a musical score becomes more detailed and complex, new kinds of predicates like mf(t_1, t_2) may be needed, but the universal quantifier ∀ and the other Boolean operators are never used. The EC subset of logic with only ∃ and ∧ is the usual version of logic for representing the specialized notations of many different fields. It is also the subset used for all the information stored in commercial database systems, both relational and object-oriented. EC logic is therefore an extremely important subset, but it has one serious limitation: it cannot represent any generalizations, negations, implications, or alternatives. For that, the operators ∀, ∼, ⊃, and ∨ are necessary.

One useful generalization is the principle that certain intervals are difficult to sing and should be avoided. In particular, the interval of three whole tones, called a *tritone*, is considered so dissonant that it was called the *diabolus in musica* in the Middle Ages. In the key of C, the tritone is the interval from B to F or from F to B; in the key of G, it is the interval from F♯ to C or from C to F♯. The next formula rules out the transition from B to F:

$$(\forall x)(\forall y)((tone(x, B) \land next(x, y)) \supset \sim tone(y, F)).$$

This formula says that for every x and y, if the tone of x is B and the next note after x is y, then the tone of y is not F. More rules like this would be needed to rule out the transition from F to B, from C to F♯, and so on. A more general rule could be stated in terms of another predicate called *tritone*:

      tritone(x, y)   Tone x and tone d form a tritone.

Then only one formula is needed to rule out all of the combinations:

$$(\forall x)(\forall y)(\forall z)(\forall w)$$
$$((next(x, y) \land tone(x, z) \land tone(y, w))$$
$$\supset \sim tritone(z, w)).$$

This formula says that for every x, y, z, and w, if the next note after x is y, the tone of x is z, and the tone of y is w, then z and w do not form a tritone. Rules like this cannot be stated in traditional musical notation because they use the operators ∀, ⊃, and ∼.

Conceptual graphs. The song "Frèere Jacques" is intended to be sung as a *round*, in which a second voice begins the melody when the first voice reaches measure 3. That kind of parallelism tends to be obscured by a linear notation, and graphs can often show the relationships more clearly. To show the third measure with two voices singing in harmony, Figure 6 uses a conceptual graph, which is a typed extension to Peirce's existential graphs (Sowa 1984, 1999). Each of the seven notes in the measure is represented by a separate concept [Note]. Each note is attached to conceptual relations that correspond to the tone, next, and dur predicates: the Tone relation links the concept of the note to a concept that indicates the type of tone; the Next relation links to the concept of the next note; and the Dur relation links to a concept of a time interval of the specified duration. Two notes that are sounded simultaneously are linked to the same concept. But at the end of the measure, the upper voice is a half note that lasts as long as the two quarter notes in the lower voice. Therefore, the interval for the half note is linked by two Part relations to the intervals for each of the quarter notes.

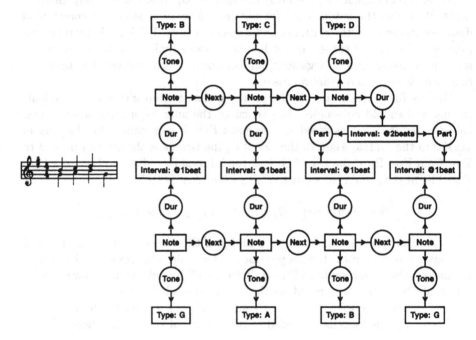

Fig. 6. Conceptual graph for two voices singing in harmony

Each concept box in Figure 6 represents something that exists: a note, an interval, or a type of tone. When the CG is translated to predicate calculus, the corresponding existential quantifiers must be shown explicitly:

$(\exists x_1, x_2, x_3, x_4, x_5, x_6, x_7 : Note)$

$(\exists y_1, y_2, y_3, y_4, y_5 : Interval)$

$(tone(x_1, B) \wedge dur(x_1, y_1) \wedge hasAmount(y_1, 1beat) \wedge next(x_1, x_2) \wedge$

$tone(x_2, C) \wedge dur(x_2, y_2) \wedge hasAmount(y_2, 1beat) \wedge next(x_2, x_3) \wedge$

$tone(x_3, D) \wedge dur(x_3, y_3) \wedge hasAmount(y_3, 2beats) \wedge$

$tone(x_4, G) \wedge dur(x_4, y_1) \wedge next(x_4, x_5) \wedge$

$tone(x_5, A) \wedge dur(x_5, y_2) \wedge next(x_5, x_6) \wedge$

$tone(x_6, B) \wedge dur(x_6, y_4) \wedge hasAmount(y_4, 1beat) \wedge next(x_6, x_7) \wedge$

$tone(x_7, G) \wedge dur(x_7, y_5) \wedge hasAmount(y_5, 1beat) \wedge$

$part(y_3, y_4) \wedge part(y_3, y_5)).$

The quantifiers at the beginning of this formula specify x_1 through x_7 as notes and y_1 through y_5 as intervals. What makes the formula difficult to read is not the quantifiers, but the proliferation of variables. In the graph, all the information about an entity is localized — either inside the concept box itself or in the relations attached directly to the box. But when the graph is mapped to a linear string, there is no way to preserve the locality of information: the variables that represent the links tend to get scattered throughout the formula.

Since Figure 6 is a direct translation from a musical score, it uses only the existential-conjunctive subset of logic. But logic, in both the graphic and linear notations, has much more expressive power for stating rules and generalizations about music. As an example, Figure 7 uses conceptual graphs as a metalanguage for stating the definition of a new relation called Simul, which states that two notes are sounded simultaneously. The graph may be read *The relation Simul has a definition (Def), which is a lambda expression that relates a note λ_1 to a note λ_2, in which both notes occur during the same interval.*

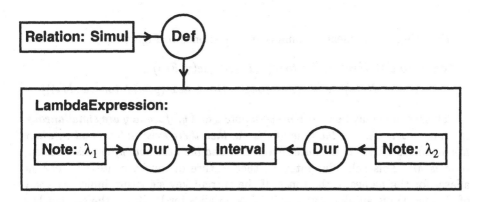

Fig. 7. Definition of the Simul relation between two notes

The definition of simultaneity in Figure 7 shows why it is important to distinguish the interval from its duration. Six of the seven notes in Figure 6 have the same duration, but only two pairs are sounded exactly simultaneously. In predicate calculus, Figure 7 corresponds to the following definition:

$$simul = (\lambda x, y : Note)(\exists z : Interval)$$
$$(dur(x, z) \land dur(y, z)).$$

The Simul relation can be used to state a rule for the harmonious resolution of a dissonance. If two notes sounded together happen to form a dissonant tritone, they can be resolved by having their successors move to a harmonious interval. In the key of G, the tritone of F# and C would be followed by the major third of G and B. In the key of C, the tritone of B and F would be followed by C and E. To avoid having to state a separate rule for every key, those rules can all be summarized by using the relative names for the types of tones: Do, Re, Mi, Fa, So, La, and Ti. Figure 8 shows a CG that says that if a note x of tone Ti is sounded simultaneously with a note y of tone Fa, then the next note after x has tone Do and the next note after y has tone Mi.

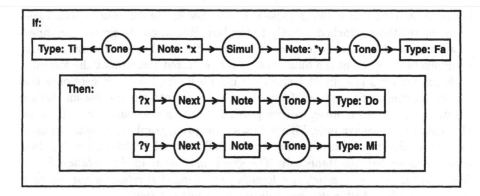

Fig. 8. Rule for the harmonious resolution of a dissonance

Following is the linear formula that corresponds to Figure 8:

$$(\forall x, y\, \mathcal{N}ote)((simul(x,y) \wedge tone(x, Ti) \wedge tone(y, Fa)) \supset$$
$$(\exists z, w \colon Note)(next(x,z) \wedge tone(z, Do) \wedge next(y,w) \wedge tone(w, Mi))).$$

This formula may be read *For every note x and y, if x and y are simultaneous, the tone of x is Ti, and the tone of y is Fa, then there exist notes z and w, where the next note after x is z, whose tone is Do, and the next note after y is w, whose tone is Mi.* This rule illustrates another feature of music: context-dependent aliases for the names of the tones. If the current key signature indicates a key of G, then Do is an alias for G and Mi is an alias for B. But if the current key is C, then Do and Mi are aliases for C and E. The rules for translating from the context-dependent to the absolute names of tones could also be expressed in logical implications.

4 Situation Calculus

Just as the graphic notations helped Peirce discover novel inference rules that other logicians had missed, graphical notations specialized for various applications can often highlight features that may be overlooked in linear notations. As an example, the notation of Petri nets suggests ways of generalizing the *situation calculus* to a distributed form that can represent a more complex and realistic problems. In introducing the situation calculus, John McCarthy (1963) proposed a metalevel operator, which treats propositions as fluents that are true in certain situations:

$$cause(\pi)(s).$$

McCarthy said that this formula is " intended to mean that the situation s will lead in the future to a situation that satisfies the fluent π. Thus $cause(\pi)$ is itself a propositional fluent". As an example, he wrote

$$(\forall s: Situation)(\forall p: Person)$$
$$[(raining \wedge outside(p)) \supset cause(wet(p))](s).$$

McCarthy's brackets enclose a propositional fluent, which is applied to the situation s to derive a proposition. The complete formula may be read *For every situation s and person p, if it is raining and p is outside, then p will become wet in a situation caused by s.*

Over the years, everybody who has used the situation calculus has adapted it to his or her preferred notation. Cordell Green (1969) used a theorem prover based on resolution, which was limited to first-order logic without metalevels. Therefore, Green translated McCarthy's notation to a form without fluents or metalevel operators. In Green's notation, every predicate had an explicit argument for the situation:

$$(\forall s: Situation)(\forall p: Person)$$
$$((raining(s) \wedge outside(p, s)) \supset getWet(p, s)).$$

This formula may be read *For every situation s and person p, if it is raining in s and p is outside in s, then p gets wet in s.* Unfortunately, Green's first-order system also required axioms to say what does not happen:

$$(\forall s: Situation)(\forall p: Person)$$
$$((raining(s) \wedge inside(p, s)) \supset \sim getWet(p, s)).$$

This formula says that every person who stays inside in a situation in which it is raining does not get wet.

The need to say what does not happen has been one of the major drawbacks of the situation calculus. For many applications, the number of axioms that say what does not happen tend to overwhelm the axioms about the changes that actually do happen. McCarthy and Hayes (1969) called such a proliferation of negative axioms the *frame problem.* That name tends to be confusing since the frame problem primarily affects the situation calculus, and it usually does not occur with frame representations.

Solving the frame problem. Leibniz's principle of sufficient reason is the key to solving the frame problem: *Nothing at all happens without some reason* (Nihil omnino fit sine aliqua ratione). That principle is a metalevel statement that cannot be used in purely first-order theorem provers. Nevertheless, it has been implemented in many systems, both logic-based and procedural. The first explicit solution to the frame problem was by Richard Fikes and Nils Nilsson (1971) with STRIPS:

> While Green's formulation represented a significant step in the development of problem solvers, it suffered some serious disadvantages connected with the " frame problem" that prevented it from solving nontrivial problems. In STRIPS, we surmount these difficulties by separating entirely

the processes of theorem proving from those of searching through a space of world models. This separation allows us to employ separate strategies for these two activities and thereby improve the overall performance of the system. Theorem-proving methods are used only *within* a given world model to answer questions about it concerning which operators are applicable and whether or not goals have been satisfied.

Each of the STRIPS world models is a collection of statements in EC logic that describes a McCarthy-style situation. The metalevel for reasoning about the models is implemented in LISP procedures that search the collection of models, generate changed models by adding or deleting propositions, and test whether the newly generated models have reached the desired goals. By copying the current world model as the first step in generating the next one, STRIPS implicitly obeys Leibniz's metalevel principle of leaving everything unchanged that is not affected by the current action. Without the metalevel, additional axioms are needed for every action and every changeable thing that is not affected by that action. With an appropriate use of metalanguage, the proliferation of axioms caused by the frame problem disappears.

Yale shooting problem. Steven Hanks and Drew McDermott (1987) posed a problem that has raised controversies about the role of logic in reasoning about time. Named after their university, the Yale shooting problem concerns a person who is alive in situation s_0. In their version of the situation calculus, they replaced McCarthy's metalevel cause operator with a function named result:

- Situation s_1 is the result of a gun being loaded in s_0:

$$s_1 = result(load, s_0).$$

- Situation s_2 is the result of waiting for some interval of time after s_1:

$$s_2 = result(wait, s_1) = result(wait, result(load, s_0)).$$

- Situation s_3 is the result of the victim being shot by the gun:

$$s_3 = result(shoot, s_2)$$
$$= result(shoot, result(wait, result(load, s_0))).$$

Figure 9 shows a finite-state machine whose states represent the situations and whose arcs represents the actions that transform one situation to the next. The problem is to determine whether the victim is alive or dead in situation s_3.

Hanks and McDermott found that the axioms of persistence in situation calculus cannot definitely predict the fate of the victim. With their representation, the state of a person being alive would normally persist, but the state of a gun being loaded would also persist. The situation calculus cannot determine whether the gun switches state from loaded to unloaded or the victim switches state from alive to dead. The length of time spent waiting between situation s_1 and s_2, for example, is not specified. If the waiting time were one minute, the

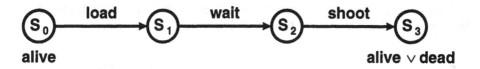

Fig. 9. A finite-state machine for the Yale shooting problem

gun would be likely to remain loaded. But if the time had been a year, it's more likely that someone would have unloaded it. The person or persons who carried the gun, loaded it, pulled the trigger, or perhaps unloaded it are not mentioned, and their motives are unknown. The type of weapon, the distance between the assassin and the victim, the victim's movements, and the assassin's shooting skills are unknown.

As someone who has long worked on logic-based approaches to AI, McDermott had hoped that logic alone would be able to give a unique answer to the Yale shooting problem and other similar, but more practical problems. He reluctantly concluded that the versions of nonmonotonic logic applied to reasoning about time cannot by themselves solve such problems:

> The whole point behind the development of nonmonotonic formal systems for reasoning about time has been to augment our logical machinery so that it reflects in a natural way the " inertia of the world." All of this effort is wasted if one is trying merely to express constraints on the physics of the world: we can solve the problem once and for all by saying " once a fact becomes true it stays true until the occurrence of some event causes it to become false." ... Many researchers, however, would not be satisfied with using logic only as a notation for expressing ontological theories.

McDermott's method of solving the problem " once and for all" is a paraphrase of Leibniz's principle of sufficient reason. But as Leibniz observed, every entity in the universe has some influence on every other entity. Only an omniscient being such as God could account for the potentially infinite number of events that might cause a change. To determine which of those events are significant, finite reasoners — human or computer — must use axioms that express the physics of the world.

5   Distributed Situations

As Figure 9 illustrates, the usual situation calculus is equivalent in structure to a finite-state machine, which can only represent a single-threaded sequence of situations and events. When multiple agents interact, however, they create distributed processes that are more naturally represented by Petri nets. Figure 10, for example, shows two representations for a robot r pushing an object k from m to n: on the left, a finite-state machine that corresponds to the situation calculus; and on the right, a Petri net. A dot or *token* in a circle indicates that the corresponding condition is true at an indexical time called *now*.

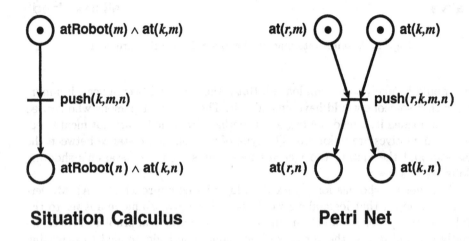

Situation Calculus   **Petri Net**

Fig. 10. Representing a robot *r* pushing an object *k*

For the situation calculus, the finite-state machine shows the preconditions and postconditions for a robot pushing an object, as Fikes and Nilsson stated them in STRIPS. Since finite-state machines correspond to Petri nets with just one token on the entire net, any version of the situation calculus that can be modeled by an FSM can only represent a single active agent, such as a robot working alone. The Petri net on the right, however, shows a distributed representation with separate input and output states for the robot *r* and the object *k*. The option of multiple tokens can support any number of active or passive entities, each with its own independent state.

For the Yale shooting problem, Figure 11 takes advantage of the greater expressive power of Petri nets to show causal links between states and events that involve different participants. Following are the mappings from Petri nets to a distributed version of the situation calculus:

- *Places.* Every place on the Petri net represents a type of condition that can be expressed by a proposition stated in predicate calculus or conceptual graphs. The seven places in Figure 11 represent seven types of conditions that might be true at some time in the past, present, or future.
- *Tokens.* A token in a place means that the corresponding condition is true at the current time *now*. Instead of representing situations by single nodes as in finite-state machines, a Petri net represents the current situation by a conjunction of the conditions for all the places that currently contain tokens. In Figure 11, the initial situation is described by a conjunction of two propositions: the assassin has a gun, and the victim is alive.
- *Events.* Every transition represents a type of event, whose precondition is the conjunction of the conditions for its input places and whose postcondition is

the conjunction of the conditions for its output places. In the example, the Misfire event has no output conditions. When it occurs, its only effect is to erase a token from the place labeled Firing-pin-struck, thereby disabling the event Gun-fires.

- *Arcs.* The arcs that link places and transitions have the effect of the add and delete lists in STRIPS. For any transition, the input arcs correspond to the delete list, because each of them erases a token from its input place, thereby causing the corresponding proposition to become false. The output arcs correspond to the add list, because each of them adds a token to its output place, thereby asserting the corresponding proposition.
- *Persistent places.* A place that is linked to a transition by both an input and an output arc is *persistent* because its condition remains true when that transition fires. In the example, the place labeled Assassin-has-gun persists after the assassin loads the gun or pulls the trigger. For all the other places in Figure 11, their preconditions become false after their tokens are used as input to some transition.

Figure 11 elaborates the Yale shooting problem with further detail. This elaboration is by no means unique, since any problem can be analyzed and extended with any amount of detail.

Questions about future situations can be answered either by executing the Petri net interpretively or by proving theorems about what states are reachable. To determine what happens to the victim, trace the flow of tokens through Figure 11:

1. If the assassin loads the gun and pulls the trigger before anyone unloads it, the gun can fire, shooting the victim, who ends up dead.
2. If somebody unloads the gun before the assassin pulls the trigger, the gun misfires, and the victim remains alive.
3. Even if the gun is loaded when the assassin pulls the trigger, there is a slight chance of a misfire because of some other malfunction. In that case, the victim also remains alive.

With these possibilities, the most that can be concluded is a disjunction:
    Misfire ∨ Victim-dead.

A conclusion of this form is inevitable unless further information can be obtained that would eliminate the possibility that the gun misfires or somebody unloads it.

Causal networks Network notations that resemble Petri nets have been used in many AI systems for representing cause and effect. Chuck Reiger (1976) developed a version of *causal networks*, which he used for analyzing problem descriptions in English and translating them to a network that could support metalevel reasoning. Judea Pearl (1988, 1996), who has developed techniques for applying statistics and probability to AI, introduced *belief networks*, which are causal networks whose links are labeled with probabilities.

To resolve the indeterminism that occurs at disjunctive nodes, Pearl would compute or estimate the probabilities of each of the options. When one option

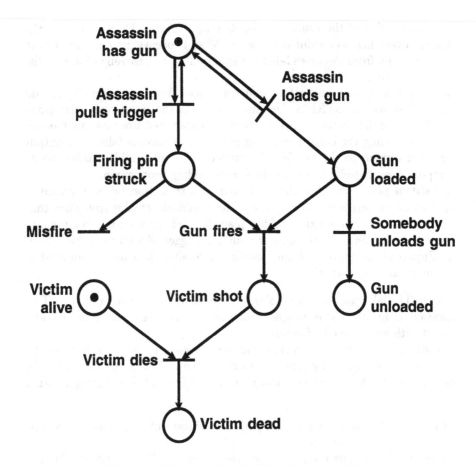

Fig. 11. A Petri net for the Yale shooting problem

is much more likely than the other, he would derive a qualitative solution by assigning a small value ϵ to them unlikely option and the complementary value $(1-\epsilon)$ to the more likely option. For the network shown in Figure 11, there are three disjunctive nodes, each of which has one likely path and one unlikely path.

1. The first disjunction occurs at the top, where the order of loading the gun or pulling the trigger is not specified. Unless the assassin were grossly incompetent, the probability of pulling the trigger before loading the gun would be a small value ϵ_1, and the option of loading first would be $(1-\epsilon_1)$.
2. After the gun is loaded, the probability that someone might happen to unload it shortly thereafter is another small number ϵ_2.
3. If the gun is unloaded, the probability of a misfire is 100%, since the transition labeled Gun-fires would not be enabled. But if the gun is loaded, the likelihood of a misfire is a small value ϵ_3.

If the network correctly captures the relevant causal dependencies, the probabilities at different disjunctive nodes would be independent. Therefore, the probability of any possible outcome would be the product of all the options along the path from start to finish. The primary path, which takes each of the more likely options, would have a probability that corresponds to informal intuitions:

$$(1 - \epsilon_1)(1 - \epsilon_2)(1 - \epsilon_3).$$

If each of the ϵ options has a probability of 10% or less, the probability that the victim dies would be at least 72.9%. For a variety of problems in temporal reasoning, Peter Grünwald (1997) compared the solutions obtained with Pearl's belief networks to other proposed methods. For each of them, he showed that Pearl's approach was equivalent to, more general than, or intuitively more convincing than the others.

As this example illustrates, Petri nets are causal networks that can be executed interpretively, be compiled to efficient procedures, or serve as the basis for metalevel analysis. Another way is to map the Petri nets to *linear logic*, in which the proof procedures mimic the firing of Petri net transitions by moving truth markers from the inputs to the outputs of an implication. Although some versions of linear logic are not decidable, Anne Troelstra (1992) showed that Petri nets are equivalent to a version of linear logic whose outcomes are decidable.

6 Bilingualism in Logic

Knowing a second language helps people distinguish the fundamental linguistic structures from the provincial features of a particular language or culture. In the same way, learning a second notation for logic enables people to see fundamental structures from a new perspective and helps them discover patterns in one notation that might be invisible or obscure in another. Peirce was fluent in several different notations for logic, most of which he invented himself. They enabled him to discover techniques that other logicians never saw because they were blinded by the limitations of their notations. The application of Petri nets to the situation calculus is another example of the way that a second notation can clarify relationships that are obscure or invisible in the first. Music shows that a notation can be precise enough to be automatically translated to logic while being readable at high speed by human experts in the domain.

Besides Peirce, Rudolf Carnap was a brilliant logician who had the good fortune to learn two different notations early in his career. Like Peirce, Carnap had greater success than most logicians in learning to overcome the limitations of a single formalism and invent new formalisms for different purposes. In his autobiography, he discussed the influence of his early education:

> When I became acquainted with Frege's symbolic system, which was for me the first system of symbolic logic, the question of planning did not immediately occur to me, because Frege simply exhibited his kind of notation and the structure of his language, proved theorems and showed applications, but said very little about his motivation for the choice of this particular language form. Only later, when I became acquainted

with the entirely different language forms of *Principia Mathematica*, the modal logic of C. I. Lewis, the intuitionistic logic of Brouwer and Heyting, and the typeless systems of Quine and others, did I recognize the infinite variety of possible language forms. On the one hand, I became aware of the problems connected with the finding of language forms suitable for given purposes; on the other hand, I gained the insight that one cannot speak of " the correct language form," because various forms have different advantages in different respects. The latter insight led me to the principle of tolerance. Thus, in time, I came to recognize that our task is one of *planning* forms of languages. Planning means to envisage the general structure of a system and to make, at different points in the system, a choice among various possibilities, theoretically an infinity of possibilities, in such a way that the various features fit together and the resulting total language system fulfills certain given desiderata.

This influence appears throughout Carnap's many books and articles. It even shows in his textbook (1954), in which he introduces several different versions of logical notations with different expressive power and with many applications of different ontologies to specialized domains. Unfortunately, the modern curriculum in computer science barely teaches the rudiments of one notation for logic and seldom, if ever shows the connections between logic and the ever growing numbers of user interfaces. Graph logics can be especially useful in building a bridge between formal methods of reasoning and the art of explaining them in a humanly readable form. In his stimulating book *Visual Explanations*, Edward Tufte (1997) has presented various techniques that could be used to visualize logic.

Bibliography

E. W. Beth. *Semantic Entailment and Formal Derivability*. North-Holland Publishing Co., Amsterdam, 1955.

R. Carnap. Autobiography. In P. Schilpp, editor, *The Philosophy of Rudolf Carnap*, pages 3–84. Open Court Press, La Salle, IL, ????

R. Carnap. *Einf"uhrung in die symbolische Logik*. Dover Publications, New York, 1954. translated as *Introduction to Symbolic Logic and its Applications*.

R. E. Fikes and N. J. Nilsson. Strips: A new approach to the application of theorem proving to problem solving. *Artificial Intelligence*, 2:189–208, 1971.

G. Gentzen. *Untersuchungen über das logische Schliessen I II*. North-Holland Publishing Co., Amsterdam, 1935. English translation in *The Collected Papers of Gerhard Gentzen*, pp. 68-131.

P. Gr"unewald. Causation and nonmonotonic temporal reasoning. In G. Brewka, C. Habel, and B. Nebel, editors, *KI-97: Advances in Artificial Intelligence*, LNAI 1303, pages 159–170. Springer Verlag, Berlin, 1997.

S. Hanks and D. McDermott. Nonmonotonic logic and temporal projection. *Artificial Intelligence*, 33:379–412, 1987.

H. Kamp. Events, discourse representations, and temporal references. *Langages*, 64:39–64, 1981.

J. McCarthy. Situations, actions, and causal laws. In M. Stanford AI Memo No. 2. Reprinted in Minsky, editor, *Semantic Information Processing*, pages 410–418. MIT Press, Cambridge, MA, 1963.

J. McCarthy and P. Hayes. *Some philosophical problems from the standpoint of artificial intelligence*. Edinburgh University Press, 1969.

J. Pearl. Fusion, propagation, and structuring in belief networks. *Artificial Intelligence*, 29:241–288, 1986.

J. Pearl. *Probabilistic Reasoning in Intelligent Systems*. Morgan Kaufmann Publishers, San Mateo, CA, 1988.

C. S. Peirce. On the algebra of logic. *American Journal of Mathematics*, 7: 180–202, 1985.

C. Rieger. An organization of knowledge for problem solving and language comprehension. *Artificial Intelligence*, 7:89–127, 1976.

D. D. Roberts. *The Existential Graphs of Charles S. Peirce*. Mouton, The Hague, 1973.

J. A. Robinson. A machine oriented logic based on the resolution principle. *Journal of the ACM*, 12:23–41, 1965.

J. F. Sowa. *Conceptual Structures: Information Processing in Mind and Machine*. Addison-Wesley, Reading, MA, 1984.

J. F. Sowa. *Knowledge Representation: Logical, Philosophical, and Computational Foundations*. PWS Publishing Co., Pacific Grove, CA, 1999.

A. S. Troelstra. *Lectures on Linear Logic*. CSLI, Stanford, CA, 1992.

E. R. Tufte. *Visual Explanations: Images and Quantities, Evidence and Narrative*. Graphics Press, 1997.

Thinking in Agents

Heinz Jürgen Müller

Deutsche Telekom AG
Technologiezentrum Darmstadt FE14k
PO 10 00 03
D-64276 Darmstadt
GERMANY
muellerhj@tzd.telekom.de

Abstract

Agents and Agencies do change the development processes for complex intelligent systems. Like Artificial Intelligence influences the way of tackling hard problems via knowledge processing, Distributed Artificial Intelligence attacks real world problems by modeling interacting intelligent agents as a mapping of higher human problem solving abilities. While classical AI is interested in studying the autistic mechanisms of single knowledge based systems, DAI is concerned with the social aspects of intelligent systems and electronic societies.

The talk will present central techniques and stepping stones for the development of distributed intelligent systems. New views an agent designer has to take and the relating research questions will be discussed. Main topics of the "technology and design" section will be:

- conflict management,
- negotiation techniques,
- goal directed behavior,
- social structure modeling, and
- cooperative learning.

In the theory section different approaches for modeling multi-agent systems will be demonstrated. The following theoretical frameworks will be used to specify multi-agent systems.

- extended abstract data types,
- dynamic logic,
- enhanced temporal logic, and
- graph grammars

Eventually a brief overview of current applications as well as an outlook for future research will be given.

Finding Regions for Local Repair in Partial Constraint Satisfaction

Harald Meyer auf'm Hofe

German Research Center for Artificial Intelligence
Postfach 2080
D-67608 Kaiserslautern, Germany

Abstract. Yet, two classes of algorithms have been used in partial constraint satisfaction: local search methods and *branch&bound* search extended by the classical constraint-processing techniques like e.g. *forward checking* and *backmarking*. Both classes exhibit characteristic advantages and drawbacks. This article presents a novel approach for solving partial constraint satisfaction problems exhaustively that combines advantages of local search and extended *branch&bound* algorithms. This method relies on repair based search and a generic method for an exhaustive enumeration of repair steps.

1 Introduction

Algorithms for solving *constraint satisfaction problems (CSP)* have been successfully applied to several fields including scheduling, design, and planning. Extending the standard CSP by a representation of constraint importance led to the class of *partial constraint satisfaction problems (PCSP)* [2] which provides new opportunities for solving several problems of combinatorial optimization more efficiently. A *PCSP* is the task of labeling each variable of a given variable set with a value of a certain domain. Constraints of an explicitly represented importance state restrictions on combinations of some variables' labels. The solution of a *PCSP* is a labeling complying with as important constraints as possible.

Yet, two classes of algorithms have been applied to partial constraint satisfaction: local search methods [9] and systematic *branch&bound* search extended by classical constraint-processing techniques like *forward checking* and *backmarking* [2,4,7]. Both paradigms exhibit characteristic advantages and drawbacks. Theoretically, the *branch&bound* algorithm is guaranteed to terminate with an optimal solution. However, tree search algorithms retract early decisions only after searching large portions of the search space exhaustively. As a consequence, minor differences in the constraint problem can result in a completely different run time behavior — especially if the number of variables is larger. In contrast, local search procedures try to improve a labeling without respecting a certain systematic in search. Thus, they are applicable to dynamic constraint problems, where variables and constraints are added resp. removed. However, the computed result is of a questionable quality. Proving the optimality of a result is not possible by use of local search algorithms. Local minima are processed by heuristics which either make use of noise strategies (*mincon-walk* and *mincon-retry* [12]), exploit information on the search history (e.g., tabu search [3]), or change more than one variable at each step of repair (e.g., EFLOP-heuristics [13] or the *lc*–algorithm [11]).

This paper presents a novel approach for solving partial constraint satisfaction problems that combines the advantages of local search and tree search algorithms. This approach is based on iterative improvement of an initially chosen labeling repeating the following steps: A region (a set of variables) in the constraint problem is chosen by an exhaustive enumeration strategy. Then, an extended *branch&bound* is used to optimize the labels in this region. This method organizes the search space flexibly like local search algorithms, i.e. the algorithm is able to change any assignment at any time if this promises to lead to an improvement in the quality of the labeling. Generally, iterative improvement algorithms have to be tailored to the application. Exhaustive enumeration of regions for local repair turns iterative improvement into a generic algorithm and provides the ability to prove optimality of a solution.

The paper is organized as follows: After providing some basic definitions on partial constraint satisfaction, the second section describes iterative improvement algorithms. A section on exhaustive enumeration of iterative repair steps follows, which starts with a small theory on enumerating improvement steps and ends with an enumeration algorithm. Then, first empirical results are presented in order to prove the relevance of the approach. A concluding section sums up the results.

2   Partial Constraint Satisfaction

In order to clarify notations, which are especially required in section 4, some basic definitions are given here.

Definition 1. *A CSP is a tuple* (V, D, C) *where V is a set of variables, the domain D is a set of values which can be assigned to the variables, and C is a set of constraints, where each $c \in C$ is defined by: $V(c) \subseteq V$ is a set of variables which are directly affected by c. The extension of c, ext(c), is a set of labelings of all variables in $V(c)$ with values of D which comply with c.*

$$l \downarrow_{V'} = \{v_i \leftarrow d_i \in l | v_i \in V\}$$

denotes the selection of labels which concern the variables in V'. A labeling l complies with a constraint c iff $l \downarrow_{V(c)} \in$ ext(c).

$$\bar{C}(l) = \{c \in C \mid l \downarrow_{V(c)} \notin \text{ext}(c)\}$$

denotes the set of constraints being violated by l. A labeling l of all variables in V is a solution of $CSP = \{V, D, C\}$ iff

$$l \in \text{ext}(C) \iff \forall c \in C : l \downarrow_{V(c)} \in \text{ext}(c)$$

$$\Longleftrightarrow \bar{C}(l) = \{\}$$
$$\Longleftrightarrow l \in \bowtie_{c \in C} \text{ext}(c).$$

Hence, a solution of a CSP is a labeling of all variables which complies with all constraints.

In partial constraint satisfaction[1], the relative importance of constraints is given by a partial ordering among constraint sets where $C' \succ C''$ means intuitively: *The constraints in C' are more important than the constraints in C''.* The solution of a $PCSP$ satisfies as important constraints as possible.

Definition 2. *A $PCSP = (V, D, C, \succ)$ extends a $CSP = (V, D, C)$ by a preference ordering $\succ$, which is a partial ordering among subsets of C. A labeling l of all variables in V is a solution of a $PCSP$ iff there is no labeling $l' \neq l$ with $\bar{C}(l) \succ \bar{C}(l')$.*

This notion of PCSPs forms the domain of the *enumerating global revisions* method. The well known algorithms for solving $PCSP$s like the *branch&bound* [2] as well as *mincon* [9] and *mincon-walk* [12] can be adopted easily to these definitions [6].

3 Iterative Improvement

Fig. 1 presents a scheme for searching by *iterative improvement* which forms the basis for our novel approach. A labeling l of all variables is modified iteratively repeating the improvement step within the rows 2 to 5. This method may be considered as a generalization of the *mincon* algorithm [9] where, in contrast to *mincon*, local minima are passed conducting more than one change in the current labeling l within a single step of repair.

Therefore, a procedure `choose-bad-region` is used to determine a set of variables whose labels will be changed in the following improvement step (row 2). The constraint graph of the problem, the domains of the variables[2], the current labeling, and the set of violated constraints are useful parameters of this procedure. In practical applications of such algorithms, e.g., in our commercial nurse scheduling system [8, 5], `choose-bad-region` is tailored to the current application. In contrast, this paper introduces a generic algorithm for this procedure.

Then, the improvement step is conducted by a variant of the *branch&bound* in row 4 that changes the labels of the variables V' in labeling l to improve the overall quality of l. The current set of violated constraints is used as initial bound because the new labeling l (after the improvement step) is not allowed to be worse than the old one (before the improvement step). Constraint propagation like *forward checking* can be employed in order to increase performance of the improvement step.

---

[1] In the sense of this paper.

[2] These domains can be the result of an initial arc-consistent filtering that has been conducted before search.

```
iterative-improvement(V, D, C, ≻)
```

1. Compute an initial labeling l of all variables in V;
2. $V' = \text{choose-bad-region}(V, C, \succ, l, \bar{C}(l))$;
3. if $V' = \emptyset$ then go to 7;
4. unassign the variables in V', propagate all constraints c with
   $V(c) \cap V' \neq \{\}$ and run *branch&bound* on the variables in V' with
   $\bar{C}(l)$ as initial bound in order to compute a new labeling l;
5. add temporary hard constraint

$$\bigvee_{v \in V \setminus V'} v \neq l \downarrow_v$$

6. go to 2;
7. remove temporary constraints. return l as result.

Fig. 1. Searching by iterative improvement.

Branch&bound searches all possible labelings of V' exhaustively. Consequently, further improvement steps have to consider a change in $V \setminus V'$ in order to prevent the search algorithm from visiting labelings more than once. This condition is enforced in row 5 by an additional temporary compulsory constraint.

As all local search algorithms, *iterative improvement* is applicable to *dynamic constraint satisfaction problems (DCSP)*, where constraints and variables are added to or removed from the current constraint problem between two calls of the search procedure. Applications of dynamic constraint satisfaction usually require consecutive search processes on related problems to result in similar solutions which share as many labels is possible. This notion of stability is provided for free by local search algorithms like *iterative improvement* that accept only an improvement of current labeling as valid repair steps.

This algorithm — enhanced by an heuristic `choose-bad-region` procedure — does a pretty good job, e.g. on nurse scheduling problems, where *mincon-walk* as well as EFLOP-like heuristics failed at producing solutions of sufficient quality [8, 5]. Nevertheless, applying heuristics to the selection of *bad regions* in partial solutions of a PCSP exhibits some remarkable drawbacks. Firstly, the applied heuristics consider only a few constraints when choosing variables for reselection. Secondly, the heuristics heavily rely on assertions on the constraint model which makes the adoption of the system to slightly different applications a non-trivial problem. These deficiencies motivated to investigate opportunities for deriving similar heuristics directly from the constraint model.

4 Exhaustive Enumeration of Improvement Steps

A naive method for avoiding the application of search heuristics in *iterative improvement* would enumerate *all possible* regions by the `choose-bad-region` procedure called in `iterative-improvement` (cf. Fig. 1). When called by the

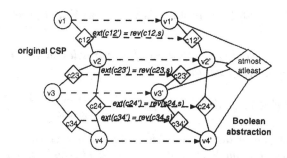

Fig. 2. Local revision sets form constraints on possible revisions of the whole problem with reference to the current labeling S.

overall search algorithm, this procedure first returns all sets of only one variable. If all of these variable sets have been enumerated, then all sets of two variables are returned and so on. Finally, after trying to improve $V' = V$, one knows that a global solution has been computed. However, this method neglects all information that can be retrieved from the constraint graph and the deficiencies of the current solution.

Our idea about a generic procedure for finding bad regions in partial solutions of a PCSP is to constrain this naive enumeration of regions for solution improvement by the available information. In the following, promising regions for solution improvement are called to form global revision sets. The problem of finding global revisions is formulated as a Boolean PCSP whose constraint graph is very similar to the original problem (cf. Fig. 2). If a solution of the Boolean problem assigns a 1 to a variable v_i', the corresponding variable v_i in the original problem is considered to be a part of a promising region for improvement. Each of the constraints c_{ij}' in this Boolean problem represents a necessary condition on promising regions that only depends on *one* constraint c_{ij} in the original problem and a partial solution S. In the following, the regions complying with the condition concerning a single constraint are called to define a set of local revisions. The constraints *atmost* and *atleast* are well known from scheduling systems and count here the occurrences of 1 in the solution of the binary problem. These constraints can be used to control the size of the regions. Hence, it is possible to return small regions first in order to conduct cheap improvement steps first.

4.1 Local Revision Sets

Firstly, the relation of the original problem to the abstract problem of finding regions for local repair according to Fig. 2 needs to be defined. In the following, v' always denotes the variable in the abstract Boolean problem that corresponds to variable v in the original problem. Analogously, c' represents the constraint in the abstract problem referring to constraint c in the original problem. The whole set of variables in the abstract problem is written as V_{rev}, the set of constraints as C_{rev}.

Definition 3. *Let l_1 and l_2 be labelings of all variables in V. Then $\text{diff}(l_1, l_2)$ returns a labeling of V_{rev} such that*

$$\forall v' \in V_{rev} : \text{diff}(l_1, l_2) \downarrow_{v'} = \begin{cases} 0 & \text{iff } l_1 \downarrow_v = l_2 \downarrow_v \\ 1 & \text{otherwise.} \end{cases}$$

Let l be a labeling of the variables in V and c be a constraint in the original problem. Then, the smallest local revision set of l respecting c is defined as follows:

$$\text{rev}(c,\, l) := \bigcup_{l' \in \text{ext}(c)} \{\text{diff}(l \downarrow_{V(c)},\, l')\}.$$

All extensions comprising $\text{rev}(c,\, l)$ are called local revision sets of l respecting c.

Local revision sets cover all differences of a current labeling l from all labelings complying with constraint c. Although defined extensionally here, intensional definitions for common constraints, which are typically defined by propagation methods in a constraint library, are possible.

4.2 Global Revision Sets

Global revision sets consider all opportunities to satisfy a set of constraints instead of single constraints.

Definition 4. *The smallest revision set of a partial solution l respecting constraint set C' is defined as*

$$\text{rev}(C',\, l) := \bigcup_{l' \in \text{ext}(C')} \{\text{diff}(l,\, l')\}.$$

All extensions comprising $\text{rev}(C',\, l)$ are called revision sets of l respecting C'. Revision sets respecting all constraints in C are called global revision sets.

Lemma 1.
$$\bowtie_{c \in C'} \text{rev}(c,\, l) \supseteq \text{rev}(C',\, l).$$

Obviously, the join of local revisions above denotes exactly the set of all solutions to the abstract problem in Fig. 2. Hence, the lemma claims that the solutions of this abstract constraint problem form a global revision set of labeling l. However, this global revision set is generally not minimal.

Proof. One can prove by a few equations that for any $l' \in \text{ext}(C')$ the difference from the current label $\text{diff}(l', l)$ is in $\bowtie_{c \in C'} \text{rev}(c, l)$ presupposing that all variables in l are directly affected by a constraint in C':

$$\bowtie_{c \in C'} \text{rev}(c, l)$$
$$= \bowtie_{c \in C'} (\{\text{diff}(l' \downarrow_{V(c)}, l \downarrow_{V(c)})\} \cup \text{rev}(c, l))$$
$$= \{\text{diff}(l', l)\} \cup \bowtie_{c \in C'} \text{rev}(c, l).$$

The first equation follows from the definition of local revision sets. The second presupposes that all variables in V are directly affected by the constraints in C' and

$$\mathrm{diff}(l' \downarrow_{V(c)}, l \downarrow_{V(c)}) \in \mathrm{rev}(c,\, l).$$

$\square$

Proposition 1.

$$\bowtie_{c \in C} \mathrm{rev}(c,\, l) \supseteq \mathrm{rev}(C',\, l)$$

holds true for all most important constraint sets $C' \subseteq C$ *in a PCSP which can be satisfied.*

Proposition 1 claims in other words that each globally optimal solution can be reached changing the regions as indicated by the global revision sets.

Proof. The inclusion $\bowtie_{c \in C} \mathrm{rev}(c,\, l) \supseteq \mathrm{rev}(C,\, l)$ follows from the lemma. $C \supseteq C' \implies \mathrm{rev}(C,\, l) \supseteq \mathrm{rev}(C',\, l)$ is implied by definition 4. $\square$

4.3 Searching Global Revisions

The basic idea for applying these results is to search the original problem by algorithm `iterative-improvement` (according to Fig. 1) controlled by an exhaustive search of the abstract problem that enumerates global revisions. The resulting hybrid algorithm still is an anytime-algorithm because partial solutions are available all the time. Additionally, proving optimality is possible due to the results of the previous section. If all global revisions have been searched without improving the current partial solution l, then l is optimal. Fig. 3 describes the idea of an enumeration algorithm for partial constraint satisfaction problems. $PCSP_{rev}$ holds the constraint problem for finding global revisions. As mentioned above, *atmost* and *atleast* constraints are used to enumerate global revisions according to their size in order to conduct cheap improvement steps first in algorithm `iterative-improvement`. The variable n, occurring in the rows 1 and 5, controls the number of assignments to be retracted. In row 1, $PCSP_{rev}$ is built up again after improving l because the constraints in C_{rev} typically depend on l. Variable δ_{rev}, which is set in row 2, serves as an initial bound in the following call of the *branch&bound* procedure. Only revisions promising to improve l are returned by the enumeration in row 4. If the *branch&bound* fails to find a new partial solution of $PCSP_{rev}$ better than δ_{rev} then, occasionally, larger revisions are required (row 5). If no larger revisions are available then l is optimal. Search in `iterative-improvement` terminates because `choose-bad-region` returns an empty variable set.

Enumerating regions ordered by their size is only one example for an enumeration strategy. There are many alternative strategies conceivable which for instance may try to find revisions first that promise to repair the most important currently violated constraints [6]. Additionally, the degree of prospective constraint processing, which is used searching the abstract problem by

---

```
choose-bad-region(V, C, ≻, 1, δ)
```

1. if $PCSP_{rev}$ has no value (this function is called for the first time) or δ has been improved by the last improvement step in iterative-improvement then begin
    (a) $PCSP_{rev} := (V_{rev}, \{0,1\}, C_{rev}, \succ')$ with $C_{rev} = \bigcup_{c \in C} \text{rev}(c,\ l)$ and
        $C_1 \succ' C_2 \Longleftrightarrow$
        $\{c\ |\ c' \in C_1\} \succ \{c\ |\ c' \in C_2\};$
    (b) $n := 1;$
    (c) add the following constraint to $PCSP_{rev}$:
        atleast and *atmost* n occurrences of 1
    end;
2. $\delta_{rev} := \bigcup_{c \in \delta} \text{rev}(c,\ l);$
3. call *branch&bound* with δ_{rev} as bound on $PCSP_{rev}$ for the *next* partial solution better than δ_{rev};
4. if a partial solution l has been found return $V' = \{v\ |\ l \downarrow_{v'} = 1\}$ and exit;
5. if no partial solution is available and $n \leq |\ V\ |$ then do begin
    (a) $n := n + 1;$
    (b) reset $PCSP_{rev}$ and remove *atleast* and *atmost* constraints;
    (c) add the following constraints to $PCSP_{rev}$: *atleast* and *atmost* n occurrences of 1;
    (d) goto row 3
    end;
6. l is optimal. Hence, return $V' = \{\}$ and exit.

Fig. 3. Enumerating global revisions (egr).

branch&bound, is obviously relevant for the performance of the enumeration. If the *branch&bound* looks ahead deeply into the search space, it will find that global revisions first which promise to repair strong deficiencies. However, the overhead for searching global revisions is increased.

5   Experiences

Enumeration of global revisions (egr) comprises a whole family of algorithms where instances differ in the used enumeration strategy and the applied constraint techniques. The major drawback of this method is the overhead which is caused by the effort of searching the abstract constraint problem. Experiments on unstructured randomly generated constraint problems are presented here to give a first answer to the question: *Is the effort of enumerating global revisions acceptable?*

A comparative analysis of *egr* has to consider the two major tasks in partial constraint satisfaction: finding optimal solutions (exhaustive search) and finding as good solutions as possible within a limited amount of time (approximative optimization).

Table 1. Empirical comparison of *bb+FC* and *enumerating global revisions (egr)* searching exhaustively. Each row presents results of 10 runs on random problems for each algorithm.

no.	den.	sat.	algo.	time/s			checks/10^6			assignments/10^3		
				⊘	min.	max	⊘	min.	max	⊘	min.	max
30 variables, domains of 10 values, 6 hierarchy levels												
1	0.44	0.7	egr+FC	5282	1744	24083	111	34	535	119	38	564
			egr+MACall	4019	704	11777	146	26	508	153	30	535
			bb+FC	4348	28	12785	139	62	336	133	62	323
2	0.44	0.5	egr+FC	7002	396	15926	168	82	371	228	13	489
			egr+MACall	7022	854	21397	174	20	529	232	28	654
			bb+FC	10537	2678	31590	284	76	857	385	100	1182
3	0.22	0.5	egr+FC	824	92	3169	14.8	1.7	52.8	44	5	161
			egr+MACall	755	208	2522	15.7	4.2	57.9	44	12	156
			bb+FC	1047	547	2294	61.4	16.7	304.6	145	46	635

In the following, variants of *egr* are compared to standard algorithms due to experiments on *hierarchical constraint satisfaction problems (HCSP)*. An HCSP is simply a special kind of a PCSP where constraints are grouped into the hierarchy levels C_0 (comprising compulsory constraints) to C_n [1,5,6]. Additionally, $\omega(c)$ assigns a real number as a constraint weight to each constraint c. To decide whether $C' \succ C''$ holds for the constraint sets C' and C'', one considers the weight sum of the constraints in $C' \cap C_1$ and $C'' \cap C_1$ first. If C' has got more important constraints in hierarchy level 1 then $C' \succ C''$ holds. If C' comprises less important constraints in level 1 then the opposite holds. Otherwise, the next hierarchy level is concerned. Hierarchy levels may be considered as a categorical degree of a constraint's importance whereas the weight is a gradual measure of importance. HCSPs turned out to be useful for representing real world problems [8,5] and, additionally, enable the use of certain *looking ahead* techniques and *dynamic variable orderings (DVO)* [6,7]. As usual, constraint problems are classified according to the number of variables, constraint density (den.) and the constraint's satisfiability (sat.).

Exhaustive search: Table 1 presents empirical results on two variants of *egr* in comparison with the *branch&bound* algorithm *bb+FC*. Algorithm *bb+FC* uses *forward checking* equivalently to the P-FC3 procedure in [2] combined with a dynamic variable ordering heuristic, which is especially appropriate to constraint hierarchies [6,7]. Forward checking results are used to assign best values first as value assignment strategy. Both *egr* procedures, *egr+FC* and *egr+MACall*, deploy *bb+FC* within the improvement step. Whereas, *egr+FC* also uses *bb+FC* searching the abstract problem, *egr+MACall* additionally applies a MAX-MIN-algorithm [10] after each assignment in the abstract problem which labels each value with the most important hierarchy level that cannot be satisfied completely assigning that value. The results of constraint propagation are used to inform the

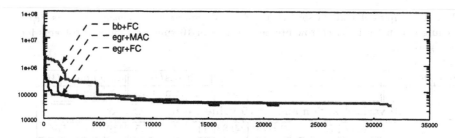

Fig. 4. Performance curve to experiment 2. Improvement in solution quality over time.

value selection strategy and the dynamic variable ordering heuristic (for details refer to [6]). This method has been included into the experiments to assess the effect of a larger amount of constraint propagation in the abstract problem which presumably increases the merit of the returned regions but causes additional costs in searching the abstraction.

Additional experiments, which are not listed in Fig. 1, turned out that *egr* algorithms are usually not recommended when searching smaller optimization problems comprising 20 variables. On problems of about 30 variables, *egr* algorithms are competitive to *bb+FC*. Apparently, spending more effort on looking ahead while searching for promising global revisions like in *egr+MACall* pays for itself when searching for optimal solutions of problems of this size.

Fig. 4 shows the major advantage that *egr* methods had in all experiments we have conducted. Solutions are improved more quickly. Fig. 4 displays the improvement in solution quality (y-axis) over time (x-axis). Therefore, the constraint hierarchy is transformed into an equivalent system of weighted constraints. A point (x, y) in a curve of Fig. 4 reports that constraints of weight y have been violated by the best yet found labeling at time x. Very similar curves result from the other experiments.

Approximative optimization: Approximative optimization of unstructured randomly generated problems is the domain of *mincon-retry* and *mincon-walk*. Fig. 5 presents the performance of *egr+FC* in comparison with *bb+FC*, *mincon-retry*, and *mincon-walk*. Forward checking results have been used to improve the initial labeling of local search algorithms in order to provide the same starting point as used in the *egr* algorithms.

Diagrams a) and b) in Fig. 5 show results on problems comprising 40 variables with a time limit of 5 minutes for each experiment. The diagrams c) and d) report the performance on larger problems comprising 100 variables with a time limit of 15 minutes for each experiment[3].

Obviously, *egr* behaves similar to *mincon-retry* and *mincon-walk*. The best yet found labeling is improved continuously without necessity to respect a certain systematic in search. Although searching two constraint problems instead of one, *egr* is more or less as fast as the standard algorithms in local search. However,

---

[3] A more detailed report on experiments of this kind can be found in [6].

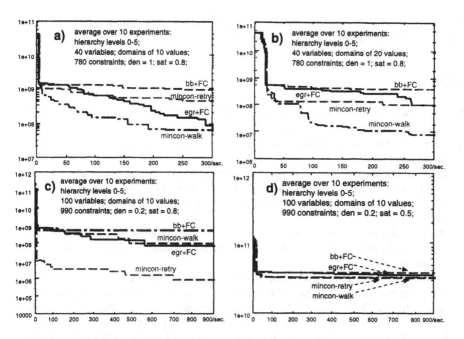

Fig. 5. Comparison of the decrease in the weight of violated constraints over time achieved by distinguished algorithms. The constraint problems vary in their size, density and the satisfiability of constraints.

on unstructured problems *mincon-retry* and *mincon-walk* perform often better than *egr*.

6 Summary

This paper introduced a novel method for turning repair-based search of partial constraint satisfaction problems into an exhaustive search procedure obtaining the advantages of local search: flexible improvement of the best yet found labeling and applicability to dynamic constraint satisfaction. This method, named *enumeration of global revisions (egr)*, relies on an enumeration of promising repair steps which is informed only by information which follows straightforward from the given constraint problem. First empirical evaluation on unstructured randomly generated constraint problems proves a general applicability of this method to both, exhaustive search of larger problems comprising about 30 variables and approximative optimization of even larger problems.

Further research aims at verifying this promise by practical application of *egr* to real world problems. Therefore, the major drawback of this method has to be attacked: the large implementation effort. For each constraint, which is used in the target application, a Boolean abstraction has to be implemented, which restricts the enumeration of revisions. As soon as constraint libraries of

68

the required expressiveness exist, *egr* will have to prove its applicability in time tabling and knowledge-based configuration.

References

1. Alan Borning, Bjorn Freeman-Benson, and Molly Wilson. Constraint hierarchies. *Lisp and Symbolic Computation*, 5:233–270, 1992.
2. Eugene C. Freuder and Rick J. Wallace. Partial constraint satisfaction. *Artificial Intelligence*, 58:21–70, 1992.
3. Philippe Galinier and Jin-Kao Hao. Tabu search for maximal constraint satisfaction problems. In *CP-97: Proceedings of the Third International Conference on Principles and Practice of Constraint Processing*, volume 1330 of *LNCS*. Springer Verlag, pages 196–208, 1997.
4. Manfred Meyer. *Finite Domain Constraints: Declarativity meets Efficiency, Theory meets Application*. Dissertation, Universität Kaiserslautern, Infix Verlag, Sankt Augustin, 1994.
5. Harald Meyer auf'm Hofe. ConPlan/ SIEDAplan: Personnel assignment as a problem of hierarchical constraint satisfaction. In *PACT-97: Proceedings of the Third International Conference on the Practical Application of Constraint Technology*, pages 257–272, London, UK, April 1997. Practical Application Company, Ltd.
6. Harald Meyer auf'm Hofe. Finding regions for local repair in hierarchical constraint satisfaction. Research Report RR-97-05, Deutsches Forschungszentrum für Künstliche Intelligenz, December 1997.
7. Harald Meyer auf'm Hofe and Andreas Abecker. Zur Verarbeitung "weicher" Constraints. *KI - Künstliche Intelligenz*, (4):31–36, 1997.
8. Harald Meyer auf'm Hofe and Enno Tolzmann. ConPlan/ SIEDAplan: Personaleinsatzplanung als Constraintproblem. *KI - Künstliche Intelligenz*, (1):37–40, 1997.
9. Steven Minton, Mark Johnston, Andrew Philips, and Philip Laird. Minimizing conflicts: a heuristic repair method for constraint satisfaction problem and scheduling problems. *Artificial Intelligence*, 58:161–205, 1992.
10. Paul Snow and Eugene C. Freuder. Improved relaxation and search methods for approximate constraint satisfaction with a maximin criterion. In *Proc. of the 8th biennal conf. of the canadian society for comput. studies of intelligence*, pages 227–230, May 1990.
11. G. Verfaillie and T. Schiex. Solution reuse in dynamic constraint satisfaction problems. In *AAAI-94: Proceedings of the 12th national conf. on AI*, pages 307–312, Seattle, WA, August 1994. AAAI Press/ The MIT Press.
12. Richard J. Wallace. Analysis of heuristic methods for partial constraint satisfaction problems. In *CP-96: Proceedings of the Second International Conference on Principles and Practice of Constraint Processing*, volume 1118 of *LNCS*. Springer Verlag, pages 482–496, 1996.
13. N. Yugami, Y. Ohta, and H. Hara. Improving repair-based constraint satisfaction methods by value propagation. In *AAAI-94: Proceedings of the 12th National Conference on Artificial Intelligence*, pages 344–349, 1994.

Needle's Eyes – A General Decomposition Principle for Practical Uses

Fritz Mädler and Karsten Knorr

Hahn-Meitner-Institut, Postfach 39 01 28, D-14 091 Berlin, Germany
{maedler, knorr}@hmi.de
http://www.hmi.de/people/

Abstract. If efficient control knowledge is available, search in the state space is a practical way of solving non-toy problems. For many applications the structure of the state space itself offers a reliable means of control: Certain states called "needle's eye" can be used as partial goals so that less complex problems remain to be solved. Originally, we formalized the "needle's eye principle" for the acquisition and representation of control knowledge for a model-based planner. We show that it is equally useful for a highly complex configuration task arising in the material sciences. From the crystallographical problem setting a natural problem decomposition is derived, such that a hierarchical configuration procedure can be used as an implicit model of "disorder". After a brief, informal review of the needle's eye principle we show that the control knowledge inferred on the top level of our knowledge-based configuration program is, in essence, a chain of needle's eyes.

1 A Complex Problem from the Material Sciences

We present some background to the application and state the problem.

Crystalline materials which can absorb molecular substances are drawing increasing interest. They are used in the chemical industries as microporous filters or catalytic converters for exhaust emission in plants or motor vehicles. Refraction properties of optical materials can be influenced deliberately by targeted inclusions. Washing powders are used world-wide; their detergent properties and their compatibility with nature and environment critically depend on the interactions of organic substances with the surfaces of the crystalline cage structures.

Fig. 1 shows dioxolane-silica-sodalite, $[Si_{12}O_{24}] \cdot 2(CH_2)_3O_2$, which is an outstanding prototype of a simple "host-guest structure": All-corner connected tetrahedra consisting of four oxygen atoms in their corners and a silicon atom in their center build the silica-sodalite framework which is able to host a dioxolane ring-molecule. The molecule does not take a unique position in the host lattice. Due to different symmetry between host and guest, the molecule is free to occupy a variety of spatial positions, orientations and conformations, where the latter are the different energetically stable formations the molecule's atoms can adopt in space. In the simplest situation, the static case, the guest molecule takes one of the possible positions in each host cell and stays there during observation.

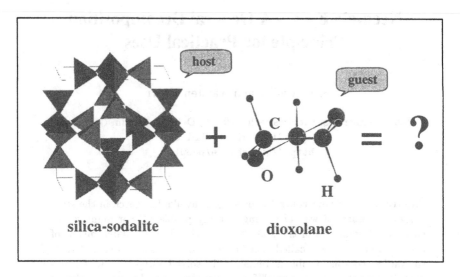

Fig. 1. The two components that form the prototypical, simple host-guest structure dioxolane-silica-sodalite $[Si_{12}O_{24}] \cdot 2(CH_2)_3O_2$: The silica-sodalite framework (*left*) is built by all-corner connected tetrahedra consisting of oxygen and silicon atoms and can enclose the dioxolane molecule (*right*) in various positions and formations which make up the molecule's disorder in the host framework

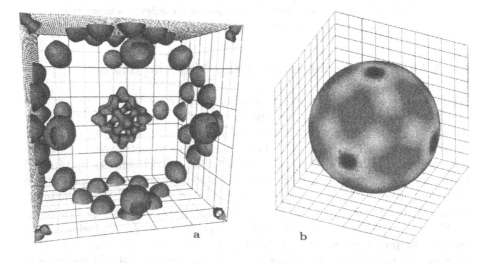

Fig. 2. Two views of the electron-density distribution reconstructed from the diffraction pattern which is detected from a powder diffraction-experiment of our prototype material: In fig. 2a (*left*), an iso-surface for the density value of 1.2 electrons / $Å^3$ is shown; the outer part belongs to the host, the central part to the time and space average of the guest in full disorder. In fig. 2b (*right*), an intersecting sphere - suitably placed in the molecule's part of the host cell - reveals, in this case, a spherical and symmetrical density distribution with six global maxima (*darker spots*), each of which is surrounded by four local maxima (*lighter spots*)

At the other extreme, the purely dynamic case, the molecule quickly changes its admissible positions or even its conformations. This static and dynamic indefiniteness (and its intermediate stages) is referred to as "disorder" of the guest molecule in the host lattice. Since the localization of the molecules in the voids of the framework structures is essential to an understanding of their properties, research into this disorder helps to explain the host-guest interactions and, we hope, will support a specific synthesis of host-guest compounds with desirable, industrially usable properties.

One way of investigating the phenomenon are high-resolution synchrotron powder diffraction-experiments. A diffraction pattern is detected, from which the spatial electron-density distribution of the host-guest structure is reconstructed with the aid of entropy maximizing methods [5]. Fig. 2a shows an iso-surface of the density distribution for our prototype material. Note that this is not the electron density of a single guest in a single host cell; experiments of this kind can only produce a space and time average of many cells with the molecule in full disorder. The question is: How can a statistical superposition of many instances of the molecule explain the detected diffraction pattern, and what is the contribution of the individual instances to the shape of the electron density? In the first place this is the problem of how to compatibly embed the molecule into the reconstructed density distribution, in full disorder and in a way that makes sense chemically as well as crystallographically. We contributed to the solution using a knowledge-based configuration procedure.

2 Knowledge-based, Hierarchical Configuration

We derive the problem decomposition and sketch the hierarchical configurator.

Even if the density distribution supplies only information which is averaged over many cells in space and time, it does contain knowledge about the individual manifestations of the molecule we search for, knowledge that should be used to embed the molecule into the density distribution. In addition to general expert knowledge from chemistry, spatial geometry, etc. which is needed to construct the molecule, this hidden information is the authoritative source of knowledge for a physically meaningful link between the molecule and the data resulting from the experiment. The essential task of the configuration program is to exploit this source and to generate a wealth of dioxolane instances, in their disorder and in acceptable time, which as a whole can serve as an explanatory model for the data measured.

For our prototype substance the extremes of the electron density provide a starting-point. In fig. 2b an intersecting sphere is positioned in the data in such a way that the distribution of the density maxima becomes visible.

One might hope that a smart selection of five (global or local) maxima could represent a valid instance of the guest molecule. But even the most similar five-rings (see fig. 3a) are too different in their dimensions - e.g. in their edges or in their spatial formation - from the stereochemical parameters of dioxolane rings to be taken as an instance of the guest molecule that is to be found.

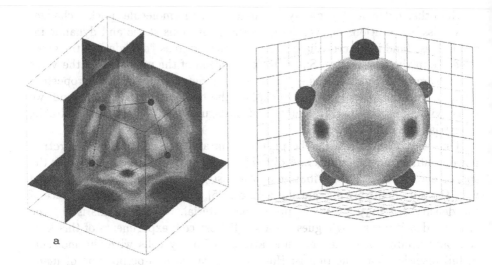

Fig. 3. In fig. 3a (*left*), a five-ring of density maxima is chosen which is the closest possible to dioxolane, but it differs too much in the stereochemical parameters to be taken as a valid instance of the molecule we search for. In fig. 3b (*right*) variance balls of chemically justified radii around the maxima are used to model the "nearness" of averaged dioxolane settlements to the maxima which they produce in a statistical superposition

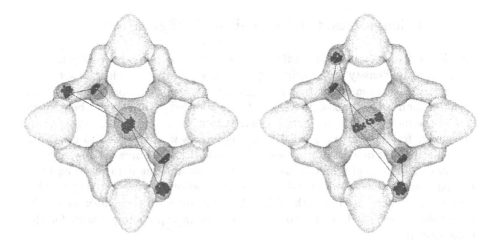

Fig. 4. The two conformations revealed for our prototype material are shown embedded in an iso-surface of the electron-density distribution. The program configured 300 instances each of "envelope" (*left*) and of "twist" conformation (*right*). Both samples are equi-distributed near their maxima-ring and belong to the same variance radii. Note that the two rings that controlled the configuration are very similar to each other (*top view along z-axis shown*): The conformations differ only in the location of one ring corner that changed from one of the local maxima to a neighbouring one (*compare top sections left and right*), a result which had not been seen before

However, such maxima-rings that are somewhat similar to dioxolane can be produced by averaged dioxolane settlements near them, generally in an ambiguous way. For example, the instances of the guest molecule could use up remaining space of the host in equi-distribution, or they could appear in normal distribution caused by thermal oscillation of their atoms around the density maxima. In both cases the maxima do not represent atom positions, but result from statistical superposition of the molecule's different manifestations within the host framework.

In our (simple) prototype case it sufficed to model "nearness" by variance balls, that is by balls around the maxima with radii which are justified by chemical knowledge. This way the positions of the atoms that are looked for - and therewith location and shape of the guest molecule - are restricted by expertise and, above all, the search is significantly restrained without pruning away the molecule's freedom, that is its tendencies towards disorder. Fig. 3b shows a maxima-ring with five suitably chosen variance balls through which the molecule is to be "threaded", in a geometric construction during the configuration, whereby its characteristic parameters such as atom sequence, bond lengths, spatial puckering[1] and pseudo-rotation angle[2], etc. must become those of a valid dioxolane instance. Any non-determinism emerging during this construction is fixed by assigning values according to a preselected statistical distribution.

All in all, this hierarchical situation - the existence of maxima-rings somewhat "similar" to dioxolane in its various instances on the one hand, and on the other hand the promising chance to constructively meet the stereochemical characteristics of dioxolane "near" such a ring - very naturally lead to a two-level configuration procedure which can be sketched informally in the following way.

---

[1] For five-rings in the three-dimensional space the "puckering amplitude"

$$q = \left(\sum_{i=1}^{5} z_i^2 \right)^{1/2}$$

is represented by means of the displacements $z_i = z_i(E^*(S(V_i)))$ of the ring corners V_i with respect to the mean ring plane $E^* = E^*(S)$: Among all planes passing through the mass center $S = S(V_i)$ of the ring corners, E^* is uniquely determined by the "non-rotation" conditions [2]

$$\sum_{i=1}^{5} z_i \cos[2\pi(i-1)/5] = 0 \quad \text{and} \quad \sum_{i=1}^{5} z_i \sin[2\pi(i-1)/5] = 0 .$$

[2] The "pseudo-rotation angle" Φ of a spatial five-ring is uniquely determined by the equations

$$z_i = q\sqrt{2/5} \cos[4\pi(i-5) + \Phi], \quad 1 = 1, \ldots, 5 .$$

A certain range of angles Φ models "rotational isomerism" : For a fixed atom sequence (e.g. C-O-C-C-O) molecules may exist belonging to the same conformation and with equal puckering amplitude q but with a different sign distribution in the corner displacements z_i.

Together the q and Φ coordinates grasp "conformational isomerism". For example: Either of the two conformations shown in fig. 4 has its characteristic (q, Φ)-pair that identifies the conformation of a molecule's instance.

Configuration Algorithm (*Sketch*):

- **Level 1.** Generate a ring candidate of five maxima that *roughly* meets the following demands:

  (i) the lengths of the ring edges are in the magnitude of dioxolane bondlengths, (ii) the ring exhibits a puckering amplitude comparable to known values of dioxolane, (iii) the ring conformation is similar to known dioxolane conformations.

- **Level 2.** Select for the ring candidate inferred at level 1:

  (i) an atom sequence (i.e. C-C-O-C-O) and its literature values for the bondlengths, (ii) variance balls with radii depending on the maxima that form the ring corners and on the atoms C or O, (iii) bounds for puckering amplitude q and rotation phase Φ depending on their ring counterparts and on theoretical values, (iv) a statistical distribution for the atom positions in the variance balls, and construct a chemically meaningful instance of the molecule.

- Backtrack to level 1 if necessary (no solution was found) or desired (alternative solutions requested).

On both levels expert knowledge is available in order to test the required properties. But unavoidably, for the stereochemical parameters there are only coarse numerical bounds to express "similarity", "nearness" etc. for the guiding maxima-ring and the molecule to be configured. Even worse, prior to the configuration, there is no explicit knowledge about a physically meaningful relation between the concrete instances of the guest molecule and the diffraction pattern or the reconstructed density distribution. No human expert, who knows the 30 density maxima shown in fig. 2b and who has access to the explicit knowledge that the program uses, could possibly generate valid instances of the molecule that could explain the shape of the electron density; for this meticulous and exacting task statistical distributions are necessary, and (rotational and conformational) isomerism is to be detected systematically. But problem decomposition and bounds for the stereochemical parameters, coarse as they are, drastically reduce the complexity, so that our Prolog program is able to configure many guest instances in acceptable time. For that part of the knowledge which is lacking Prolog substitutes exhaustive search in the remaining "combinatorial rest-space": its predicate-logic theorem prover systematically generates the desired instances by producing admissible combinatorial results and proving them with respect to the part of the knowledge which is represented explicitly.

Thus the configurator may be seen as an implicit, computer-based explanatory model for disorder. Fig. 4 renders the two conformations revealed for our prototype material. A critical discussion of results with respect to material sciences can be found in [5].

This knowledge-based configuration procedure is general and will serve as an implicit model for other host-guest structures, especially in less symmetrical or more dynamical cases when there is virtually no hope for an explicit model in the form of a mathematical law.

3   The Decomposition as a Chain of Needle's Eyes

The control knowledge inferred by the program is seen as a chain of needle's eyes.

It is not by chance that planning and configuration tasks are assigned to the same problem class *construction* [3], [11]. Their common aspects emerge clearly, if *state* and *action* are suitably formalized [12]; then both problem types lead to very similar solution graphs which are subgraphs of the state space and show a remarkable shape. In [6], [9] we used the special structure of such graphs for an axiomatic outfit of a general "needle's eye principle" that served for the acquisition and representation of control knowledge for the prototype of a planning system. Here we give an informal sketch of how the control of the above two-level configuration - the "threading" of the molecule through a sequence of variance balls which significantly reduces the complexity - can be seen as an application of control knowledge in the sense of a chain of needle's eyes.

An action, for example[3],

$$A = \text{action}(\ A_{name}, P_0, P_1, S_0, S_1\ )$$

produces an effect on domain features by moving an actuator or "switch" named A_{name} from its actual position P_0 into a new position P_1, thus transferring the actual domain state S_0 into a successor state S_1. The states consist of position values $X_1, \ldots, X_m$ for the switches and of feature values $X_{m+1}, \ldots, X_n$ for "derived parameters"[4] that is

$$S = \text{state}(\ X_1, \ldots, X_m; X_{m+1}, \ldots, X_n\ ).$$

In Prolog the state transition $S_1 = A(S_0)$ can be represented in the form

action($A_{name}, P_0, P_1, S_0, S_1$)
    <=
        update_1($A_{name}, \ldots, X_i, \ldots$),$\cdots$,update_r($A_{name}, \ldots, X_j, \ldots$).

An action succeeds if the body clauses update_1,$\cdots$,update_r can be proved by Prolog's inference mechanism with respect to the knowledge base.

The graph in fig. 5 is directed downwards. Each numbered node represents a state S, each edge A_1 between nodes S_0 and S_1 renders a state transition $S_1 = A_1(S_0)$ and every (whole or partial) path consisting of such transitions stands for a shortest, "optimal" linear plan $L = (A_1, \ldots, A_k)$, that transfers an initial state S_0 into a goal state $S_k = L(S_0)$, passing through the states $S_i = A_i(S_{i-1})$, $i = 1, \ldots, k$.

---

[3] The example is taken from a process-control prototype-application in the Hahn-Meitner-Institut, where optimal plans for intricate and expensive rinsing and cleansing procedures of a plasma-deposition device used to produce photo-voltaic layers were generated by the model-based SOLEIL planner [6].

[4] In our example they are variables for gas and pressure states of deposition chambers and feed pipes. They are effected or controlled by the switches and represent critical values of the deposition device that decide the legality of an action and can become part of the planning goals like any other feature of the application.

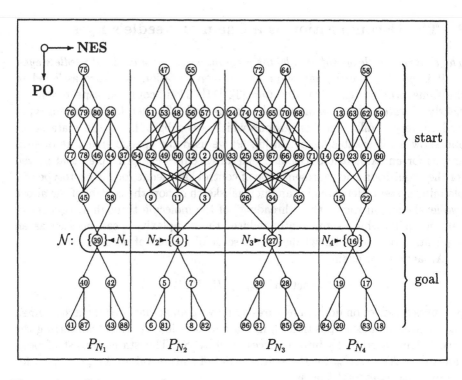

Fig. 5. A needle's eyes set $\mathcal{N}$ as an extensional representation of an abstract planning operator. (See section 3 for the explanation)

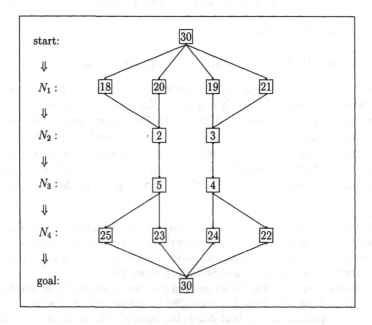

Fig. 6. One of the chains of needle's eyes which control the configuration in section 2

The existence of several plans $L_j = (A_1, \ldots, A_k)$ that connect the same state pair S_0 and $S_k = L_j(S_0)$ and that are built from two or more permutations of the same ground set H of actions, $H = \{A_1, \ldots, A_k\}$, is a necessary condition for a parallelized plan P in the form of a series-parallel partial order [10] for H, whose linear extensions L_j then form a subset of all linear plans $L_i(S_0) = S_k$ with optimal length [6], [7].

The special shape of the graph is not limited to the example given, but is inherent in the concept of optimal (linear or parallel) acting and emerges as soon as a more or less complete description of optimal acting is asked for. The structure is closed under concatenation in the following sense: If two optimal linear plans, say $(S_0, \ldots, S_i^\star, \ldots \ldots, S_k)$ and $(S_0', \ldots \ldots, S_i^\star, \ldots, S_{k'}')$, have a state $S_i^\star$ in common, their "crossing-over"

$$(S_0, \ldots, S_{i-1}, S_i^\star, S_{i+1}', \ldots, S_{k'}') \text{ and } (S_0', \ldots \ldots, S_{i-1}', S_i^\star, S_{i+1}, \ldots \ldots, S_k)$$

produces optimal plans for the "crossed-over" problems $(S_0, S_{k'}')$ and (S_0', S_k). For this reason the states of a plan belong to subsequent node layers and no layer can be skipped by an optimal linear plan. Axiomatically seen, fig. 5 renders the diagram of a Jordan-Dedekind order with depth function (see [1], e.g.). For this type of order the distance between a node and its predecessors (or successors) does not depend on the path.

In such a structure it is possible to decompose problems in a well-defined way: In a partial order $(\mathcal{P}, \prec)$ it can be stated precisely for each element *what precedes* and *what follows*. Ideally - as it is the case for the state of node 39 in the left column of fig. 5 - a single element suffices to completely decompose the partial substructure that is built by its predecessors and successors in the order diagram. If the former are taken to be initial states S_0 and the latter to be goal states S_g, then state 39 is an unavoidable *needle's eye state*, which can act as a complexity-reducing partial goal for all planning problems (S_0, S_g) with $S_0 \prec 39 \prec S_g$. In a less "narrow" case - take for example node 45 - the set $N := \{45, 38\}$ of the two states 45 and 38 could serve as a *needle's eye* and produce the desired logarithmic reduction in the complexity. On the layer of any state S there is always a minimally extended state set $N \subset \mathcal{P}$ with $S \in N$ which can be used as a decomposing needle's eye.

Furthermore, needle's eyes N_i can be assembled to a *set* $\mathcal{N} = \{N_1, \ldots, N_m\}$ *of needle's eyes* (a "NES") which decomposes the whole structure in the form of a complete and disjoint partitioning of the states involved. An example of this is the set system $\mathcal{N} = \{\{39\}, \{4\}, \{27\}, \{16\}\}$. Note that the needle's eyes of a NES do not have to belong to the same layer of states; systems such as $\mathcal{N} = \{\{45, 38\}, \{4\}, \{30, 28\}, \{16\}\}$ or $\mathcal{N} = \{\{45, 38\}, \{4\}, \{30\}, \{28\}, \{16\}\}$ are covered by the formalism. If necessary, even decomposition in a single needle's eye consisting of all the states of a layer is permitted.[5]

Fig. 5 renders control knowledge in its *extensional* form, in the sense that a variety of planning problems (S_0, S_g) and their decomposing needle's eyes N_i are

---

[5] Decomposition in a needle's eye that consists of all the states of its layer is a kind of "last resort" this principle offers for poorly structured applications.

expressed as a structured list of domain states. But we can make use of "structural abstraction" and apply machine-learning techniques in order to translate the structural representation into an *intensional* description, which expresses this knowledge in less redundant and more manageable terms of domain features [8]. If the two classifications inherent to the needle's eye principle are used - on the one hand the vertical classification along the partial order into start and goal sets, and on the other hand the well-defined horizontal partitioning along the needle's eyes set $\mathcal{N}$ -, then two inductive-learning steps will generate a classic abstract planning operator (in the sense of, e.g., [4], [13]) with pre- and post-conditions and an expansion instruction in the form of partial or intermediate goals for optimal forward chaining.

In order to interpret the problem decomposition in section 2 as an application of the needle's eye principle we start again from *state* and *action*, now in the context of configuration.

A configuration state in section 2 is a stepwise instantiated term of the form

$$\text{state}(A_1, A_2, \ldots, A_5),$$

with atoms

$$A_i = \text{atom}(C_i, P_i, M_i, R_i), \quad i = 1, \ldots, 5,$$

that have a name $C_i = oxygen$ or $C_i = carbon$, a spatial location

$$P_i = P_i(x, y, z), \quad x, y, z \text{ real numbers},$$

a location for their guiding maximum, $M_i = M_i(x, y, z)$, and a positive real number as radius R_i for their variance ball around M_i. Then an action or configuration step - such as, for example, the construction of the location P_2 of the second atom after a value has already been assigned to P_1 - in essence can be modeled by a Prolog clause of the form

```
c_step( state( atom( C_1, P_1, M_1, R_1 ), atom( C_2, P_2, M_2, R_2 ), A_3, A_4, A_5 ) )
    <=
        bond_length( C_1, C_2 ),
        position( C_1, C_2, P_1, P_2, M_2, R_2 ).
```

The concatenation of such configuration steps on level 2 of the above configuration procedure along a guiding maxima-ring $M_1 M_2 M_3 M_4 M_5 M_1$ from level 1 produces a candidate for a molecule instance $A_1 A_2 A_3 A_4 A_5 A_1$ that in the case of a successful configuration is a valid dioxolane instance near the density maxima M_i (to which it contributes with its electrons).

Fig. 6 depicts all the maxima-rings $M_1 M_2 \cdots M_5 M_1$ which run through maximum $M_1 = "30"$ and control the configuration of that part of the disorder that consists of all valid dioxolane instances with an atom near M_1. The node numbers refer to the maxima involved as well as to their variance ball. We show that the graph also represents the states and steps of the valid configurations:

The balls (M_i, R_i) contribute to every instance of the molecule with one of their points which becomes an atom position P_i for the state of that instance in the ith configuration step. Thus, in fig. 6 all those instances of the disordered molecule are represented whose first atom A_1 (with $C_1 = oxygen$ or $C_1 = carbon$) lies in a variance ball around maximum M_1 and whose other four atoms $A_2, \ldots, A_5$ are chained along a path of the graph and belong to the variance balls $M_2, \ldots, M_5$ of consecutive layers.

We may finally identify that ball point P_i which becomes an atom position in state $S = (\ldots, \text{atom}(C_i, P_i, M_i, R_i), \ldots)$ with S. Then the ith layer of the graph also represents the states that valid instances through (M_1, R_1) can adopt in the ith step of the configuration procedure $(i = 1, \ldots, 5)$.

As in the case of the above representation of the optimal plans, this graph of all valid instances of the disordered molecule near M_1 also is a "graph of states and actions" which is closed under concatenation, and as before it is the diagram of a Jordan-Dedekind order. These structural properties were the crucial prerequisites for the definitions and decomposition theorems of the needle's eye formalism. Thus, controlling the above configuration procedure by moving stepwise from one variance ball to the next, i.e. along an edge to the subsequent layer in the graph, one basically follows a chain of needle's eyes $N_1, \ldots, N_4$, because in terms of the needle's eye concept one moves through four single-element needle's eyes sets $\mathcal{N}_i = \{N_i\}$ consisting of infinite state sets N_i which in this case are made up by all the configuration states of their layer.[6] The width of the graph's layers and the close neighborhood of the decomposition sets only seemingly contradict one's intuition of a needle's eye: Outside the variance balls there is more than ample space for "combinatorial hyper-explosion"; note that most of the features of this domain are not discrete, but are defined by real-valued coordinates. Without the variance balls - the decomposing needle's eyes of this application - the most costly features, i.e. the coordinates of the atoms which must be statistically distributed in space, would take their values from the full three-dimensional cube underlying the data measured.

The problem decomposition by variance balls was derived in a natural way from the crystallographical problem setting; for this application it is not necessary to consult the needle's eye formalism consciously in order to achieve sufficient reduction in complexity. But the interpretation of the hierarchical configuration procedure in terms of the solution graph which exhibits the control knowledge in its extensional form shows that we basically followed a structure-given, highly abstract decomposition principle. The universality and efficiency of the needle's eye principle clearly points beyond the applications presented here.

4 Summary

If efficient control knowledge is available, real world-problems can be attacked successfully. We used a hierarchical configuration program to model some aspects of the disorder of molecules included in a host structure, which is a highly complex problem occurring in the material sciences. The hierarchy of the knowledge-

---

[6] We took up what the principle offers and made use of its "last resort" for this poorly structured domain, cf. the preceding footnote.

based approach reflects a problem decomposition which is derived from the chemical and crystallographical setting of the problem in a natural way.

A closer look at the structural aspects of the decomposition reveals its general decomposition principle which we have used before as an effective means for the acquisition and representation of control knowledge for a model-based planning system: An assembly of narrows in parts of the state space that carry a Jordan-Dedekind order acts as "needle's eye" and can be used as an intermediate goal during a planning or configuration process, thus reducing the complexity significantly. According to this "needle's eye principle" the control knowledge which is generated on the upper level of our configuration program and which guides the configuration on the base level is, in essence, a chain of needle's eyes.

Acknowledgements

We would like to thank Helmar Gust, Ulrich Nielsen and Claus Rollinger for fruitful discussions and helpful comments on an earlier draft of this paper.

References

1. Birkhoff, G.: *Lattice Theory.* Am. Math. Soc., Colloquium Publ. XXV (1961)
2. Gilli, G.: *Molecules and molecular crystals.* In: C. Giacovazzo (ed.), Fundaments of Crystallography. Oxford Univ. Press (1994)
3. Günter, A.: *Flexible Kontrolle in Expertensystemen zur Planung und Konfigurierung in technischen Domänen.* DISKI vol. 3, infix, St. Augustin (1992)
4. Hertzberg, J.: *Planen - Einführung in die Planerstellungsmethoden der Künstlichen Intelligenz.* BI Reihe Informatik 65, Mannheim (1989)
5. Knorr, K., Mädler, F., Papoular, R.: *Model-free Density Reconstruction of Host-Guest-Compounds from High-Resolution Powder Diffraction Data.* J. Micro- and Mesoporous Materials, Elsevier (in print)
6. Mädler, F.: *Problemzerlegung durch Nadelöhrmengen - Ein modellbasierter Ansatz zur Akquisition von Kontrollwissen für Planungssysteme.* DISKI vol. 74, infix, St. Augustin (1994)
7. Mädler. F.: *Seriell-parallele Ordnung als Lösungsbegriff für Planungsaufgaben.* In: A. Horz (ed.), 7. Workshop Planen und Konfigurieren: 74-85. Arbeitspapiere GMD 723, Inst. f. Angewandte Informationstechnologie, St. Augustin (1993)
8. Mädler, F.: *Towards Structural Abstraction.* In: J. Hendler (ed.), First Int. Conf. on AI Planning Systems (AIPS-92): 163-171. M. Kaufmann, San Mateo (1992)
9. Mädler, F.: *Problemzerlegung als optimalitätserhaltende Operatorabstraktion.* In: Th. Christaller (ed.), Proc. GWAI-91: 74-83. IFB 285, Springer (1991). Also in: KI 2/92: 37-41 (1992)
10. Möhring, R.H.: *Computationally Tractable Classes of Ordered Sets.* In: I. Rival (ed.), Algorithms and Order: 105-194. Kluwer, Dordrecht (1989)
11. Puppe, F.: *Problemlösungsmethoden in Expertensystemen.* Studienreihe Informatik, Springer (1990)
12. Russel, S., Norvig, P.: *Artificial Intelligence - a Modern Approach.* Prentice Hall, International Editions, Englewood Cliffs, NJ (1995)
13. Wilkins, D.E.: *Practical Planning.* Morgan Kaufmann, San Mateo, Ca (1988)

OBDDs in Heuristic Search

Stefan Edelkamp[1] and Frank Reffel[2]

[1] Institut für Informatik, Albert-Ludwigs-Universität, Am Flughafen 17, D-79110
Freiburg; eMail: edelkamp@informatik.uni-freiburg.de
[2] Institut für Logik, Komplexität und Deduktionssysteme, Universität Karlsruhe,
Am Fasanengarten 5, D-76128 Karlsruhe; eMail: reffel@ira.uka.de

Abstract. The use of a lower bound estimate in the search has a tremendous impact on the size of the resulting search trees, whereas *OBDDs* can be used to efficiently describe sets of states based on their binary encoding. This paper combines these two ideas into a new algorithm *BDDA**. It challenges both the breadth-first search using *OBDDs* and the traditional *A** algorithm. The problem with *A** is that in many application areas the set of states is too huge to be kept in main memory. In contrast, brute-force breadth-first search using *OBDDs* unnecessarily expands several nodes. Therefore, we exhibit a new trade-off between time and space requirements and tackle the most important problem in heuristic search, the overcoming of space limitations while avoiding a strong penalty in time. We evaluate our approach in the $(n^2 - 1)$-Puzzle and within Sokoban.

1 Introduction

In *heuristic search* we explore the state space by generating the successor set over and over again. The choice of the node next to be expanded is based on two criteria: the length of the path up to that node and the estimate for the shortest path to the desired goal. In the A^* algorithm [7] this estimate has to be a lower bound to the optimal solution length. All generated nodes are stored in a hash table and all horizon nodes are kept in a priority queue data structure ordered according to the combined merit $f = g + h$ of generating path length g and heuristic estimate h. The merit of a node is calculated dynamically by storing the minimum value found on all paths up to that node in a hash table. If the estimate h is set to zero we establish a breadth-first traversal of the search tree.

The search spaces considered in heuristic search tend to exceed the memory resources by several magnitudes, such that it is difficult to maintain the full set of explored nodes. Almost all ideas for handling this problem are based on the *IDA** algorithm [10]. *IDA** (for iterative deepening *A**) performs several depth first traversals while increasing a threshold value for the combined merit. The space requirements of *IDA** are linear in the depth of the search tree, but, unfortunately, *IDA** has to explore several nodes more than once.

For a more extensive use of the main memory a lot of solutions have been proposed. Memory bounded algorithms [6,14] try to store the maximal number of nodes of the search tree and to investigate which node to expand and which node to delete next. Finite state machine pruning [15] detects and generalizes transition sequences that have abbreviations and pattern database techniques [4] try to improve the heuristic function by maintaining a huge hash table of the estimation. The algorithm *IDA** and its variants have been successfully applied to solve difficult problems, especially in solitaire games like the $(n^2 - 1)$ Puzzle [12], Rubik's Cube [11] and the Sokoban Puzzle [8,9].

In this paper we utilize a compressed description of the set of nodes in the search tree. The idea is based on a data structure to describe Boolean functions. We represent a given set by its characteristic function. In section 2 and 3 we explain the basic properties of *OBDDs* and how to use them for a breadth-first search, while in section 4 we describe the main contribution: the algorithm *BDDA**. In section 5 some examples for the application of *BDDA** are presented and in section 6 we investigate the complexity of *BDDA**.

2 OBDDs

Ordered binary decision diagrams (*OBDDs*) introduced by Bryant [3] are a graphical representation of Boolean functions. An *OBDD* $G(f, \pi)$ with respect to the function f and the variable ordering π is an acyclic graph with one source and two sinks labelled with 0 and 1. All other (internal) nodes are labelled with a Boolean variable x_i of f and have two outgoing edges *left* and *right*. For all edges from an x_i labelled node to an x_j labelled node we have $\pi(i) < \pi(j)$, such that on every path in G each variable is tested at most once. In the sequel we omit π if the ordering is clear from the context.

There are two rules in reducing an *OBDD*, called the *deletion rule* and the *merging rule*, respectively. The first one eliminates a node when its two outgoing edges lead to the same successor. The *merging rule* eliminates one of two same labelled nodes with the same pair of sucessors. For every *OBDD* $G(f, \pi)$ there exists an equivalent reduced *OBDD* $G^*(f, \pi)$ which arises from the successive application of the reduction rules, until no other rule can be applied.

The variable ordering π has a huge influence on the size of an *OBDD*, e.g. the function $f = x_1 x_2 \vee x_3 x_4 \vee \ldots x_{2n-1} x_{2n}$ has linear size $(2n + 2$ nodes) if π is the trivial permutation and exponential size $(2^n + 1$ nodes) if π is given by $(1, 3, \ldots 2n - 1, 2, 4, \ldots 2n)$. Unfortunately, the problem of finding the best ordering π for a given function f is *NP*-hard. There are heuristics used to find good orderings for a lot of practical relevant examples [1] where exponentially growing sets of states can be represented by only linearly growing *OBDD*-sizes.

Since a reduced *OBDD* is unique the satisfiability test is trivial (the *OBDD* consists of more than the singleton 0 sink). Evaluating $f(a)$ for $a \in \{0, 1\}^n$ can be done in linear time by simply traversing the *OBDD* downwards. The most important operation on *OBDDs* is the procedure *Apply*. Given two *OBDDs* G_f and G_g and a Boolean operator $\otimes$, $Apply(G_f, G_g, \otimes)$ computes the *OBDD* $G_{f \otimes g}$ in $O(|G_f||G_g|)$ time and space. The reduced *OBDD* can be constructed directly, integrating the two reduction rules in the postorder traversal of *Apply*. In the future we will only speak of *OBDDs*, however we always mean reduced *OBDDs*.

3 Breadth-First Search with *OBDDs*

OBDDs are successfully used in the model checking domain [13], where an important task is to determine the set of reachable states. This is done by a simple breadth-first search, starting from an initial set of states until no new states can be added to the transitive closure. In our case, however, we terminate the search when a goal position is reached. Let us consider a very simple example. We are given an array containing four squares in a row (see Fig. 1). On one of the squares a tile is found, which can be slid onto adjacent squares. In the goal state the tile has to be at position three.

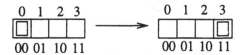

Fig. 1. A simple sliding game.

Obviously, at least three moves are necessary to solve the problem. A characteristic function Φ_S for a set of states S is a Boolean mapping from $\{0,1\}^n$ into $\{0,1\}$ that evaluates to true exactly for all states s in S and to false otherwise. Since we only have four different situations two variables are sufficient to uniquely describe the characteristic function of a state in the example. For the goal position (11) we get the minterm $x_0 \wedge x_1$. The characteristic function for combining two or more positions is given by the disjunction of the characteristic functions of the single ones.

Next we try to build a transition function T to represent the rules in our game. The transition function should have twice as many variables than the encoding of the board: if and only if x is the encoding of a given position and x' is the encoding of a successor position $T(x, x')$ should be true. Therefore, T is the disjunction of all rules. In our case we have the six movements $(00) \rightarrow (01)$, $(01) \rightarrow (00)$, $(01) \rightarrow (10)$, $(10) \rightarrow (01)$, $(10) \rightarrow (11)$ and $(11) \rightarrow (10)$. The *OBDD* according to the transition function corresponds to the disjunction of these rules and is depicted in Fig. 2.

In the sliding game, we determine the characterstic function of all situations reachable from the initial position s in a single step by applying T to the characteristic function of s. That is we ask for any successor x' such that the conjunction of T with the characteristic function of s gets true. Let Φ_S be the characteristic function of a set S and S^0 be initialised to $\{s\}$. Our aim is to calculate $\Phi_{S^{i+1}}$ given Φ_{S^i}. This is done by using existential quantification. We can describe $\Phi_{S^{i+1}}(x')$ to be the evaluation of the formula $\exists x \ (T(x, x') \wedge \Phi_{S^i}(x))$, and, starting with Φ_{S^0}, we can iterate the procedure to get the functions $\Phi_{S^1}, \Phi_{S^2}, \Phi_{S^3}$ and so on, until one of the characteristic functions has a non-empty intersection with the goal situation. In this case we have found a solution. Since the domain of $\Phi_{S^{i+1}}$ is x' we have to change the variables between x and x' in each step, which corresponds to a simple substitution of indices without a change of the structure

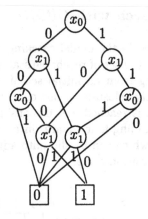

Fig. 2. The *OBDD* for the transition function.

of the *OBDD*. The set S^i contains all states that are reachable in i steps from the initial state, such that this approach reflects a breadth-first traversal of the search tree.

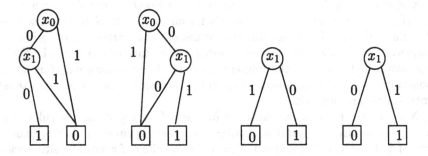

Fig. 3. *OBDDs* of Φ_{S^0}, Φ_{S^1}, Φ_{S^2} and Φ_{S^3}.

The remaining question is how to implement the existential quantifier. In Boolean algebra we have $\exists x_i f(x) = f|_{x_i=0} \vee f|_{x_i=1}$. In a naive approach we need $O(|x'|)$ *Apply* invocations, since replacement of x_i by a constant c can be done by using the reduction rules in the *OBDD*, in which for every node with index i, the $(1-c)$ successor is linked to the 0-sink. In Fig. 2 we recognize that we can do even better by computing directly the disjunction of all root nodes of the lower half in the *OBDD*. Last but not least, we can combine the application of the conjunction of $T(x, x')$ and Φ_{S^i} with the quantification in one step, since Φ_{S^i} only restricts the set of root nodes to the satisfiability set of Φ_{S^i}.

For a tractable size of the *OBDDs* the variable ordering of the transition function consists of interleaving the variables of x and x'. Therefore, the recursive calculation of the conjunction with the disjunction of subtrees has to be mixed as in function *ExistAnd* shown in Table 1 (see [1] for a detailed discussion).

This program differs from the single conjunction of T and Φ by the return value in the second line and the surplus of the second last line only. The function $xindex(var)$ is true if and only if var is an element of the set of x-variables. For the sake of clarity we have omitted the two hash tables, which have to be used in the implementation, and which contain the already computed results and the unique $OBDD$ nodes. The first one prevents us from computing the same calculations several times, whereas the second is necessary to construct *reduced* $OBDDs$, avoiding the creation of isomorphic $OBDD$ nodes.

---

function $ExistAnd(G_T, G_\Phi)$
    if $(sink_0(G_T)$ **or** $sink_0(G_\Phi))$ **return** $sink_0$
    if $(sink_1(G_T))$ **return** $sink_1$
    if $(\pi(top(G_T)) < \pi(top(G_\Phi)))$
        $s_0 \leftarrow ExistAnd(left(G_T), G_\Phi)$
        $s_1 \leftarrow ExistAnd(right(G_T), G_\Phi)$
    else if $(\pi(top(G_T)) > \pi(top(G_\Phi)))$
        $s_0 \leftarrow ExistAnd(G_T, left(G_\Phi))$
        $s_1 \leftarrow ExistAnd(G_T, right(G_\Phi))$
    else
        $s_0 \leftarrow ExistAnd(left(G_T), left(G_\Phi))$
        $s_1 \leftarrow ExistAnd(right(G_T), right(G_\Phi))$
    $min \leftarrow min\{\pi(top(G_T)), \pi(top(G_\Phi))\}$
    if $(s_0 = s_1)$ **return** s_0
    if $(xindex(min))$ **return** $Apply(s_0, s_1, \vee)$
    return $new(s0, s1, min)$

Table 1. Existential quantifying x in the conjunction of $OBDD$ $T(x, x')$ and $\Phi(x)$. Input: $OBDDs$ G_T, G_Φ Output: $OBDD$ $G_{\exists x(T(x,x') \wedge \Phi(x))}$.

4 Heuristic Search with $OBDDs$

In heuristic search we try to find the solution path with minimal length within the problem graph. In most cases this graph is uniformly weighted, i.e., each move has the cost one. With every state in the search space we associate a lower bound estimate, which can be determined efficiently.

A* differs from breadth-first search in ranking the states next to be expanded. The rank is given by the combined merit $f = g + h$ of generating path length g and the estimate h. The information h allows us to search in the direction of the goal and its quality influences mainly the number of nodes to be expanded until the goal is reached. A priority queue is used, in which the states are ordered with respect to an increasing f value. Initially, it contains only the start state together with its estimate. In each step the state with the minimum merit f is dequeued and expanded. Then the successor states have to be inserted into the queue according to their newly determined f value. The algorithm terminates when the dequeued element is a goal state. The f value of this state is the length of the minimal solution path and its estimate is zero.

In A^* the states in the priority queue are expanded one after another. *OBDDs*, however, allow sets of states to be represented very efficiently. This suggests the representation of all states with the same f value in one *OBDD*. The algorithm *ExistAnd* determines all successor states of this set in one evaluation step. It remains to determine their merits. For the dequeued state x we have $f(x) = g(x) + h(x)$. Since we can access $f(x)$, but usually not $g(x)$, the new value $f(x')$ of a successor x' has to be calculated in the following way:

$$f(x') = g(x') + h(x') = g(x) + 1 + h(x') = f(x) + 1 - h(x) + h(x'). \quad (1)$$

The estimator h can be seen as a relation of tuples (*estimate, state*) which is true if and only if $h(state)=estimate$. We assume, that h can be represented as an *OBDD* for the entire problem space which is realistic if an h-function is used which is not too complicated.

The priority queue *Open* itself can also be represented by an *OBDD*, realizing a relation based on tuples of the form (*merit, state*). The variables should be ordered in a way which allows the most significant variables to be tested at the top. Thus, the variables for the encoding of the *merit* have smaller indices than the variables encoding the *state*. This encoding leads to small *OBDDs* and enables us to simulate several steps of A^*. Furthermore, it allows an intuitive understanding of the *OBDD* and its association with the priority queue.

Next, we are going to explain our main state space search algorithm *BDDA** (for A^* with *OBDDs*) shown in Table 2. Initially, the *OBDD Open* is set to the heuristic function h of the initial state.

---

procedure *BDDA**
  $Open(f, x) \leftarrow h(f, x) \land \Phi_{S0}(x)$
  while ($Open \neq \emptyset$)
    $(f_{\min}, Min(x), Open'(f, x)) \leftarrow goLeft(Open)$
    if ($\exists x \ (Min(x) \land \Phi_G(x))$) **return** $f_{\min}$
    $VarTrans_{x,x'}(Min(x))$
    $Open''(f, x) \leftarrow \exists x' \ Min(x') \land T(x', x) \land$
      $\exists e' \ h(e', x') \land \exists e \ h(e, x) \land (f = f_{\min} + e - e' + 1)$
    $Open(f, x) \leftarrow Open'(f, x) \lor Open''(f, x)$

Table 2. The A^* algorithm using *OBDDs*.

The function *goLeft* determines the minimal f value $f_{\min}$, the *OBDD Min* of all states in the priority queue with value $f_{\min}$, and the *OBDD* of the remaining set. To fix the minimal value $f_{\min}$ it is sufficient to traverse the path from the root-node of *Open* to the first state variable, choosing always the left branch, unless it leads directly to the 0-sink. The node found is the root of the *OBDD Min*. To extract *Min*, the edge leading to *Min* has to be linked to the 0-sink for a remaining *OBDD Open'*. We might reduce *Open'* since it is not minimal.

Let Φ_G be the characteristic function of the set of goal states G. The set *Min* contains a goal state if the *OBDD Min* $\wedge\ \Phi_G$ is not the trivial zero function. If no goal state is found, the variables of x have to be substituted with the variables of x' (*VarTrans*) in the *OBDD* of *Min* before the transition function T can be applied to achieve the *OBDD Open''* for the set of successor states. To attach the new f values to this set we have to retain the old f value and the old and new h value and perform the calculations of equation 1. Finally, the *OBDD Open* for the next iteration is obtained through the disjunction of *Open'* with *Open''*.

To see how the algorithm *BDDA** works, let us consider our simple sliding game example once more. The *OBDD* for the estimate h is depicted in Fig. 4, where the estimate is set to one for state zero and one, and set to zero for state three and four.

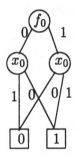

Fig. 4. The *OBDD* for the heuristic function.

Since the minimal and maximal f value turn out to be one and four, respectively, we need only two variables to encode the merit (add one to the binary encoding in the variables f_0 and f_1).

After the initialization step, the priority queue *Open* is filled with the initial state represented by minterm $\overline{x}_0\overline{x}_1$. The h value is one and so is the initial f value. There is only one successor to the initial situation, namely $\overline{x}_0 x_1$, which has an h value of one and, therefore, an f value of two. Applying T to the resulting *OBDD* we get the combined characteristic function of the states with number zero and two. Their heuristic values differ by one. Therefore, minterm $x_0\overline{x}_1$ is associated with an f value two and $\overline{x}_0\overline{x}_1$ is assigned to the merit three. The status of the priority queue is depicted to the left of Fig. 5. In the next *while* iteration we extract $x_0\overline{x}_1$ with value two and find the successor set, which in this case consists of the two positions one and three. By combining the characteristic function x_1 with the estimate h we split the *OBDD* of x_1 into two parts, since $x_0 x_1$ relates to the heuristic value zero, whereas $\overline{x}_0 x_1$ relates to one. The resulting priority queue is shown on the right hand side of Fig. 5. Since *Min* has a non-empty intersection with the characteristic function of the goal state we have found a solution. The minimal solution length is three as expected.

How to perform the arithmetics using *OBDDs*? Since the f values are restricted to a finite domain, we can build up a Boolean function *add* with param-

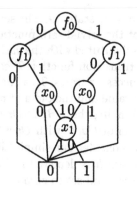 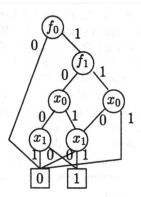

Fig. 5. The priority queue *Open* after two and after three steps.

eter a, b and c which is true if c equals the sum of a and b. Therefore, we have to build the disjunction of the characteristic functions of all such triples (a, b, c). The *minus* operator can easily be obtained by swapping the variable a and c in *add*.

5 Experiments

Though there are already various efficient *OBDD* packages which are mainly used in the model checking domain, our interest was to utilise such an implementation for our purposes. Thus we chose the *OBDD* package of the μ-calculus model checker μcke [2] and replaced the classical breadth-first search with our *BDDA** algorithm. Since the model checker does not support special functions like *goLeft*, the function had to be simulated by standard *OBDD* operations, causing some overhead that can be avoided by a suitable implementation.

Our first example is the Eight Puzzle, the 3×3 version of the well-known sliding-tile puzzles (see Fig. 6). There are eight numbered square tiles, and one empty position, called the "blank". Any tile horizontally or vertically adjacent to the blank can be swapped with the blank. The goal is to rearrange the tiles from some random initial configuration into a particular goal configuration, such as shown in Fig. 6.

We experimented with several initial configurations solvable in 20 to 27 moves, comparing *BDDA** using the well-known Manhattan distance heuristic as a lower bound with a breadth-first search approach (*BFS*). In 26 to 63 iterations *BDDA** finds the solution 4 to 7 times faster than *BFS*, which expanded up to 100 times more nodes. The number of *OBDD* nodes needed to represent the reachable states with *BFS* is 6 to 30 times higher than the number of nodes necessary for the priority queue. So obviously the *BDDA** algorithm leads to a great economy of memory usage, which is particularly important in handling examples with larger search spaces.

We also solved some configurations of the related Fifteen Puzzle. For example a minimal solution of 45 moves was found within 176 iterations with a maximal

Fig. 6. The Eight Puzzle.

OBDD-size of 215.000 nodes representing 136.000 states. With a breadth-first search approach it was impossible to find a solution because of memory limitations. Already after 19 steps more than 1 million *OBDD*-nodes were needed to represent more than 1.4 million states.

Our second example is Sokoban, one of the remaining one-person games in which the quality of the human solution quality is still better than that of all attempts at automatic solving strategies. In Sokoban *n* balls are placed somewhere in a maze containing *n* goal fields which they must eventually reach. The player controls a man which can traverse the board and push the balls onto adjacent empty squares. The initial position of one Sokoban instance is shown in Fig. 7. Solving Sokoban with the classical A^* or IDA^* algorithm turns out to be difficult, since a very refined heuristic has to be devised leading to an immense blow-up of code.

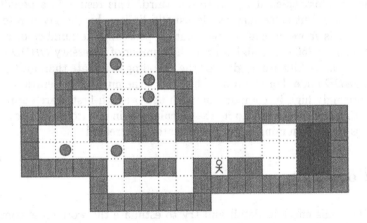

Fig. 7. Instance to the Sokoban Puzzle.

Minimizing the number of pushes in Sokoban has been studied by Junghanns and Schaefer [8,9]. Their program manages to solve 29 positions (of the benchmark set of 90 positions provided at http://xsokoban.lcs.mit.edu/xsokoban.html) in the optimal number of pushes. In our opinion, the subpattern dictionary in their approach can best be realized by using *OBDDs*. To find the minimal number of moves is by far more difficult. Doppelhamer and Lehnert [5] use *OBDDs* in a bidirectional breadth-first search to solve six positions.

To find the minimal solution of the depicted instance an efficient encoding is essential. There are 56 different fields available for the man, resulting in a binary encoding of six bits. For the balls 23 positions are either not reachable or the configuration becomes unsolvable. Therefore, 33 bits are sufficient to represent the ball positions as a bitmap. We have found a minimal solution with the breadth-first search approach, but with a high memory consumption. The *BDDA** algorithm was invoked with a very poor heuristic (h_1), counting the number of balls not on a goal position and with a better but still very simple heuristic (h_2). The results of these two approaches are compared in Table 3.

	breadth-first search	*BDDA** (h_1)	*BDDA** (h_2)
number of iterations	230	419	1671
max. size of states in Open	8.400.000	4.300.000	4.200.000
max. number of *OBDD* nodes	75.000	68.000	50.000
time consumption	0h37min	6h12min	5h16min

Table 3. Comparision of the results in Sokoban

Note that even with such poor heuristics, the number of nodes *BDDA** expands is half the number of nodes in breadth-first-search and their representation is more memory efficient by up to one third. This results in a penalty of time consumption, but since memory is usually limited by the given resources this parameter is more crucial in the solution process. The number of represented states is up to 250 times higher than the number of necessary *OBDD* nodes. Additionally, more bits are needed for the encoding of a state than for the encoding of an *OBDD* node. For elaborated heuristics the number of iterations of *BDDA** is surprisingly high in comparision with the breadth-first search approach. But comparing the effect of h_1 to h_2 the calculations in one iteration become simpler and less time consuming, since fewer states are treated.

6 Complexity

We study this effect in detail and try to estimate the worst-case complexity of the number of iterations within *BDDA**. Let f^* be the optimal solution length to a given instance s and h be the lower bound estimate. We assume that for every node u and every successor v of u the equation $h(u) \leq h(v) + 1$ is true. In other words, h is consistent, and, using Equation 1, on every path f is non-decreasing.

For an optimal heuristic, i.e., a heuristic that estimates the shortest path distance, we have at most $h(s) = f^*$ iterations in *BDDA**. On the other hand, if the heuristic is equivalent to the zero function (breadth-first search), we need f^* iterations, too. This leads to the hypothesis that the number of iterations in *BDDA** is f^*. Unfortunately, this is not true. Consider Fig. 8, in which the g

values are plotted with respect to the h value, such that nodes with the same g and h value appear on the diagonals $f = g + h$.

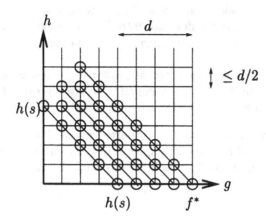

Fig. 8. The number of iterations in $BDDA^*$.

The number of noughts for each diagonal is an upper bound on the number of iterations within that slot. Therefore, we have to count the total number of noughts. Let d be the distance $f^* - h(s)$ between f^* and $h(s)$. Below the $h(s)$ value there are at most $dh(s) + h(s)$ nodes. The "roof" above $h(s)$ has at most $1 + 3 + \ldots + 2(d/2) - 1$ nodes. Since the sum evaluates to $d^2/4$ we need at most $dh(s) + h(s) + d^2/4$ iterations altogether. The maximal number of iterations $(f^{*2} + f^* + 1)/3$ is reached for $h(s) = (f^* + 2)/3$. Since f^* is not known in advance, a good upper bound to f^* is necessary to predict the search efforts. If the difference of h values to adjacent nodes is of absolute value 1, only every second f value is encountered in the search, halving the number of iterations.

7 Conclusion

The A^* algorithm has been outperformed by IDA^* methods in several application areas, since for its admissibility it has to keep all ever expanded nodes in memory. We have shown how to overcome the problem, by using $OBDDs$ that are capable of storing a huge set of positions through a binary encoding of the problem states.

States found by applying a few moves often have only small local changes in their encodings. Therefore, we take advantage of the fact that a huge number of states are similar and can be represented very efficiently. In heuristic search the set of generated states is not far away from the states on the minimal solution path. However, a simple state enumeration does not take profit from this circumstance.

A big advantage of $BDDA^*$ over existing approaches is that the use of a very simple heuristic already suffices to achieve solutions for problems that cannot be solved with A^* without introducing additional problem-specific knowledge.

The design of a non-trivial heuristic always increases the iteration depth. The memory consumption on the other hand decreases because less nodes have to be expanded. An estimate near the optimum is hard to find and usually requires a time consuming calculation, too. Thus, the aim should be to use a rather simple lower bound, which does not introduce a big penalty in iteration depth, but allows the saving of as much memory as is needed in respect to the limited resources.

In A^* each node is represented at most once, whereas in our approach we detect duplicates in the search tree only if they have the same f value. Combining our method with existing pruning schemes is addressed to further research.

Acknowledgments S. Edelkamp is supported by DFG within the graduate program on human and machine intelligence. F. Reffel is supported by DFG within the graduate program on controlability of complex systems.

References

1. A. Biere. *Efficient model checking with binary decision diagramms.* PhD thesis, Computer Science Department, University of Karlsruhe, 1997.
2. A. Biere. μcke - efficient μ-calculus model checking. In *Computer Aided Verification*, volume 1254 of *LNCS*, pages 468–471, 1997.
3. R. E. Bryant. Symbolic manipulation of boolean functions using a graphical representation. In *Proceedings of the 22nd ACM/IEEE Design Automation Conference*, pages 688–694, Los Alamitos, Ca., USA, 1985. IEEE Computer Society Press.
4. J. C. Culberson and J. Schaeffer. Searching with pattern databases. In *Proceedings of the Eleventh Biennial Conference of the Canadian Society for Computational Studies of Intelligence on Advances in Artificial Intelligence*, volume 1081 of *LNAI*, pages 402–416, Berlin, 1996. Springer.
5. J. Doppelhamer and J. K. Lehnert. Optimal solution for sokoban using OBDDs. University of Trier, available from the authors, 1998.
6. J. Eckerle and S. Schuierer. Efficient memory-limited graph search. *LNCS*, 981:101–112, 1995.
7. P. E. Hart, N. J. Nilsson, and B. Raphael. A formal basis for heuristic determination of minimum path cost. *IEEE Trans. on SSC*, 4:100, 1968.
8. A. Junghanns and J. Schaeffer. Single agent search in the presence of deadlocks. To appear in: *Proceedings AAAI-98*, 1998.
9. A. Junghanns and J. Schaeffer. Sokoban: Evaluating standard single-agent search techniques in the presence of deadlock. To appear in: Proceedings CSCSI-98, Vancouver, Canada, LNCS, Springer, 1998.
10. R. E. Korf. Depth-first iterative-deepening: An optimal admissible tree search. *Artificial Intelligence*, 27(1):97–109, 1985.
11. R. E. Korf. Finding optimal solutions to Rubik's cube using pattern databases. In *Proceedings AAAI-97*, pages 700–705. AAAI Press, 1997.
12. R. E. Korf and L. A. Taylor. Finding optimal solutions to the twenty-four puzzle. In *Proceedings AAAI-96*, pages 1202–1207. AAAI Press, 1996.
13. K. McMillan. *Symbolic Model Checking.* Kluwer Academic Press, 1993.
14. S. Russell. Efficient memory-bounded search methods. In *Proceedings of ECAI-92*, pages 1–5. Wiley, 1992.
15. L. A. Taylor and R. E. Korf. Pruning duplicate nodes in depth-first search. In *AAAI-93*, pages 756–761. AAAI Press, 1993.

Handling Negative Assumptions in a Generic User Modeling Framework

Wolfgang Pohl

GMD – National Research Center for Information Technology
Human-Computer Interaction Research Group (FIT.MMK)
Wolfgang.Pohl@gmd.de

Abstract. Traditionally, there have been two approaches to powerful logic-based user modeling: First, in the modal logic approach, there is one knowledge base that consists of formulas of one (modal) logic formalism. Second, the partition approach divides the user model into partial knowledge bases, mainly to distinguish between different types of assumptions about the user. For the user modeling shell system BGP-MS an approach to integrate partitions with modal logic was developed and later refined to become the user model representation and reasoning framework AsTRa, which is also applicable in the more general case of agent modeling. In this framework, however, there is a representational gap between partitions and modal logic. A specific kind of user model contents, which we call negative assumptions, falls into this gap. Since negative assumptions have been quite frequently used with BGP-MS, we developed specialized mechanisms for dealing with them. This paper gives a brief overview of AsTRa, and formally presents the above-mentioned mechanisms. Like the whole AsTRa framework, they are semantically related to modal logic, which is proven.

1 Introduction

Generic user modeling techniques have been implemented into user modeling shell systems in order to relieve user-adaptive applications from the several burdens of the user modeling task. Central among these burdens are user model representation and reasoning. Ideally, a user modeling shell system provides representation and reasoning mechanisms that are powerful enough to be useful to complex applications, and are flexible enough to appropriately fit the needs of less sophisticated systems. In [Poh97], we present a logic-based framework for user model representation and reasoning (called AsTRa), which combines power and flexibility by integrating partition-based representation with modal logic.

There is a specific class of user model contents, namely assumptions about what users do *not* believe, want, etc., which we call *negative assumptions*. As our experience with the user modeling shell BGP-MS [KP95] shows, negative assumptions are relevant to many user modeling systems. In AsTRa, however, they cannot be handled by standard partitions, and full modal logic is inappropriately complex. Therefore, we developed special representation and reasoning facilities for negative assumptions. They are based on partitions but semantically consistent with modal logic, so that they neatly fit into the AsTRa framework.

In the rest of this paper, we will first discuss the main logic-based approaches to user modeling, briefly sketch the AsTRa framework, and then present our specialized mechanisms for handling negative assumptions.

2 Logic-Based Approaches to User Model Representation

2.1 Assumption Type and Content

What does a typical content of a user model look like? Let us have a look at the following simple example, concerning a user belief:

(The system assumes that) The user believes that sharks are dangerous. (1)

The first approach to represent this user model content is to formulate the whole sentence (including the—redundant—part in parentheses or not) as a logical expression. However, if the user model is to contain assumptions about user beliefs only, it is sufficient to have an expression for

Sharks are dangerous.

in the user model in order to represent the first sentence. But also if different kinds of assumptions need to be considered, this second approach is possible: Divide the user model into partial knowledge bases (often called partitions), one for each *assumption type* (in the example: assumption about user beliefs), and store the *assumption content* (here: sharks are dangerous) only within these knowledge bases. In this case, user model contents can be regarded as consisting of two components, namely the assumption type AT and the assumption content ac. Then, $AT{:}ac$ is the general form of assumptions about the user.

In the following, we will look at the mentioned approaches in more detail and suggest to integrate both approaches in order to combine their advantages.

2.2 Partition Approach

The explicit distinction of assumption type and content has been pursued in the *partition approach* to user modeling. This approach is based on the use of partial knowledge bases (also called partitions) within a user model. Partitions were introduced by [Coh78], while Kobsa further developed the approach [Kob85, Kob90]. Partitions are typically used to distinguish between different kinds of knowledge. In user modeling, they correspond to different types of assumptions about the user, and are typically labeled with sequences of agent-modality pairs. Examples are SBUB (System Beliefs about User Beliefs), SBUW (System Beliefs about User Wants), SBUBSB (System Beliefs about User Beliefs about System Beliefs) etc.

On the left of Figure 1, there is a partition representation of the example assumption (1). A partition SBUB stores assumptions about user beliefs.

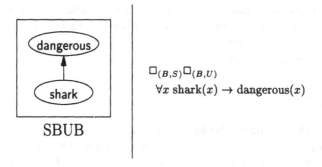

Fig. 1. Partition-based and modal logic user model representation

Within SBUB, a KL-ONE-like graphical notation is used to represent "sharks are dangerous". Using our *AT:ac* notation with a linear terminological formalism, this reads SBUB:shark ⊑ dangerous. This example shows the advantages of a partition-based representation. First, no logical means need to be employed to code the assumption type. Second, within partitions, assumption contents may be coded in appropriate special-purpose formalisms.

2.3 Modal Logic Approach

In the *modal logic approach,* user model contents are fully coded as formulas of a modal logic or of FOPC with specific, modal-operator-like predicates. The standard modal operator is $\Box$. However, for user modeling specialized operators (like B for belief or W for wants) are needed, which may also carry agent indices (like B_U for "the user believes"). Such operators can be regarded as parameterized variants of $\Box$: B_U can be written $\Box_{(B,U)}$. The generic form is $\Box_{(m,a)}$, with m short for "modality", and a short for "agent". Thus, our example assumption can be written as shown on the right of Figure 1. The sequence of modal operators $\Box_{(B,S)}\Box_{(B,U)}$ corresponds to the partition label SBUB, and the non-modal part of the formula, $\forall x\ \text{shark}(x) \rightarrow \text{dangerous}(x)$, represents the assumption content.

The modal logic approach was suggested and supported mainly in [AOR92, Hus94]. Its main advantage is the expressive power of modal logic, which exceeds the possibilities of "partition expressions" *AT:ac.* E.g., the formula

$$\Box_{(B,S)}\neg\Box_{(B,U)}\, p$$

expresses that a proposition p is assumed not to be believed by the user. Similar assumptions about what is *not* believed, wanted, etc. will we called *negative assumptions* further on. The formula

$$\Box_{(B,S)}\Box_{(W,U)}\, q\ \rightarrow\ \Box_{(B,S)}\Box_{(B,U)}\, p$$

expresses that assuming goal q implies an assumption about belief in p.

Both examples show that modal logic is more powerful than partition-based representation. However, handling of modal formulas is more complex than handling partition contents; and with modal logic, special purpose formalisms cannot be used to represent assumption contents.

2.4 Integration

Since both partitions and modal logic have their advantages, it is a straightforward idea to integrate both approaches. For instance, the user modeling shell BGP-MS [KP95] implements modal logic as uniform interface language, while internally partitions are preferred. In [PH97], an alternative *bottom-up* integration is suggested based on experiences with BGP-MS applications: Partitions and content formalisms are directly accessible, since they are sufficient for many user modeling purposes. Modal logic is additionally available and includes partition contents into its reasoning procedures. This approach offers more flexibility, which is particularly relevant to user modeling shell systems with their ambition to satisfy the user modeling needs of different systems.

In the next section, we will sketch a framework for logic-based user model representation and reasoning with a bottom-up integration of modal logic and partition-based representation.

3 AsTRa: A Representation Framework for User Modeling Shells

The AsTRa (Assumption Type Representation) framework for logic-based user model representation and reasoning was developed to provide powerful and flexible representation and reasoning facilities to user modeling shell systems. AsTRa was introduced in [PH97] and presented in full detail in [Poh97].

3.1 Basic Facilities

The basic representation entity of AsTRa is the assumption type (AT), which essentially is a partition-like partial knowledge base (KB_{AT}). AsTRa assumption types are labeled like partitions (cf. Section 2.2): SBUB, SBUW, SBUBSB, etc. An AsTRa implementation should however permit the use of more modalities than B and W only, like I (for "interests"), Pref (for "preferences"), etc.

Within assumption types, assumption contents can be represented using logic-based formalisms. "Logic-based" means that expressions of a content formalism F can be translated into first-order predicate calculus (FOPC) with a translation function t_F, and that reasoning in F is at least sound with respect to FOPC: $KB_{AT} \vdash_F ac \implies t_F(KB_{AT}) \models t_F(ac)$. Note that $t_F(KB_{AT})$ means the application of t_F to all F-expressions in KB_{AT}. Further on, we will simply say t instead of t_F, unless the detail is necessary. In addition, content formalisms are required to offer the basic reasoning functions *derivable*$_F$ (which is assumed to soundly and correctly implement $\vdash_F$), *forward$_F$*, and *consistent$_F$* for backward derivability checks, forward inferences, and consistency checks.

So far, $AT{:}ac$ expressions can be represented in an AsTRa user modeling knowledge base (UMKB) by maintaining a content expression ac in an assumption type knowledge base KB_{AT}. Since it is not possible to express relationships between assumption types, basic AsTRa reasoning is *type-internal*. I.e., global AsTRa reasoning functions can be reduced to applying the functions of the appropriate content formalism $F(ac)$ to KB_{AT} and ac, e.g.:

$$\mathbf{derivable}(\text{UMKB}, AT{:}ac) := derivable_{F(ac)}(\text{KB}_{AT}, ac)$$

3.2 Extended Facilities: Modal Logic

$AT{:}ac$ expressions, which the basic AsTRa facilities deal with, are syntactically related to modal formulas: an assumption type label AT corresponds to a modal operator sequence $\mathcal{M}(AT)$, and assumption contents ac can be translated into FOPC formulas $t(ac)$. Thus, an $AT{:}ac$ expression corresponds to a modal formula $\mathcal{M}(AT)\,t(ac)$. An example was presented in Section 2: The expression

$$\text{SBUB} : \text{shark} \sqsubseteq \text{dangerous}$$

corresponds to the modal formula

$$\Box_{(B,S)}\Box_{(B,U)} \; \forall x \, \text{shark}(x) \rightarrow \text{dangerous}(x)$$

The logic that is syntactically restricted to $\mathcal{M}(AT)\,t(ac)$ expressions is called AL (short for "assumption logic"). Then, all KB_{AT} within a UMKB can be translated into an AL knowledge base KB_{AT}^{AL}. The union of all KB_{AT}^{AL} is the AL version of the UMKB, UMKB^{AL}.

Beyond being syntactically related, the basic AsTRa facilities are also semantically consistent with modal logic. Under certain conditions on content formalisms, it can be proven that type-internal reasoning is sound and complete with respect to modal logic (see [Poh97]):

$$\mathbf{derivable}(\text{UMKB}, AT{:}ac) \iff \text{UMKB}^{AL} \models \mathcal{M}(AT)\,t(ac)$$

Based on these syntactic and semantic correlations, modal logic is integrated into AsTRa as follows: The full version of AL (i.e., a full modal logic with $\Box_{(m,a)}$ operators) is called AL^+. Then, an *extended* AsTRa UMKB, in addition to assumption types and contents, contains a set $\mathcal{MF}$ of AL^+ modal formulas. Such a UMKB can be transformed into an AL^+ knowledge base $\text{UMKB}^{AL^+} := \text{UMKB}^{AL} \cup \mathcal{MF}$.

For modal logic reasoning purposes, functions $\mathbf{derivable}_{AL^+}$, $\mathbf{forward}_{AL^+}$, and $\mathbf{consistent}_{AL^+}$ are required, which operate on AL^+ formulas and knowledge bases. By applying these functions to UMKB^{AL^+}, they consider both the modal logic part $\mathcal{MF}$ of an (extended) AsTRa UMKB as well as its basic $AT{:}ac$ contents. The semantic equivalence of basic AsTRa and AL guarantees that, if only type-internal expressions $AT{:}ac$ need to be considered, type-internal reasoning can be used equivalently to AL^+ reasoning.

AL^+ is a normal, multi-modal, multi-agent logic. Assuming a standard possible worlds semantics [Kri63], for any possible operator $\Box_{(m,a)}$ of AL axiom K holds and the necessitation rule (NR) and modus ponens (MP) are inference rules:

$$\models \Box_{(m,a)}(\phi \to \psi) \to (\Box_{(m,a)}\phi \to \Box_{(m,a)}\psi) \text{ (K)}$$
$$\phi \models \Box_{(m,a)}\phi \qquad\qquad \text{(NR)}$$
$$\phi, \phi \to \psi \models \psi \qquad\qquad \text{(MP)}$$

In specific AsTRa implementations, however, AL^+ reasoning may be based on a more specific semantics. For instance, for the user modeling shell BGP-MS, AL^+ reasoning was implemented based on the modal logic axiom D ($\Box\phi \to \neg\Box\neg\phi$) [Poh96]. In the next section, we will describe special mechanisms for reasoning with negative assumptions which also rely on axiom D.

4 Handling Negative Assumptions

4.1 Negative Assumptions Are Special

The notion of negative assumptions was introduced in Section 2 in order to refer to assumptions about what is *not* believed, wanted, etc. by the user. Such assumptions can be represented by AL^+ formulas. An example is

$$\Box_{(B,S)}\neg\Box_{(B,U)} \text{ dangerous(dolphin21)} \qquad\qquad (2)$$

This formula states that the user is assumed not to believe that the object 'dolphin21' is classified as 'dangerous'.

For several reasons, it makes sense to deal with negative assumptions in a special way. Syntactically, negative assumption formulas differ from AL formulas (i.e., type-internal knowledge) only in the possible negation of modal operators, thus inducing an AL extension AL^-. Moreover, several user modeling systems made use of negative assumptions without needing other type-external representation or reasoning methods [HMGN91, KMN94, PHFK95].

The first step towards special handling of negative assumptions is to organize them in assumption types: By using the negation symbol $\sim$ in assumption type labels, we can introduce negative assumption types like SB~UW (assumptions about what is not a user goal) etc. Then, Formula 2 corresponds to the type-internal expression SB~UB:dangerous(dolphin21).

As a second step, reasoning mechanisms are needed that operate on such negative assumptions (and perhaps take other UMKB contents into account). Unfortunately, type-internal reasoning based on content formalisms is not applicable, due to the modal logic semantics of negative assumptions. For positive types, if an assumption type knowledge base entails a content expression, $\mathrm{KB}_{AT} \models ac$, an entailment will also hold for the corresponding AL expressions: $\mathrm{KB}_{AT}^{AL} \models \mathcal{M}(AT)\,t(ac)$. For negative assumption types and AL^-, this *entailment correspondence* does not exist. In terms of modal logic: $\phi \models \psi$ is *not* equivalent to $\neg\Box_{(m,a)}\phi \models \neg\Box_{(m,a)}\psi$.

4.2 Reasoning with Negative Assumptions

Since type-internal reasoning does not apply to negative assumption types, we invented specialized reasoning methods for dealing with negative assumptions. In modal logics, one of the classical characterizing axioms is axiom D:

$$\Box\phi \rightarrow \neg\Box\neg\phi \text{ (D)}$$

D is often taken to be characteristic for logics of belief. In this case, it says that if something is believed, its contrary is not believed. D obviously allows for inferences that involve negated modal operators. For our reasoning procedures for negative assumptions, we take advantage of that.

Box-Diamond Forms. Our task is to specify inference procedures which efficiently imitate modal logic reasoning that is based on axiom D. For this purpose, we will make use of the "diamond" operator $\Diamond$ of modal logic. This operator can replace negated $\Box$ ("box") operators, since $\Diamond\phi \equiv \neg\Box\neg\phi$ holds. In particular, axiom D can be rewritten $\Box\phi \rightarrow \Diamond\phi$. This suggests that inferences based on D might be mechanically executed by simply replacing $\Box$ operators with $\Diamond$ operators. In the following we will pursue this idea, making use of the fact that, using $\Diamond$, any $AL^\neg$ formula can be written without negations in front of modal operators. For example:

$$\Box_{(B,S)}\neg\Box_{(W,U)}\,\phi \equiv \Box_{(B,S)}\Diamond_{(W,U)}\,\neg\phi$$

We will call such a negation-free form *box-diamond form* (BDF). It consists of a *box-diamond sequence* (BDS) of box and diamond operators and a non-modal part, which is equal to the original non-modal part or its negation. The BDF of a negative assumption in AT:ac form (short: BDF(AT:ac)) is defined as the BDF of its corresponding $AL^\neg$ formula $\mathcal{M}(AT)\,t(ac)$.

An example is: BDF(SB~UW:ϕ) = $\Box_{(B,S)}\Diamond_{(W,U)}\,\neg\phi$. This example indicates that transformation into BDF does not modify assumption contents besides possibly negating it. Hence, transforming AT:ac into BDF can be reduced to determine (a) the box-diamond sequence of AT and (b) whether ac needs to be negated or not. That is, with

$$BDF(AT{:}ac) = O_{1(m_1,a_1)} \ldots O_{n(m_n,a_n)}\,sig\,ac$$

where $sig \in \{\neg, \varepsilon\}$ (and ε being the empty word), we define BD(AT) as a pair that consists of the box-diamond sequence of AT and an indication whether contents need to be negated:

$$BD(AT) := \langle O_{1(m_1,a_1)} \ldots O_{n(m_n,a_n)}, sig \rangle$$

Example: BD(SB~UW) = $\langle \Box_{(B,S)}\Diamond_{(W,U)}, \neg \rangle$.

Below, we will define relations between box-diamond sequences (the first part of BD(AT) pairs), which will lead to inference procedures for negative assumptions. Finally, however, we will need assumption types again to take the place of box-diamond sequences. The corresponding transformation is called BD^{-1}; e.g., BD$^{-1}(\langle \Box_{(B,S)}\Diamond_{(W,U)}, \neg \rangle) = \langle$SB~UW$, \varepsilon \rangle$.

Inference Relations. The reason for introducing BDF was that inferences might be realizable using BDF formulas and the negation-free version of axiom D,

$$\Box\phi \to \Diamond\phi$$

With axiom K, the necessitation rule, and modus ponens (cf. Section 3.2), axiom D entails similar implications also for BDF formulas with more than one operator. In case of two operators, all valid implications are $\Box\Box\phi \to \Box\Diamond\phi$, $\Diamond\Box\phi \to \Diamond\Diamond\phi$, $\Box\Diamond\phi \to \Diamond\Diamond\phi$, and $\Box\Box\phi \to \Diamond\Diamond\phi$. In all these implications the conclusion is obtained by replacing at least one $\Box$ operator of the antecedent with a $\Diamond$ operator. This observation can be generalized to operator sequences of any length, so that we obtain the following proposition:

Theorem 1. *Let* $O_{1(m_1,a_1)}\ldots O_{n(m_n,a_n)}\phi$ *and* $O'_{1(m_1,a_1)}\ldots O'_{n(m_n,a_n)}\phi$ *be* $AL^\neg$ *formulas in BDF (i.e.,* $O_i(') \in \{\Box,\Diamond\}$, *and* ϕ *is an arbitrary FOPC formula). Assume axiom D for all operators of* $AL^\neg$ *(i.e.,* $\Box_{(m,a)}\phi \to \Diamond_{(m,a)}\phi$ *holds for all* m, a). *Then:*

$$\models O_{1(m_1,a_1)}\ldots O_{n(m_n,a_n)}\phi \to O'_{1(m_1,a_1)}\ldots O'_{n(m_n,a_n)}\phi$$

if (*) $O'_i = \Diamond$ *if* $O_i = \Diamond$, *and* $O'_i \in \{\Box,\Diamond\}$ *if* $O_i = \Box$.

Proof. (by induction over the length n of the operator sequence. We omit the modality indices m_i and a_i for sake of readability.)

$n = 1$: (a) If $O_i = \Box$ then $O'_i \in \{\Box,\Diamond\}$: $\models \Box\phi \to \Box\phi$ is obvious, $\models \Box\phi \to \Diamond\phi$ since axiom D is assumed. (b) If $O_i = \Diamond$, then $O'_i = \Diamond$: $\models \Diamond\phi \to \Diamond\phi$ is obvious.

$n \to n+1$: Let $O_1\ldots O_n$ and $O'_1\ldots O'_n$ be BDSs such that (*) is satisfied. Induction assumption: $\models O_1\ldots O_n\phi \to O'_1\ldots O'_n\phi$. Then also

$$\models \Box O_1\ldots O_n\phi \to \Box O'_1\ldots O'_n\phi \tag{3}$$

(because of NR, K, and MP). Applying axiom D, we get

$$\models \Box O'_1\ldots O'_n\phi \to \Diamond O'_1\ldots O'_n\phi \tag{4}$$

Together, 3 and 4 yield:

$$\models \Box O_1\ldots O_n\phi \to \Diamond O'_1\ldots O'_n\phi \tag{5}$$

From the induction assumption, we further can derive

$$\models \neg(O'_1\ldots O'_n\phi) \to \neg(O_1\ldots O_n\phi)$$
$$(\text{NR, K, MP}) \Rightarrow \models \Box\neg(O'_1\ldots O'_n\phi) \to \Box\neg(O_1\ldots O_n\phi)$$
$$\Rightarrow \models \neg\Box\neg(O_1\ldots O_n\phi) \to \neg\Box\neg(O'_1\ldots O'_n\phi)$$

In BDF, the last implication reads

$$\models \Diamond O_1\ldots O_n\phi \to \Diamond O'_1\ldots O'_n\phi \tag{6}$$

3, 5, and 6 cover all possibilities for the $n+1$th operators (O_0 and O'_0) that are permissible according to (*). $\qquad\Box$

From Theorem 1, we can obtain several corollaries, which are more directly applicable for inference procedures. First, a mere reformulation of Theorem 1 is (we leave out the preconditions)

Corollary 1.

$$O_{1(m_1,a_1)} \cdots O_{n(m_n,a_n)} \phi \models O'_{1(m_1,a_1)} \cdots O'_{n(m_n,a_n)} \phi$$

if $O'_i = \diamond$ *if* $O_i = \diamond$, *and* $O'_i \in \{\square, \diamond\}$ *if* $O_i = \square$.

An immediate application of this corollary is forward reasoning. We define a relation FOR between box-diamond sequences bds_i:

$$\text{FOR}(bds_1, bds_2) \iff bds_1 \phi \models bds_2 \phi \text{ and } bds_1 \neq bds_2$$

for all content formulas ϕ. The condition $bds_1 \neq bds_2$ is to exclude the trivial case that a formula entails itself.

Example 1. $\square_{(B,S)} \square_{(W,U)} \phi$ entails $\square_{(B,S)} \diamond_{(W,U)} \phi$, $\diamond_{(B,S)} \square_{(W,U)} \phi$, $\square_{(B,S)} \diamond_{(W,U)} \phi$, and itself. Therefore,

$$\text{FOR}(\square_{(B,S)} \square_{(W,U)}, \square_{(B,S)} \diamond_{(W,U)}), \text{FOR}(\square_{(B,S)} \square_{(W,U)}, \diamond_{(B,S)} \square_{(W,U)}), \text{ and}$$
$$\text{FOR}(\square_{(B,S)} \square_{(W,U)}, \diamond_{(B,S)} \diamond_{(W,U)}).$$

Corollary 1 is also relevant in case of queries to the UMKB. For a query that concerns a (negative) assumption type, it is crucial to know by which UMKB contents the queried expression is implied. Hence, we also define a backward derivation relation DER between box-diamond sequences:

$$\text{DER}(bds_1, bds_2) \iff bds_2 \phi \models bds_1 \phi \text{ and } bds_1 \neq bds_2$$

for all content formulas ϕ. The condition $bds_1 \neq bds_2$ is to exclude the trivial case that a formula is entailed by itself.

Example 2. $\square_{(B,S)} \diamond_{(W,U)} \phi$ is entailed by $\square_{(B,S)} \square_{(W,U)} \phi$ and itself. Hence,

$$\text{DER}(\square_{(B,S)} \diamond_{(W,U)}, \square_{(B,S)} \square_{(W,U)})$$

Also inconsistency relationships between positive and negative assumptions exist. Note that $\neg \square \phi \equiv \diamond \neg \phi$ so that $\square \phi$ is inconsistent with $\diamond \neg \phi$. Furthermore, $\neg \square \neg \phi \equiv \diamond \phi$ so that $\square \neg \phi$ is inconsistent with $\diamond \phi$. In general, the negation of a BDF is a BDF with switched operators and negated inner formula:

$$\neg O_{1(m_1,a_1)} \cdots O_{n(m_n,a_n)} \phi \equiv O'_{1(m_1,a_1)} \cdots O'_{n(m_n,a_n)} \neg \phi \qquad (7)$$

where $O'_i = \diamond$ if $O_i = \square$, and $O'_i = \square$ if $O_i = \diamond$.

Now, an $AL^\neg$ formula is not only inconsistent with its own negation, but also with the negation of all its implications. Hence, we combine (7) with Corollary 1 to derive a statement about inconsistencies:

Corollary 2.

$$O_{1(m_1,a_1)} \cdots O_{n(m_n,a_n)}\phi \wedge O'_{1(m_1,a_1)} \cdots O'_{n(m_n,a_n)}\neg\phi \models \perp$$

where $O'_i = \square$ if $O_i = \diamond$, and $O_i \in \{\square, \diamond\}$ if $O_i = \square$.

Analogous to the FOR and DER relations, a relation INC between box-diamond sequences is defined:

$$\text{INC}(bds_1, bds_2) \iff bds_1\phi \wedge bds_2\neg\phi \models \perp \text{ and } bds_1 \neq bds_2$$

for all content formulas ϕ. The condition $bds_1 \neq bds_2$ is to exclude the trivial case of the type-internal inconsistency of an assumption content ac with its negation, which may occur in case of a positive assumption type.

Example 3. $\square_{(B,S)}\square_{(W,U)}\phi$ is inconsistent with $\square_{(B,S)}\diamond_{(W,U)}\neg\phi$, $\diamond_{(B,S)}\square_{(W,U)}\neg\phi$, $\diamond_{(B,S)}\diamond_{(W,U)}\neg\phi$, and $\square_{(B,S)}\square_{(W,U)}\neg\phi$. Hence,

$\text{INC}(\square_{(B,S)}\square_{(W,U)}, \square_{(B,S)}\diamond_{(W,U)})$, $\text{INC}(\square_{(B,S)}\square_{(W,U)}, \diamond_{(B,S)}\square_{(W,U)})$, and
$\text{INC}(\square_{(B,S)}\square_{(W,U)}, \diamond_{(B,S)}\diamond_{(W,U)})$

The relations FOR, DER, and INC can be employed to establish forward derivation, backward derivation, and inconsistency relations, respectively, between assumption types. The following principle is applied: An $AL^\neg$ formula ϕ is equivalent to its box-diamond form ϕ'. ϕ' entails (can be derived from, is inconsistent with) a number of box-diamond forms ψ'_i according to FOR (DER, INC), which are equivalent to $AL^\neg$ formulas ψ_i. Hence, ϕ entails (can be derived from, is inconsistent with) all ψ_i. More formally, for an assumption type AT we define forward(AT), derivable(AT), and inconsistent(AT) as sets of pairs $\langle AT', sig \rangle$ such that $\mathcal{M}(AT) ac$ entails (can be derived from, is inconsistent with) $\mathcal{M}(AT') sig ac$. sig can be $\neg$ or ε; it indicates if ac needs to be negated or not.

Let bds, bds' be box-diamond sequences, and $sig \in \{\neg, \varepsilon\}$. Then, we define:

1. forward(AT) :=
   $\{\text{BD}^{-1}(\langle bds', sig \rangle) \mid \text{BD}(AT) = \langle bds, sig \rangle \text{ and } \text{FOR}(bds, bds')\}$
2. derivable(AT) :=
   $\{\text{BD}^{-1}(\langle bds', sig \rangle) \mid \text{BD}(AT) = \langle bds, sig \rangle \text{ and } \text{DER}(bds, bds')\}$
3. inconsistent(AT) :=
   $\{\text{BD}^{-1}(\langle bds', \overline{sig} \rangle) \mid \text{BD}(AT) = \langle bds, sig \rangle \text{ and } \text{INC}(bds, bds')\}$

$\overline{sig}$ is the complement of sig, i.e. $\overline{\neg} = \varepsilon$ and $\overline{\varepsilon} = \neg$. forward($AT$), derivable($AT$) and inconsistent($AT$) may contain pairs $\langle AT', sig \rangle$ where AT' does not start with SB. Since that is not permitted in AsTRa, such pairs are removed.

Example 4. $\text{BD}(\text{SB}\sim\text{UW}) = \langle \square_{(B,S)}\diamond_{(W,U)}, \neg \rangle$

1. $\text{FOR}(\square_{(B,S)}\diamond_{(W,U)}, \diamond_{(B,S)}\diamond_{(W,U)})$, $\text{BD}^{-1}(\langle \diamond_{(B,S)}\diamond_{(W,U)}, \neg \rangle = \langle \sim\text{SBUW}, \varepsilon \rangle$
   $\implies$ forward(SB$\sim$UW) = $\emptyset$

2. $\text{DER}(\Box_{(B,S)}\Diamond_{(W,U)}, \Box_{(B,S)}\Box_{(W,U)})$, $\text{BD}^{-1}((\Box_{(B,S)}\Box_{(W,U)}, \neg) = \langle \text{SBUW}, \neg \rangle$
   $\implies$ derivable(SB~UW) = $\{\langle \text{SBUW}, \neg \rangle\}$
3. $\text{INC}(\Box_{(B,S)}\Diamond_{(W,U)}, \Box_{(B,S)}\Box_{(W,U)})$, $\text{BD}^{-1}((\Box_{(B,S)}\Box_{(W,U)}, \varepsilon)) = \langle \text{SBUW}, \varepsilon \rangle$
   $\text{INC}(\Box_{(B,S)}\Diamond_{(W,U)}, \Diamond_{(B,S)}\Box_{(W,U)})$, $\text{BD}^{-1}((\Diamond_{(B,S)}\Box_{(W,U)}, \varepsilon)) = \langle \sim\text{SB}\sim\text{UW}, \varepsilon \rangle$
   $\implies$ inconsistent(SB~UW) = $\{\langle \text{SBUW}, \varepsilon \rangle\}$

From the definitions of the inference relations, the following statements can be deduced for any given assumption type AT and all assumption contents ac:

- For all $\langle AT', sig \rangle \in$ forward(AT), AT:ac entails AT':$sig\,ac$.
- For all $\langle AT', sig \rangle \in$ derivable(AT), AT:ac is derivable from AT':$sig\,ac$.
- For all $\langle AT', sig \rangle \in$ inconsistent(AT), AT:ac is inconsistent with AT':$sig\,ac$.

These statements can almost immediately be transformed into reasoning procedures for negative assumptions. Due to Theorem 1, these procedures are sound with respect to modal logic semantics (with axiom D presumed). The most important reasoning information for these procedures are the forward, derivable, and inconsistent relations, which can be computed a priori for any assumption type. This makes the presented special mechanisms for reasoning with negative assumptions quite efficient.

Example 5. 1. derivable(SB~UW) = $\{\langle \text{SBUW}, \neg \rangle\}$; hence, SB~UW:$ac$ is derivable from SBUW:$\neg ac$.
2. inconsistent(SB~UW) = $\{\langle \text{SBUW}, \varepsilon \rangle\}$; hence, SB~UW:$ac$ is inconsistent to SBUW:ac.
3. forward(SBUB) = $\{\langle \text{SB}\sim\text{UB}, \neg \rangle\}$; hence, SBUB:$ac$ entails SB~UB:$\neg ac$.

5 Conclusions

In this paper, we addressed the demand for user modeling shell systems that provide powerful representation and reasoning mechanisms in a flexible way to developers of adaptive application systems. We briefly sketched an approach to integrating partitions (assumption types) and modal logic for this purpose. In this approach, negative assumptions can in principle be handled using modal logic. However, as our experience with the user modeling shell system BGP-MS indicates, negative assumptions are needed in a number of user modeling systems that otherwise would not make use of modal logic.

In order to offer such systems an appropriate solution for handling negative assumptions, we introduced negative assumption types for a partition-based representation of negative assumptions. In addition, we presented special reasoning mechanisms for this representation. They are consistent with modal logic semantics, which we proved. They are also efficient, since they are based on information which can be computed a priori for all assumption types. Moreover, like the whole AsTRa framework, the introduced mechanisms are not specific to user modeling and hence applicable also in the more general case of agent modeling.

References

[AOR92]   J. Allgayer, H. J. Ohlbach, and C. Reddig. Modelling agents with logic. In *Proc. of the Third International Workshop on User Modeling*, pages 22–34, Dagstuhl, Germany, 1992.

[Coh78]   P. R. Cohen. On knowing what to say: Planning speech acts. Technical Report 118, Department of Computer Science, University of Toronto, Canada, 1978.

[HMGN91]   X. Huang, G. I. McCalla, J. E. Greer, and E. Neufeld. Revising deductive knowledge and stereotypical knowledge in a student model. *User Modeling and User-Adapted Interaction*, 1(1):87–115, 1991.

[Hus94]   U. Hustadt. A multi-modal logic for stereotyping. In *Proceedings of the Fourth International Conference on User Modeling*, pages 87–92, 1994.

[KMN94]   A. Kobsa, D. Müller, and A. Nill. KN-AHS: An adaptive hypertext client of the user modeling system BGP-MS. In *Proc. of the Fourth International Conference on User Modeling*, pages 99–105, Hyannis, MA, 1994.

[Kob85]   A. Kobsa. *Benutzermodellierung in Dialogsystemen*. Springer-Verlag, Berlin, Heidelberg, 1985.

[Kob90]   A. Kobsa. Modeling the user's conceptual knowledge in BGP-MS, a user modeling shell system. *Computational Intelligence*, 6:193–208, 1990.

[KP95]   A. Kobsa and W. Pohl. The user modeling shell system BGP-MS. *User Modeling and User-Adapted Interaction*, 4(2):59–106, 1995.

[Kri63]   S. Kripke. Semantic considerations on modal logic. *Acta Philosophica Fennica*, 16:83–94, 1963.

[PH97]   W. Pohl and J. Höhle. Mechanisms for flexible representation and use of knowledge in user modeling shell systems. In A. Jameson, C. Paris, and C. Tasso, editors, *User Modeling: Proceedings of the Sixth International Conference*, pages 403–414, Wien, New York, 1997. Springer-Verlag.

[PHFK95]   W. Pohl, J. Höhle, J. Fink, and D.-W. Kim. Building adaptive applications on widely-used platforms with BGP-MS. In C. Stephanidis, editor, *Proc. ERCIM Workshop "Towards User Interfaces for All: Current Efforts and Future Trends"*, Heraklion, Greece, October 1995.

[Poh96]   W. Pohl. Combining partitions and modal logic for user modeling. In D. M. Gabbay and H. J. Ohlbach, editors, *Practical Reasoning: Proceedings of the International Conference on Formal and Applied Practical Reasoning*, pages 480–494, Berlin, Heidelberg, 1996. Springer.

[Poh97]   W. Pohl. *Logic-Based Representation and Reasoning for User Modeling Shell Systems*. PhD thesis, University of Essen, 1997.

From Theory to Practice in Multiagent System Design: The Case of Structural Co-operation

Sascha Ossowski [1], Ana García-Serrano[2] and José Cuena[2]

[1] School of Engineering, Rey Juan Carlos University,
Camino de Humanes 63, 28936 Móstoles (Madrid), Spain
S.Ossowski@escet.urjc.es

[2] Department of Artificial Intelligence, Technical University of Madrid,
Campus de Montegancedo s/n, 28660 Boadilla del Monte (Madrid), Spain
{agarcia, jcuena}@dia.fi.upm.es

Abstract. In Distributed Problem-solving (DPS) systems a group of purpose-fully designed computational agents interact and co-ordinate their activities so as to jointly achieve a global goal. Social co-ordination is a decentralised mechanism, that sets out from non-benevolent agents that interact primarily to improve the degree of attainment of their local goals. One way of ensuring the effectivity of social co-ordination with respect to global problem-solving is to rely on self-interested agents and to coerce their behaviour in a desired direction. In this paper we describe the decentralised co-ordination mechanism of structural co-operation that follows this approach, and present its formalisation within bargaining theory. We then show how this theoretical model is trans-ferred to a practical real-world application: within the experimental TRYSA$_2$ system autonomous traffic control agents co-ordinate their activities by means of structural co-operation, so as to jointly perform road traffic management in an urban motorway network.

1. Introduction

Distributed Problem-Solving (DPS) rely on a purposefully designed architecture of computational agents that interact in order to jointly achieve a desired global functionality. The traditional DPS design philosophy of *reductionism*, that relies on a top-down decomposition of the global task, the assignment of subtasks to agents and co-ordination based on pre-established interaction patterns among *benevolent* agents [6], often turns out to be too rigid for large-scale agent systems [7]. Instead, a *constructionist* approach, based on the metaphor of societies of *autonomous problem-solving agents*, has become popular: agents are primarily interested in their local goals and interact to increase the degree of their attainment. This *decentralised* interaction [5] is termed *social co-ordination*. In order that the DPS system copes with the global task, social co-ordination must be based on agent behaviour that lies between benevolence and self-interest [11]. A popular solution to this problem consists in building a model of purely self-interested behaviour (e.g. [16,14]) and designing a coercive external context to modify it (e.g. [15,14]).

We have developed a social co-ordination mechanism called *structural co-operation*, which follows this approach [9]. Elsewhere [11] we show how this mechanism combines quantitative [14] and qualitative [16] models of self-interested action in a multiagent world within the frame of social co-ordination. The purpose of this paper, however, is not a detailed description of our abstract mechanism. We rather aim to point out how theoretical models in multiagent system research can be turned into practical results: we show how the rather abstract formalisation of structural co-operation leads to the real-world multiagent application of urban road traffic management.

Section 2 presents a model of the type of domains that structural co-operation has been designed for. Section 3 describes and formalises the mechanism of structural co-operation and its operationalisation. Section 4 presents the TRYSA$_2$ experimental system, that uses structural co-operation to co-ordinate autonomous traffic management agents, while concluding remarks are presented in section 5.

2. The problem: reactive social co-ordination

Many real-world domains are highly dynamic: perceptions are error-prone, actions fail, contingencies occur. A common way to deal with this problem is to build systems that only plan their actions for a short-time horizon, in order to assess the effects of their interventions as early as possible, and to adapt future behaviour accordingly [3]. When such systems are modelled on the basis of a multiagent architecture, two essential constraints have to be taken into account: first, agents need to cope with the fact that their plans and actions interfere because they share an environment with only limited resources; second, agents should be prepared to consider actions that attain their goals only *partially* due to resource limitation and environmental contingencies. In the sequel we formalise essential features of this type of problems.

Let S be a set of *world states* and Π a finite set of *plans*. The execution of a plan π changes the state of the world which is modelled as a partially defined mapping

$$res: \Pi \times S \rightarrow S.$$

A plan is *executable* in s, if only if *res* is defined for a certain world state s, fact which we express formally by the predicate $exec(\pi,s)$. At least one *empty plan* π_ε is required to be included in the set of plans Π; it is modelled as identity.

There is a set of agents A, each of which can act in the world thereby modifying its state. An agent $\alpha \in A$ is characterised by the following notions:

- a predicate $can(\alpha,\pi)$, determining the *individual plans* $\pi \in \Pi$ that α is able to execute. An agent α is always capable of executing the empty plan π_ε;
- a predicate $ideal(\alpha,s)$, expressing the states $s \in S$ that the agent $\alpha \in A$ would ideally like to bring about;
- a metric function d_α, which maps two states to a real number, representing agent α's estimation of "how far" one state is away from another. It usually models the notion of (relative) "difficulty" to bring about changes between world states.

In the scenarios that we are interested in, an agent usually cannot fully reach an ideal state. So, we will use the notion of ideal states together with the distance measure d_α to describe an agent's preferences respecting world states. Note that the agents in A

may have different (partially conflicting) ideal states and may even measure the distance between states in different scales.

We now introduce a notion of interdependent action. The set M of *multiplans* comprises all multisets over the individual plans Π, i.e. $M = bagof(\Pi)$. A multiplan $\mu \in M$ models the simultaneous execution of all its component plans, i.e. of the individual plans $\pi \in \mu$ that are contained in the multiset μ. The commutative operator $\circ$ denotes multiset union and hence states that its operands are executed together. By identifying an individual plan with a multiplan that contains it as its only element, the partial function *res* is extended to multiplans:

$$res : M \times S \rightarrow S \ .$$

The function *res* is undefined for a multiplan μ and a state s, if some of the individual plans that it contains are *incompatible*, i.e. in case that in a state s of a modelled domain it is impossible to execute them simultaneously. Otherwise, μ is said to be *executable* in s (formally: $exec(\mu,s)$). The empty plan π_ε is compatible with every multiplan and does not affect its outcome.

The notion of capability for executing a multiplan is also a natural extension of the single agent case. We define the set of groups Γ as the powerset of the set of agents, i.e. $\Gamma = \wp(A)$. A group $\gamma \in \Gamma$ is capable of executing a multiplan μ, if there is an assignment such that every agent is to execute exactly one individual plan and this agent is capable of doing so, i.e. there is a bijective mapping ψ from individual plans to agents, such that

$$can(\gamma,\mu) \equiv \forall \pi \in \mu. \ can(\psi(\pi),\pi) \ .$$

Definition 1. A co-ordination setting D is defined by the sets of individuals S, Π, A, M and Γ, the functions *res*, d_α and $\circ$ as well as the predicates *exec*, *can* and *ideal*.

3. The mechanism: structural co-operation

The outcome of a co-ordination process within a co-ordination setting D can be conceived as a multiplan. When it represents the result of social co-ordination, the multiplan reflects the self-interested choice of all agents, i.e. agents do *not* refer to a notion of joint utility and do *not* care for whether the multiplan contributes to the overall functionality of the DPS system or not. Structural co-operation provides a model of such self-interested action, and introduces a mechanism to bias the outcome of co-ordination among social DPS agents[1]. The designer is supposed to use that mechanism so as to make the outcome of social co-ordination instrumental with respect to the desired functionality of the DPS system [10].

In the sequel, we will sketch both, a model of multiagent rational action as well as a biasing mechanism. Subsequently, we model these ideas within bargaining theory. Finally, we show how the outcome of social co-ordination in a co-ordination setting D can be determined and computed.

---

[1] As will be outlined below, we conceive a "social" agent to be norm-abiding.

3.1 Social Agents

In the above co-ordination setting, the need for co-ordination is expressed by the fact that, when an individual plan π is executed in conjunction with a multiplan μ, the resulting world state changes (i.e. $res(\pi,s) \neq res(\pi \circ \mu,s)$). When an agent α is able to execute π and a group γ is able to execute μ, then the group γ has the power to influence α: the agent *depends* on γ with respect to π. There are different types and degrees of dependence. The strongest degree is *feasibility* dependence (used in section 4), in the presence of which a group γ can turn down or enable an agent's *possibility* to execute its individual plan π (in the frame of a multiplan μ) [10].

We model self-interested choice within a co-ordination setting on the basis of this notion of dependence: the less an agent *depends* on the choices of others with respect to the outcome of its plans, the better is its position in society. And the better an agent's position in the agent society, the more weight will have its preferences in the outcome of social co-ordination; if an agreement is reached, it will be biased towards that agent.

In consequence, the outcome of social co-ordination is determined by the network of social dependence relations. We now introduce the notion of *normative prescription* [2]: if in a situation s it is forbidden for a group γ to enact a multiplan μ we write

$$forbidden_s(\gamma, \mu)$$

Our *social* agents are norm-abiding: they do not even consider executing plans that are forbidden for them. So, we introduce the notion of *preparedness* as capability plus the absence of such prohibitions

$$prep_s(\gamma,\mu) \Leftrightarrow can(\gamma,\mu) \wedge \neg forbidden_s(\gamma,\mu)$$

Reconsidering the above model of self-interested action on the basis of the notion of preparedness instead of capability, it becomes clear that by issuing prohibitions, a designer can modify the social dependence structure and, in consequence, also the outcome of social co-ordination. These ideas will be formalised in the sequel, taking into account that prescriptions are conceived to worsen the position of the involved agents, potentially improving the position of the remaining agents.

3.2 Social Co-ordination as a Bargaining Scenario

In a first step, a quantitative notion of preference over *agreements* is introduced. Agent α's preference for a world state s is expressed by its distance to some ideal state, which can be written as

$$|s|_\alpha = min\{d_\alpha(s,\bar{s}) \mid ideal(\alpha,\bar{s})\}$$

The set X of *legally enactable* multiplans in a situation s comprises all plans that are executable in s and for which there is a group of agents prepared to do so:

$$X = \{\mu \in M \mid exec(\mu,s) \wedge \exists \gamma \in \Gamma. \, prep_s(\gamma,\mu)\}$$

On this basis we can define a quantitative preference over multiplans.

Definition 2. The *utility* for an agent α_i of a legally enactable multiplan $\mu \in X$ is

$$U_i(\mu) = |s|_{\alpha_i} - |res(\mu,s)|_{\alpha_i}.$$

The utilities that each agent obtains from a multiplan can be comprised in a vector. The set of utility vectors that are realisable over X is denoted by $U(X)$.

When agents have different points of view respecting which multiplan to agree upon, they may "flip a coin" in order to choose between alternative agreements. A probability distribution over the set of legally enactable multiplans is called a *mixed multiplan*. Let m be the cardinality of X, then a mixed multiplan is a m-dimensional vector

$$\sigma = (p_1, \ldots, p_m), 0 \le p_i \le 1, \sum_{i=1}^{m} p_i = 1 .$$

The set of mixed multiplans is denoted by Σ. The *expected* utility of a mixed multiplan is given by the sum of each legally enactable multiplan's utility weighed by its probability:

Definition 3. The utility for an agent α_i of a mixed multiplan $\sigma \in \Sigma$ is given by

$$U_i(\sigma) = \sum_{k=1}^{m} p_k U_i(\mu_k) .$$

The set of expected utility vectors that are realisable over Σ is denoted by $U(\Sigma)$.

When agents co-ordinate their strategies and agree on some mixed multiplan, the corresponding vector of utilities is what each agent expects to obtain. Still, agents are autonomous and not forced to co-operate. So, it remains to model what happens in case of conflict.

In a conflict situation we define the *response* of the set of agents γ to a single agent α's plan π to be the multiplan μ that they are capable of executing and that minimises α's utility from $\pi \circ \mu$, i.e.

$$response_s(\pi, \alpha_i, \mu, \gamma) \Leftrightarrow \mu = \min_{U_i(\pi \circ \mu')} \{ \mu' \in X \mid prep_s(\mu', \gamma) \} .$$

This models that in case of disagreement an agent must account for the unpleasant situation that all its acquaintances jointly try to harm it. As the possibility of reaching an incompatible multiplan has to be excluded, α can only choose from the set $FEAS_s(\alpha)$ of plans that are feasible regardless what others do. The empty plan π_ε is contained in $FEAS_s(\alpha)$ by definition [11].

Agent α will choose the plan π out of $FEAS_s(\alpha)$, that maximises its individual utility value when combined with the response of its acquaintances.

Definition 4. The *conflict utility* of the agent α is

$$U_i^d = max \{ U_i(\pi \circ \mu) \in R \mid \pi \in FEAS_s(\alpha_i) \wedge response_s(\pi, \alpha_i, \mu, \gamma) \} .$$

We now outline how a bargaining scenario can be defined on the basis of the above notions. For this purpose, we define the overall conflict utility as

$$\vec{d} = (U_1^d, \ldots, U_n^d) ,$$

and treat the conflict utility vector as an effectively reachable agreement, defining a set S to be the convex and comprehensive hull (*cch*) of the legally enactable multiplans plus the conflict utility vector

$$S = cch(U(X) \cup \{ \vec{d} \}).$$

The set S usually equals $U(\Sigma)$, but may also be a (convex) superset of the latter.

Definition 5. The *bargaining scenario B* associated with a social co-ordination problem is a pair $B = (S, \bar{d})$

S is called the *bargaining set* and $\bar{d}$ the *disagreement point*. B complies with the formal properties of bargaining models, so the whole mathematical apparatus of bargaining theory becomes applicable [17].

3.3 The Outcome of Social Co-ordination

In this section we rely on Bargaining Theory to find a solution to the associated bargaining scenario $(S, \bar{d})$: a vector $\bar{\varphi} \in S$ needs to be singled out upon which a bargaining process – and the social co-ordination that it models – is supposed to converge. Strategic bargaining theory relies on a sequential setting where agents alternate in making offers to each other in a pre-specified order and eventually converge on an agreement. By contrast, the axiomatic models of bargaining that we will use in the sequel first postulate desirable properties of a bargaining solution, and then seek the solution concept that satisfies them.

The five requirements of *individual rationality*, *Pareto-optimali*ty, *symmetry*, *scale invariance* and *contraction independence* that Nash bargaining models state for "fair" solutions to a bargaining scenario [18], provide an adequate model for our purposes.

Theorem 1 (due to Nash [8]). A utility vector $\bar{\varphi}$, that complies with the above axioms, maximises the function

$$N(\bar{x}) = \prod_{i=1}^{n}(x_i - d_i)$$

So, a solution $\bar{\varphi}$ maximises the *product* of gains from the disagreement point. It always exists and is unique [17].

In remains to be shown that the bargaining scenario and its solution concept capture the intention underlying normative prescriptions: a prohibition limits the agents' freedom of choice, potentially making another agent less vulnerable, i.e. less dependent on them. In consequence, the social position of the latter is strengthened and it is supposed to obtain a larger bribe in a potential compromise. In terms of the associated bargaining scenario, normative prescriptions can modify the disagreement point $\bar{d}$ by declaring the "worst responses" of an agent's acquaintances to be illegal. So, when the disagreement point is moved in the direction of only one agent, the utility that it gets from the solution should increase, i.e. the bargaining outcome should "move towards" it. Still, this is precisely the property of *disagreement point monotonicity* of the Nash solution: if $\bar{d}$ and $\bar{d}'$ are two arbitrary disagreement points for the same bargaining set S, and $\bar{\varphi}$

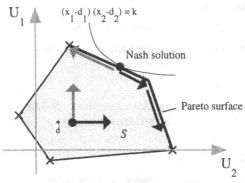

Figure 1. Disagreement point monotonicity

and $\bar{\phi}'$ denote the solutions to the corresponding bargaining scenarios, then

$$d'_i \ge d_i, \; \forall j \ne i \; d'_j = d_j \; \Rightarrow \; \varphi'_i \ge \varphi_i \; [17]$$

Figure 1 illustrates this: the bargaining solution moves on the Pareto surface in the direction of the agent that strengthens its fallback position. By adequately designing a normative prescriptions, a designer can thus bias the solution towards an agent.

3.4 Computing the Outcome

We are now endowed with a characterisation of the *outcome* of social co-ordination. So, there is no need to explicitly "simulate" the co-ordination process among norm-abiding autonomous agents. Instead, we use a distributed multistage algorithm that *directly* computes the solution [9]:

- stage 1 performs an asynchronous distributed search for Pareto-optimal multiplans; this is done by a variant of the asynchronous weak commitment search algorithm [18], which we have modified to cope with distributed constraint optimisation problems;
- stage 2 determines the *mixed* multiplan that constitutes the solution to the associated bargaining scenario;
- finally, in stage 3 a specific multiplan is chosen by means of a lottery and the corresponding individual plans are assigned to the agents.

Note that on the micro-level this algorithm requires agents to follow strict behaviour rules. Still, although this behaviour is rather benevolent, we can assure that its *outcome* corresponds to the result of social co-ordination among autonomous agents.

4. The application: urban road traffic management

The model of structural co-operation described previously remains rather abstract. In this section we describe how it is put to use in a practical real-world case: road traffic management in the motorway network around Barcelona.

4.1 The system architecture

In Barcelona, the local traffic control centre JPT is in charge of managing urban transport, so as to maintain and restore the "smooth" flow of vehicles. Traffic engineers within the JPT continuously receive information about the traffic state, identify potential problems, and act upon control devices to overcome them. It has become particularly difficult for the JPT engineers to perform this job in real time, as in the follow-up of the 1992 Olympic Games the traffic management infrastructure in Barcelona has become increasingly complex. Nowadays, information about the traffic state of the urban motorway network, consisting of one ring-road and seven adjacent motorways, is provided by over 300 telemetered sensors ("loop detectors") via fibre optics communication links. Control actions can be taken by means of 52 Variable

Message Signals (VMS), 3 traffic lights for junction control, as well as by ramp metering on 7 ring-road drives.

In the sequel, we describe the TRYSA$_2$ prototype (TRYS Autonomous Agents)[2]. TRYSA$_2$ is an experimental decentralised multiagent system, which proposes traffic control actions for the Barcelona motorway network in real time. In line with the traffic engineer's logical subdivision of the road network into *problem areas*, TRYSA$_2$ relies on a set of 11 knowledge-based traffic control *agents*, each responsible for traffic management in one such area (Figure 2). Every few minutes, an agent receives information about the traffic state in its problem area and generates proposals of signal plans (i.e. sets of control actions) for control devices. Subsequently, potential conflicts between this signal plan and the control actions of other agents (problem area overlap!) are resolved by communication on the basis of structural co-operation. The agents' next reasoning cycle will just be based on the modified traffic state[3].

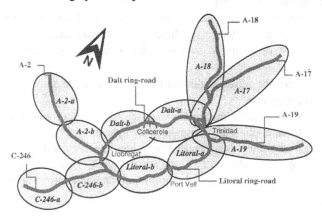

Figure 2. Autonomous traffic agents for Barcelona

In the sequel we first outline the local problem-solving model approach of TRYSA$_2$, by means of which the agents' local utility functions have been implemented.[4] We then show how decentralised co-ordination among the agents is achieved. Finally, we sketch the implementation and operation of the system.

4.2 Modelling Local Utility

The magnitude of a traffic problem in certain part of the road network can be expressed by the amount of traffic demand that exceeds the capacity of a certain road

---

[2] TRYSA$_2$ is a multiagent version of the TRYS system [4], which has actually been installed and tested at the Barcelona test site. Large parts of the code and the knowledge bases of the TRYS system have been reused in TRYSA$_2$.

[3] By not taking into account previous control action proposals, TRYSA$_2$ agents comply with the "reactivity assumption" of section 2.

[4] Current multiagent system research tends to take the existance of a utility function for granted. However, it is important to notice that the design of computational utility functions for real world applications is definately *non-trivial*.

segment (in vehicles per hour). This is called the segment's traffic *excess*. The quality of a traffic management action can be measured by the *reduction* of traffic excess, that they are expected to produce. In consequence, TRYSA$_2$ traffic management agents use the overall reduction of excess in their problem areas (i.e. the sum over all road segments that belong to their area) as a local utility measure. In the sequel we show how AI techniques can be used to build such utility functions.

Every couple of minutes, a TRYSA$_2$ agent receives temporal series of magnitudes such as traffic speed, flow and occupancy from the road sensors of its area. This raw data is initially pre-processed in order to filter out noisy and erroneous data. Subsequently, data abstraction is performed, calculating aggregate magnitudes such as temporal and spatial gradients for the different sections.

In a second step, problem identification (and also some part of problem diagnosis) is performed by matching the abstracted traffic data against a knowledge base of frames which model problem scenarios. Figure 3 shows one such frame that matches the abstracted traffic data. Suppose that as a result of data abstraction low speed and high occupancy are identified in *Ronda de Dalt en Diagonal* and medium to high speed and low occupancy in *Ronda en d'Eslugues*. These facts match the frame shown in Figure 3, so that an incident in the central lane of Diagonal road is identified, which manifests itself as a traffic excess (with respect to the road's capacity) of 2200 veh/h between *Diagonal* and *Llobregat* in the *Dalt* ring-road. Traffic from *Collcerola* to *Llobregat* and, in a minor degree, from *Diagonal* heading towards *Llobregat* contributes to this excess.

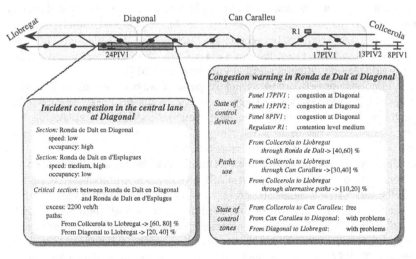

Figure 3. An example scenario

Step three, the control recommendation phase, adheres to the following line of reasoning: first, the historic traffic demand between nodes is retrieved and the contribution of each path to the problem in the critical section calculated. This is done by matching the current abstract traffic state and the state of the control devices against a knowledge base of frames, representing traffic distribution scenarios.

Finally, coherent alternative signal plans are generated by using the distribution scenario frames once again: every frame applicable to the current situation is preselected. Assume that this is the case for the frame shown in Figure 3. Its short-term effects are estimated by simulating its impact on the current traffic situation. This is done by using network structure knowledge to assign traffic demand to the road network, in accordance with the distribution of traffic volume among paths that the frame specifies. In the example about one half of the traffic volume from *Collcerola* to *Llobregat* will pass through the *Dalt* ring-road, while a smaller amount chooses a path through *Can Caralleu* or other alternative paths, if the corresponding signal plan is set. If the simulation shows a reasonable decrease of excess in the critical section, the frame's signal plan constitutes one recommendation of the system. In the example, it is suggested to display congestion warnings at *Diagonal* for panels *17PIV1*, *13PIV2* and *8PIV1*, while setting the contention level of regulator *R1* to medium. As a result of this process, a set of alternative signal plan recommendations, together with their utility (i.e. their expected reduction of local traffic excess) is produced.

4.3 Modelling Social Co-ordination

In order to choose a local signal plan, $TRYSA_2$ agents not only need to take into account their local utility, but also the effects that the control actions of their acquaintances have on it. In terms of the model presented in section 3, they need to base their decision on the utility of *multiplans* instead of individual plans. In the sequel we will consider *feasibility* relations between plans, in the presence of which an agent's acquaintances can turn down its local control plan, by threatening to take control actions that would result in an incompatible multiplan. In the domain under study, this can happen when *physical* conflicts between control actions are possible, i.e. when two agents have the possibility to set the same control device in different, incompatible states (e.g. by displaying different messages on the same VMS).

Physical relationships between plans and the possible ways of dealing with them in terms of states of control devices are expressed in the *plan interrelation* knowledge base of an agent. It is represented by rules, that obey to the following format:

$$[cdev_1 \ , \ \ldots \ , \ cdev_n \ ] \ \Rightarrow \ [cdev_m \ , \ \ldots \ , \ cdev_j \ ] \qquad \text{or}$$
$$[cdev_1 \ , \ \ldots \ , \ cdev_n \ ] \ \Rightarrow \ [nogood \ ]$$

The operational semantics of such a rule determines that the control device states of the antecedent can be substituted by those of the consequent without any important changes in the effect of the signal plans (e.g. by merging different messages "congestion at A" and "congestion at B" to be displayed on the same VMS into one "congestion at A and B" message). If control devices are merely incompatible, the consequent is the constant *nogood*.

In addition, $TRYSA_2$ agents are endowed with an *agent dependence* knowledge base, which hosts rules of the form

$$[cdev_1 \ , \ \ldots \ , \ cdev_n \ ] \ \Rightarrow \ [\alpha_1 \ , \ \ldots \ , \ \alpha_m \ ]$$

They state that if all control devices $cdev_1$ to $cdev_n$ switch to new states, then this concerns the agents α_1 to α_m. Note that these rules actually compile knowledge about the capabilities of an agent's acquaintances, upon the background of possible physical plan relations. For instance, if agent α_i may set a message M_i on VMS P, and α_j possibly displays a message M_j on the same panel, while both messages are incompatible, then the knowledge base will contain a rule stating that setting M_i on VMS P concerns agent α_j. This serves two purposes: when used with forward inference, it allows an agent to deduce which agents are "interested" in changes of its local signal plans; using backward inference, it enables an agent to determine which agents can affect the executability a certain set of control actions. On the basis of this knowledge, TRYSA$_2$ agents exchange messages in line with the algorithm sketched in section 3.3.

It remains to be shown how normative biasing is achieved. In TRYSA$_2$ normative prescriptions refer to the prohibition of setting certain control device states. These are generated by the *norm* knowledge base, which qualifies a set of prohibitions temporally by current date and time as well as by the categories *type of day* (*Working day*, *Sunday*, *Saturday* or *Holiday*) and *type of season* (*Xmas*, *Easter*, *Summer*, or *Normal*). Different such temporal qualifications essentially reflect different traffic demand patterns, which require different sets of normative prescriptions.

4.4 The system

The TRYSA$_2$ system has been implemented experimentally on networked workstations. The TRYSA agents constitute separate Prolog processes (with some extensions in C++), which communicate via sockets. The Barcelona test site is simulated by the AIMSUN traffic simulator [1]. AIMSUN is endowed with a precise description of the traffic management infrastructure at the test site, including detailed models of the road network, the sensors, control devices etc., and performs microscopic ("car by car") simulation of traffic flows. A special observer agent has been implemented in Tcl/Tk in order to visualise the problem-solving process and its results [9].

5. Discussion

In this paper we have outlined the social co-ordination mechanism of structural co-operation, by means of which the outcome of autonomous agents' self interested choice is biased by normative prescriptions, so as to make it instrumental with respect to a global problem to be solved. We have shown how this theoretical model can be applied to the practical problem of decentralised multiagent traffic management in an urban motorway network.

Some words on the adequacy of this mechanism appear convenient here, as the choice of classical bargaining theory as a vehicle to formalise structural co-operation entails a "price to be paid". Firstly, we assume that agents make joint *binding* agreements. Secondly, we do not account for the formation of coalitions. Finally, we assume agents to be perfectly rational. Still, as our aim is to build a decentralised co-ordination mechanism for *homogeneous* societies of problem-solving agents, these assumptions become less severe: law abidance can just be "build into" our artificial agents; by ignoring coalition formation, we have sacrificed some plausibility of our model in favour of efficiency, as coalition formation is a computationally complex process. The assumption of perfect rationality is justified by the fact that there exists a sound axiomatic characterisation of a solution, which allows for its direct computation without an extensive "simulation" of the bargaining process. After all, the

TRYSA$_2$ prototype indicates that the above assumptions do not necessarily limit, (but may even foster) the applicability of the mechanism to real-world problems.

With respect to the adequacy of using structural co-operation for traffic management, we suggest that the decentralised co-ordination architecture of TRYSA$_2$ promotes scalability in comparison to centralised architectures, which rely an a special co-ordinator agent [4]: the introduction of new agents in the system generates a shift in the outcome of structural co-operation, leading to a new baseline co-ordination.

In future work we will further refine the normative knowledge within the TRYSA$_2$ system. The different effects of particular types of prescriptions in real-world traffic situations will be examined by means of experimental studies. In addition, we are thinking of applying multiagent learning techniques to this task.

References

1. Barceló, J.; Ferrer, J.; Grau, R. : "AIMSUN2 and the GETRAM Simulation Environment". *13. EURO Conf*, 1994
2. Conte, R.; Castelfranchi, C.: *Cognitive and Social Action*. UCL Press, 1995
3. Cuena J., Ossowski S.: "Distributed Models for Decision Support". To appear in: *Introduction to Distributed Artificial Intelligence* (Weiß & Sen, editors). AAAI/MIT Press, 1998
4. Cuena, J.; Hernández, J.; Molina, M.: "An Intelligent Model for Road Traffic Management in the Motorway Network around Barcelona". *Proc. 14th IFIP World Congress*, Chapman&Hall, 1996, pp. 173-180
5. Demazeau, Y.: "Decentralised A.I. 2". *North Holland*, 1991
6. Durfee, E.; Rosenschein, J.: "Distributed Problem-solving and Multi-agent Systems: Comparisons and Examples". *Proc. 13th DAI Workshop*, 1994, pp. 94-104
7. Jennings, N.; Campos, J.: "Towards a Social Level Characterisation of Socially Responsible Agents". *IEE Proc. on Software Engineering, 144(1)*, 1997
8. Nash, J.: "The bargaining problem". *Econometrica 20*, 1950, pp. 155-162
9. Ossowski S. *On the Functionality of Social Structure in Artificial Agent Societies*. Monograph to appear in the LNAI series, Springer, 1998
10. Ossowski, S.; García Serrano, A.: "Social Co-ordination Among Autonomous Problem-solving Agents". To appear in: *Proc. 3rd Australian DAI Workshop*, Springer, 1997
11. Ossowski, S.; García Serrano, A.: "Social Structure in Artificial Agent Societies: Implications for Autonomous Problem-solving Agents". To appear in: *Proc. ATAL-98*, 1998
12. Ossowski, S.; García Serrano, A.; Cuena, J.: "Emergent Co-ordination of Flow Control Actions Through Functional Co-operation of Social Agents". *Proc. 12. European Conference on Artificial Intelligence (ECAI-96)*, Wiley & Sons, 1996, pp. 539-543
13. Owen, G.: *Game Theory*, 3rd edition, 1995
14. Rosenschein, J.; Zlotkin, G.: *Rules of Encounter: Designing Conventions for Automated Negotiation among Computers*. AAAI/MIT Press, 1994
15. Shoham, Y.; Tennenholz, M.: "On Social Laws for Artificial Agent Societies: Off-line Design". *Artificial Intelligence 73*, 1995, pp. 231-252
16. Sichman, J.; Demazeau, Y.; Conte, R.; Castelfranchi, C.: "A Social Reasoning Mechanism Based On Dependence Networks". *Proc. ECAI-94*, 1994, pp. 188-192
17. Thomson, W.: "Cooperative Models of Bargaining". *Handbook of Game Theory* (Auman & Hart, eds.), 1994, pp. 1238-1284
18. Yokoo, M.: "Asynchronous Weak-commitment Search for Solving Distributed Constraint Satisfaction Problems". *Proc. Constraint Logic Programming*, 1995, pp. 88-102

Distributive Concept Exploration –
A Knowledge Acquisition Tool
in Formal Concept Analysis

Gerd Stumme

Technische Universität Darmstadt, Fachbereich Mathematik
Schloßgartenstr. 7, D–64289 Darmstadt, stumme@mathematik.tu-darmstadt.de

1 Introduction

Formal Concept Analysis ([9], [1]) provides a mathematical model of the concept 'concept' which is used in data analysis for examining conceptual hierarchies in data tables. If these data tables are too large to be completely given, then the conceptual structure has to be determined in an interactive knowledge acquisition process from an expert of the domain. *Exploration tools* suggest, starting with the concepts to be examined, hierarchical relationships. The expert is asked either to confirm them or to provide typical counter-examples. The result of the exploration is a lattice that is generated by adding all largest common subconcepts and/or least common superconcepts.

In [12] and [4], an overview over different exploration tools in Formal Concept Analysis is given. While *Attribute Exploration* considers largest common subconcepts only and *Object Exploration* least common superconcepts only ([1]), *Concept Exploration* treats largest common subconcepts (*infima*) and least common superconcepts (*suprema*) equally ([3], [6], [7], [11], [12]). It determines the lattice of all combinations of infima and suprema of the starting concepts (which are also called the *basic concepts*).

A big problem of Concept Exploration is the fact that the resulting lattice (and the exploration dialogue) may be infinite. Even only three concepts can generate an infinite lattice! In practice however, this case does not appear. We can overcome this principal difficulty if general knowledge about the domain provides more information about the structure of the intended lattice. If we know in advance that the lattice is distributive, then the finiteness of the result is ensured.

Which additional assumptions imply the distributivity of the lattice? This is especially the case, if we know that the attributes which generate the conceptual hierarchy are closed under disjunction. One interesting application is within *Description Logics* where disjunction is usually used as constructor. For logics having a complete subsumption algorithm, this algorithm can be considered as 'expert' for the exploration procedure. By combining both algorithms, one obtains a completely automatic knowledge acqusition tool ([5], [7]).

With distributivity of the resulting lattice known in advance, we can use its much stronger structure in the algorithm. This is the underlying idea of *Distributive Concept Exploration*. In particular, Distributive Concept Exploration uses the tensor product of lattices ([10]), which is the co-product in the category of completely distributive complete lattices. This approach cannot be adapted to Concept Exploration, since there is no co-product in the category of complete lattices.

During the exploration the user is asked questions of the form "Is s a subconcept of t?", where s and t are lattice terms built with the basic concepts. If the user replies "No", he must justify his answer by an object belonging to s and an attribute belonging to t such that the object does not have the attribute. The result of the exploration is the concept lattice of all combinations of infima and suprema of the basic concepts, together with a list of objects and attributes which separate the concepts. The algorithm is implemented by B. Groh.

In the next section the basic notions of Formal Concept Analysis are introduced. The algorithm of Distributive Concept Exploration is described in Section 3 and illustrated by an example in Section 4. Because of space limitation, the mathematical part is quite condensed. In order to get an idea of the exploration procedure, the reader may first read the next section until the example and then have a look at Section 4 before going in the details in Section 3.

2   Formal Concept Analysis

Tensor products of lattices and congruence relations on lattices are the essential constructions for Cistributive Concept Exploration. Both can adequately be described in terms of Formal Concept Analysis. Formal Concept Analysis (cf. [9], [1]) is a mathematical approach which reflects the philosophical understanding of concepts as units of thought consisting of two parts: the extension containing all objects which belong to the concept and the intension containing the attributes shared by all those objects (cf. [8]). In Formal Concept Analysis this is modeled by *formal concepts* that are derived from a *formal context*. We briefly recall some basic definitions:

A *(formal) context* is a triple $\mathbb{K} := (G, M, I)$ where G and M are sets and I is a relation between G and M. The elements of G and M are called *objects* and *attributes*, respectively, and gIm is read *"the object g has the attribute m"*. For $A \subseteq G$ and $B \subseteq M$ we define $A' := \{m \in M \mid \forall g \in A : gIm\}$ and dually $B' := \{g \in G \mid \forall m \in B : gIm\}$. Now a *(formal) concept* is a pair (A, B) with $A \subseteq G$, $B \subseteq M$, $A' = B$ and $B' = A$. The set A is called the *extent* and the set B the *intent* of the concept. The hierarchical subconcept–superconcept–relation of concepts is formalized by $(A, B) \leq (C, D) : \iff A \subseteq C (\iff B \supseteq D)$. The set of all concepts of the context $\mathbb{K}$ together with this order relation is a complete lattice that is called the *concept lattice* of $\mathbb{K}$ and is denoted by $\mathfrak{B}(\mathbb{K})$. Each complete lattice can be viewed as a concept lattice: A complete lattice L is isomorphic to the concept lattice $\mathfrak{B}(L, L, \leq)$.

Example. Figure 1 shows a formal context about the potential of gaseous pollutants. Gases are objects, and possible perils are attributes. In the line diagram of the concept lattice, we label, for each object $g \in G$, its *object concept* $\gamma g := (\{g\}'', \{g\}')$ with the name of the object and, for each attribute $m \in M$,

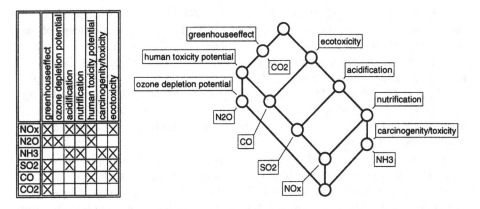

Fig. 1. Formal context and concept lattice of gaseous pollutants

its *attribute concept* $\mu m := (\{m\}', \{m\}'')$ with the name of the attribute. This labeling allows us to determine for each concept its extent and its intent: The extent [intent] of a concept contains all objects [attributes] whose object concepts [attribute concepts] can be reached from the concept on a descending [ascending] path of straight line segments. For instance, the concept labeled with CO has $\{CO, SO_2, NO_x\}$ as extent, and {human toxicity potential, greenhouse effect, ecotoxicity} as intent. The concept lattice combines the view of different pollution scenarios with the influence of individual polluants. Such an integrated view can be of interest for the planning of chimneys for plants generating specific polluants. Generally spoken, Formal Concept Analysis treats intensional and extensional aspects equally and in an integrative way.

The *tensor product* of two complete lattices L_1 and L_2 is defined to be the concept lattice $L_1 \otimes L_2 := \mathfrak{B}(L_1 \times L_2, L_1 \times L_2, \nabla)$ with $(x_1, x_2) \nabla (y_1, y_2) : \Longleftrightarrow (x_1 \leq y_1$ or $x_2 \leq y_2)$. R. Wille showed in [10] that the tensor product is the co-product in the category of completely distributive complete lattices with complete homomorphisms. Hence the tensor product of L_1 and L_2 is, in a certain sense, the largest complete distributive lattice that can be generated by L_1 and L_2.

We define the *direct product* of two contexts $\mathbb{K}_1 := (G_1, M_1, I_1)$ and $\mathbb{K}_2 := (G_2, M_2, I_2)$ to be the context $\mathbb{K}_1 \times \mathbb{K}_2 := (G_1 \times G_2, M_1 \times M_2, \nabla)$ with the incidence $(g_1, g_2) \nabla (m_1, m_2) : \Longleftrightarrow ((g_1, m_1) \in I_1$ or $(g_2, m_2) \in I_2)$. The tensor product of two concept lattices is (up to isomorphism) just the concept lattice of the direct product of their contexts: We have $\mathfrak{B}(\mathbb{K}_1) \otimes \mathfrak{B}(\mathbb{K}_2) \cong \mathfrak{B}(\mathbb{K}_1 \times \mathbb{K}_2)$.

A context is called *reduced* if each object concept is $\bigvee$-irreducible (i. e., is not supremum of smaller elements) and each attribute concept is $\bigwedge$-irreducible (i. e., is not infimum of larger elements). For a $\bigvee$–irreducible ($\bigwedge$–irreducible) element x of a finite lattice we write x_* (x^*) for its unique lower (upper) cover. If $\mathbb{K}_1$ and $\mathbb{K}_2$ are reduced, then $\mathbb{K}_1 \times \mathbb{K}_2$ is also reduced (cf. [10]).

Congruence relations of complete lattices appear in a quite natural way in Formal Concept Analysis. For finite concept lattices they can always be described by *compatible subcontexts*: A context (H, N, J) is called a *subcontext* of a context

(G, M, I) if $H \subseteq G$, $N \subseteq M$ and $J = I \cap (H \times N)$. It is called *compatible* if for each concept (A, B) of (G, M, I) the pair $(A \cap H, B \cap N)$ is also a concept of the subcontext. Factorizing a concept lattice is equivalent to providing a compatible subcontext, i.e. to deleting suitable rows and columns in the context. The rows and columns that have to be deleted can be described by using the relation $\nearrow$:

For $g \in G$ and $m \in M$ we define $g \nearrow m$ if $g \, Im$, $g' \subset h'$ implies hIm for all $h \in G$, and $m' \subset n'$ implies gIn for all $n \in M$. For two elements u and v of a complete lattice L, we write $u \nearrow v$, if u is maximal in $\{x \in L \mid x \not\geq v\}$ and v is minimal in $\{x \in L \mid x \not\leq u\}$.

For two elements u and v of a complete lattice, $u \nearrow v$ implies that u is $\bigvee$–irreducible and v is $\bigwedge$–irreducible and that $u \not\leq v$, $u_* \leq v$, and $u \leq v^*$ hold. It should not be confusing that we use $\nearrow$ at the same time as a relation between elements of a lattice and between objects and attributes of a context because $g \nearrow m$ in $\mathbb{K}$ is equivalent to $\gamma g \nearrow \mu m$ in the concept lattice $\mathfrak{B}(\mathbb{K})$.

A context is called *distributive* if its concept lattice is distributive. All the contexts needed for Distributive Concept Exploration are distributive reduced finite contexts. In these contexts the $\nearrow$-relation is a bijection between the set of objects and the set of attributes. According to [1], in a distributive reduced finite context the compatible subcontexts are exactly those of the form $(H, N, I \cap (H \times N))$ where for each $m \in N$ exists $g \in H$ s.t. $g \nearrow m$. The following theorem describes the correspondence between compatible subcontexts and congruence relations. It is a consequence of Lemmata 34 and 36 in [1].

Theorem 1. *Let (G, M, I) be a distributive reduced finite context, $g \in G$ and $m \in M$ with $g \nearrow m$. Then the kernel of the complete homomorphism*

$$\pi \colon \mathfrak{B}(G, M, I) \to \mathfrak{B}(G \setminus \{g\}, M \setminus \{m\}, I \setminus (\{g\} \times M \cup G \times \{m\}))$$

with $(A, B) \mapsto (A \setminus \{g\}, B \setminus \{m\})$ is the congruence relation on $\mathfrak{B}(G, M, I)$ that is generated by forcing $\gamma g \leq \mu m$.

3 Distributive Concept Exploration

Let $\mathfrak{b}_1, \mathfrak{b}_2, \ldots, \mathfrak{b}_n$ be names of the concepts the user wants to explore. They are called *basic concepts*. We assume that they generate (by taking greatest common subconcepts and least common superconcepts) a (yet unknown) distributive lattice L_n. Distributive Concept Exploration determines the lattice L_n together with a list of objects and attributes which are separating different concepts.

The lattice L_n is isomorphic to a quotient lattice $\mathrm{FBD}(\mathfrak{b}_1, \ldots, \mathfrak{b}_n)/\Theta$ of the free bounded distributive lattice generated by the basic concepts. The congruence relation Θ reflects the answers given by the user. We use the fact that $\mathrm{FBD}(\mathfrak{b}_1, \ldots, \mathfrak{b}_i) \cong \mathrm{FBD}(\mathfrak{b}_1, \ldots, \mathfrak{b}_{i-1}) \otimes \mathrm{FBD}(\mathfrak{b}_i)$ for splitting the determination of Θ into smaller parts: For $i = 0, \ldots, n$, the exploration algorithm subsequently determines the lattice L_i that is completely generated by the basic concepts $\mathfrak{b}_1, \ldots, \mathfrak{b}_i$ with respect to their hierarchical relationships. The lattice L_i is obtained from L_{i-1} by $L_i \cong (L_{i-1} \otimes \mathrm{FBD}(\mathfrak{b}_i))/\Theta_i$, where Θ_i reflects the hierarchical relationship between $\mathfrak{b}_i$ and the elements of L_{i-1}. The result of the exploration is then given by the lattice L_n.

For each $i \in \{0, \ldots, n\}$, the lattice L_i will be determined in two steps: First $\widetilde{L}_i$, the tensor product of L_{i-1} with $\mathrm{FBD}(\mathfrak{b}_i)$ (which is the three element chain $\bot < \mathfrak{b}_i < \top$), is calculated. Then the user is asked questions of the kind "Is s a subconcept of t?" with s and t being lattice terms built with $\mathfrak{b}_1, \ldots, \mathfrak{b}_i$. The congruence relation Θ_i on $\widetilde{L}_i$ is deduced from the answers given by the user. The factorization of $\widetilde{L}_i$ by the congruence relation yields the lattice L_i.

In the algorithm, the lattices L_i are *represented* by reduced contexts $\mathbb{K}_i := (G_i, M_i, I_i)$, i.e. the lattice L_i is isomorphic to the concept lattice $\mathfrak{B}(\mathbb{K}_i)$. As this context is the result of a repeated use of the direct product of contexts, its objects and attributes are tuples. They are of the form $\vec{x} := (x_0, \ldots, x_i) \in G_i$ with $x_0 = \top$ and $x_k \in \{\top, \mathfrak{b}_k\}$ for $k = 1, \ldots, n$ and $\vec{y} := (y_0, \ldots, y_i) \in M_i$ with $y_0 = \bot$ and $y_k \in \{\bot, \mathfrak{b}_k\}$ for $k = 1, \ldots, n$. The incidence $\vec{x} I_i \vec{y}$ represents the inequality $\bigwedge \vec{x} \le \bigvee \vec{y}$ with $\bigwedge \vec{x} := \bigwedge_{k=0}^{i} x_k$ and $\bigvee \vec{y} := \bigvee_{k=0}^{i} y_k$.

As mentioned above, the lattice $\widetilde{L}_i$ has to be calculated as intermediate step in the determination of the lattice L_i. This tensor product of L_{i-1} with the chain $\bot < \mathfrak{b}_i < \top$ will be represented by the context $\widetilde{\mathbb{K}}_i := (\widetilde{G}_i, \widetilde{M}_i, \widetilde{I}_i)$ being the direct product of $\mathbb{K}_{i-1}$ with the context $(\{\mathfrak{b}_i, \top\}, \{\bot, \mathfrak{b}_i\}, \{(\mathfrak{b}_i, \mathfrak{b}_i)\})$. The context $\mathbb{K}_i$ will then be derived from $\widetilde{\mathbb{K}}_i$ by deleting suitable rows and columns. This corresponds to finding a suitable congruence relation on the tensor product. Theorem 1 indicates the questions needed for determining these rows and columns: For all $\vec{x} \in \widetilde{G}_i$ and $\vec{y} \in \widetilde{M}_i$ with $\vec{x} \nearrow \vec{y}$ the user is asked: "Is the infimum of $\vec{x}$ a subconcept of the supremum of $\vec{y}$?" This question is equivalent to "Does each object belonging to all concepts $x_0, \ldots, x_i$ belong to at least one of the concepts $y_0, \ldots, y_i$?". If the user agrees to the question, the object $\vec{x}$ and the attribute $\vec{y}$ will be deleted, otherwise they will be kept in G_i and M_i, respectively.

Observe that the $\nearrow$-relation is inherited and can thus easily be calculated: For $\vec{x} \nearrow \vec{y}$ in $\mathbb{K}_{i-1}$, we have $(\vec{x}, \top) \nearrow (\vec{y}, \mathfrak{b}_i)$ and $(\vec{x}, \mathfrak{b}_i) \nearrow (\vec{y}, \bot)$ in $\widetilde{\mathbb{K}}_i$. Deleting corresponding rows and columns does not change the $\nearrow$-relation.

The algorithm starts with the determination of L_0 out of the two element lattice $\widetilde{L}_0 := \mathrm{FBD}(\emptyset) = (\bot < \top)$. The elements $\bot$ and $\top$ are the concepts *nothing* and *everything (in our field of interest)*. The lattice $\widetilde{L}_0$ is represented by the context $\widetilde{\mathbb{K}}_0 := (\{\top\}, \{\bot\}, \emptyset)$. As we have $\top \nearrow \bot$ in $\widetilde{\mathbb{K}}_0$, the first question in each exploration is "Is $\top$ (*everything*) a subconcept of $\bot$ (*nothing*)?" Usually, this will be denied. If however the user agrees, the exploration is terminated because he obtains $\mathbb{K}_0 = (\emptyset, \emptyset, \emptyset)$ which is the absorbing element for the direct product of contexts. Its concept lattice $\mathfrak{B}(\emptyset, \emptyset, \emptyset)$ is the one element lattice which is the absorbing element for the tensor product of lattices.

Next we introduce *separating pairs*. They are justifications for the claim that two concepts are different. More precisely, they justify that one of the concepts is not a subconcept of the other. For two concepts $\mathfrak{a}$ and $\mathfrak{b}$ with $\mathfrak{a}$ not a subconcept of $\mathfrak{b}$, a pair (g, m) is called a *separating pair* if g is an object of the concept $\mathfrak{a}$ and m is an attribute of the concept $\mathfrak{b}$ such that g does not have the attribute m.

The algorithm computes for each L_i with $i = 0, \ldots, n$ a minimal list of pairs of objects and attributes, such that for two concepts a and b of L_i with $a \not\leq b$ there is at least one pair in this list which is a separating pair for a and b. It is sufficient to have a list of separating pairs for elements c and $\mathfrak{d}$ of L_i with $c \nearrow \mathfrak{d}$, as for two elements a and b of L_i with $a \not\leq b$ there always exist such c and $\mathfrak{d}$ with $c \leq a$ and $b \leq \mathfrak{d}$, because L_i is finite and distributive. The separating pair for c and $\mathfrak{d}$ is also a separating pair for a and b. On the other hand there must be different separating pairs for different $c \nearrow \mathfrak{d}$, so that in fact this list is minimal.

During the exploration, the user is asked for separating pairs: Whenever he denies the question "Is the infimum of $\vec{x}$ a subconcept of the supremum of $\vec{y}$?", he is prompted for a separating pair for $\bigwedge \vec{x}$ and $\bigvee \vec{y}$. The pair will be denoted by $(\mathbf{g}_i(\vec{x}), \mathbf{m}_i(\vec{y}))$. Thus we obtain two mappings: $\mathbf{g}_i$ maps from G_i to the set of objects of the separating pairs, and $\mathbf{m}_i$ maps from M_i to the attributes. These mappings indicate that the object $\mathbf{g}_i(\vec{x})$ belongs to the concept $\bigwedge \vec{x}$, and that the attribute $\mathbf{m}_i(\vec{y})$ belongs to the concept $\bigvee \vec{y}$. Because of $\bigwedge \vec{x} \nearrow \bigvee \vec{y}$, we know that $\mathbf{g}_i(\vec{x})$ and $\mathbf{m}_i(\vec{y})$ form a separating pair. The mappings $\mathbf{g}_i$ and $\mathbf{m}_i$ however do not indicate whether an object or attribute does *not* belong to a concept. This information cannot be deduced from the answers given by the expert during the exploration dialogue. I. e., because the expert is not asked how objects and attributes of different separating pairs are related.

Unfortunately, $\bigwedge \vec{x} \nearrow \bigvee \vec{y}$ in L_i does not imply $\bigwedge \vec{x} \nearrow \bigvee \vec{y}$ in L_{i+1}. This means that the separating pair $(\mathbf{g}_i(\vec{x}), \mathbf{m}_i(\vec{y}))$ will in general not remain in the minimal list for L_{i+1}: If neither $\mathbf{g}_i(\vec{x})$ nor $\mathbf{m}_i(\vec{y})$ belong to b_{i+1}, then there is no $c \nearrow \mathfrak{d}$ in L_{i+1} separated by this pair. However it can be used to find new separating pairs for the minimal list: $\mathbf{g}_i(\vec{x})$ might appear in a separating pair for $\bigwedge(\vec{x}, \top)$ and $\bigvee(\vec{y}, b_{i+1})$ and $\mathbf{m}_i(\vec{y})$ might appear in a separating pair for $\bigwedge(\vec{x}, b_{i+1})$ and $\bigvee(\vec{y}, \bot)$. If the object $\mathbf{g}_i(\vec{x})$ belongs to the concept b_{i+1} and the attribute $\mathbf{m}_i(\vec{y})$ does not, then they are a separating pair for $\bigwedge(\vec{x}, b_{i+1}) \nearrow \bigvee(\vec{y}, \bot)$ in L_{i+1} and remain therefore in the minimal list. If the object $\mathbf{g}_i(\vec{x})$ does not belong to the concept b_{i+1} and the attribute $\mathbf{m}_i(\vec{y})$ does, then they are a separating pair for $\bigwedge(\vec{x}, \top) \nearrow \bigvee(\vec{y}, b_{i+1})$ in L_{i+1} and remain in the list. Because the object $\mathbf{g}_i(\vec{x})$ does not have the attribute $\mathbf{m}_i(\vec{y})$, it is not possible that both belong to the concept b_{i+1}. This justifies the following definition:

$$\widetilde{\mathbf{g}}_{i+1}(\vec{x}, b_{i+1}) := \begin{cases} \mathbf{g}_i(\vec{x}) & \text{if } \mathbf{g}_i(\vec{x}) \text{ belongs to } b_{i+1} \\ \text{undefined} & \text{else} \end{cases}$$

$$\widetilde{\mathbf{g}}_{i+1}(\vec{x}, \top) := \begin{cases} \mathbf{g}_i(\vec{x}) & \text{if } \mathbf{g}_i(\vec{x}) \text{ does not belong to } b_{i+1} \\ \text{undefined} & \text{else} \end{cases}$$

$$\widetilde{\mathbf{m}}_{i+1}(\vec{y}, b_{i+1}) := \begin{cases} \mathbf{m}_i(\vec{y}) & \text{if } \mathbf{m}_i(\vec{y}) \text{ belongs to } b_{i+1} \\ \text{undefined} & \text{else} \end{cases}$$

$$\widetilde{\mathbf{m}}_{i+1}(\vec{y}, \bot) := \begin{cases} \mathbf{m}_i(\vec{y}) & \text{if } \mathbf{m}_i(\vec{y}) \text{ does not belong to } b_{i+1} \\ \text{undefined} & \text{else} \end{cases}$$

Thus, for each separating pair $(\mathbf{g}_i(\vec{x}), \mathbf{m}_i(\vec{y}))$ in L_i, the user has to answer the two following questions: "Does the object $\mathbf{g}_i(\vec{x})$ belong to the concept b_{i+1}?" and "Does the attribute $\mathbf{m}_i(\vec{y})$ belong the concept b_{i+1}?". The algorithm uses the fact that the answer "Yes" to one of the questions implies the answer "No" to the other one.

The problem of finding the rows and columns in $\widetilde{\mathbb{K}}_i$ that have to be deleted, now turns out to be equivalent to completing the partial mappings $\widetilde{g}_i$ and $\widetilde{m}_i$: If, for $\vec{x} \in \widetilde{G}_i$ and $\vec{y} \in \widetilde{M}_i$ with $\vec{x} \nearrow \vec{y}$, at least one of $\widetilde{g}_i(\vec{x})$ and $\widetilde{m}_i(\vec{y})$ is undefined and the user is not able to find an object or attribute for completing the separating pair, then the row $\vec{x}$ and the column $\vec{y}$ have to be deleted. In two cases we can benefit from the already given knowledge:

1. If $\widetilde{g}_i(\vec{x})$ is undefined, $\widetilde{m}_i(\vec{y})$ is defined and $\vec{x} = (\top, \ldots, \top, b_i)$, then we already know that there must exist an object that belongs to b_i and that does not have the attribute $\widetilde{m}_i(\vec{y})$. The user is then asked for such an object.
2. If $\widetilde{g}_i(\vec{x})$ is defined and $\widetilde{m}_i(\vec{y})$ is undefined then there must exist an attribute of $\bigvee \vec{y}$ that $\widetilde{g}_i(\vec{x})$ does not have. The user is then asked for such an attribute.

We are now ready to list the algorithm of Distributive Concept Exploration:

Algorithm: Given is the list $b_1, b_2, \ldots, b_n$ of basic concepts.
1. $i := 0$, $\widetilde{\mathbb{K}}_0 := (\{\top\}, \{\bot\}, \emptyset)$, $\widetilde{g}_0(\top) :=$ undefined, $\widetilde{m}_0(\bot) :=$ undefined.
2. For each $(\vec{x}, \vec{y}) \in \widetilde{G}_i \times \widetilde{M}_i$ with $\vec{x} \nearrow \vec{y}$,
   where $\widetilde{g}_i(\vec{x})$ or $\widetilde{m}_i(\vec{y})$ are undefined, do:
   - If $\widetilde{g}_i(\vec{x})$ is undefined:
     - If $\widetilde{m}_i(\vec{y})$ is defined and $\vec{x} = (\top, \ldots, \top, b_i)$:
       Prompt: "Name an object belonging to b_i and not having the attribute $\widetilde{m}_i(\vec{y})$!" Set $\widetilde{g}_i(\vec{x})$ according to the answer.
     - Else do:
       Ask the user: "Is the infimum of $\vec{x}$ a subconcept
                      of the supremum of $\vec{y}$?"
       "Yes": Delete $\vec{x}$ in $\widetilde{G}_i$, $\vec{y}$ in $\widetilde{M}_i$,
                and the corresponding row and column in $\widetilde{I}_i$.
       "No": Prompt: "Give a separating pair for $\bigwedge \vec{x}$ and $\bigvee \vec{y}$!"
               If $\widetilde{m}_i(\vec{y})$ is defined, add:
               "Eventually you can use $\widetilde{m}_i(\vec{y})$ as attribute."
               Set $\widetilde{g}_i(\vec{x})$ and $\widetilde{m}_i(\vec{y})$ according to the answer.
   - Else (i.e. $\widetilde{g}_i(\vec{x})$ is defined and $\widetilde{m}_i(\vec{y})$ is undefined) do:
     Prompt: "Name an attribute of $\bigvee \vec{y}$ that $\widetilde{g}_i(\vec{x})$ does not have!"
     Set $\widetilde{m}_i(\vec{y})$ according to the answer.
3. Set $\mathbb{K}_i := \widetilde{\mathbb{K}}_i$, $g_i := \widetilde{g}_i|_{G_i}$, $m_i := \widetilde{m}_i|_{M_i}$.
4. If $i=n$, then S T O P.
5. Set $\widetilde{\mathbb{K}}_{i+1} := \mathbb{K}_i \times (\{b_{i+1}, \top\}, \{\bot, b_{i+1}\}, \{(b_{i+1}, b_{i+1})\})$.
6. For each $(\vec{x}, \vec{y}) \in G_i \times M_i$ with $\vec{x} \nearrow \vec{y}$:
   - Ask the user: "Is $g_i(\vec{x})$ a b_{i+1}?"
   - If *"No"*, ask "Has each object in b_{i+1} the attribute $m_i(\vec{y})$?" [1]
   - Set $\widetilde{g}_{i+1}(\vec{x}, b_{i+1})$ and $\widetilde{g}_{i+1}(\vec{x}, \top)$ as defined above.

---

[1] These two questions are equivalent to "Does the object $g_i(\vec{x})$ belong to the concept b_{i+1}?" and "Does the attribute $m_i(\vec{y})$ belong to the concept b_{i+1}?", resp.

- Set $\widetilde{\mathbf{m}}_{i+1}(\vec{y}, \mathfrak{b}_{i+1})$ and $\widetilde{\mathbf{m}}_{i+1}(\vec{y}, \bot)$ as defined above.

7. Set $i := i + 1$.
8. Goto Step 2.

The result of the algorithm can be shown by a line diagram of $\underline{\mathfrak{B}}(\mathbb{K}_n)$. It is not necessary to label all the object and attribute concepts in the diagram. Only the concepts $\bigvee\{\gamma\vec{x} \mid \vec{x} \in G_n,\ x_i = \mathfrak{b}_i\}$ $(= \bigwedge\{\mu\vec{y} \mid \vec{y} \in M_n,\ y_i = \mathfrak{b}_i\})$ of $\underline{\mathfrak{B}}(\mathbb{K}_n)$ have to be labeled by $\mathfrak{b}_i$, as they correspond to the basic concepts which completely generate the whole lattice. The resulting list of separating pairs can be displayed in the same diagram: For each pair $\vec{x} \nearrow \vec{y}$ in $\mathbb{K}_n$, there is exactly one separating pair $(\mathbf{g}_n(\vec{x}), \mathbf{m}_n(\vec{y}))$. We label the concept $\gamma\vec{x}$ by $\mathbf{g}_n(\vec{x})$ and the concept $\mu\vec{y}$ by $\mathbf{m}_n(\vec{y})$ and mark $\gamma\vec{x}$ and $\mu\vec{y}$ with the same symbol. An example can be seen in the next section.

4   An Exploration of Zinks

As an example, we want to explore a family of musical instruments: *Zinks* are wind instruments with a conical wide–bored tube, a shortening hole–system and a mouth piece played like a trumpet. We start the exploration with the following basic concepts: $\mathfrak{b}_1 = $ *straight zink [gerader Zink]*, $\mathfrak{b}_2 = $ *silent zink [stiller Zink]*, $\mathfrak{b}_3 = $ *curved zink [krummer Zink]*, $\mathfrak{b}_4 = $ *cornettino*, and $\mathfrak{b}_5 = $ *cornetto*. The exploration is based on information given by the catalogue of the museum of musical instruments of the University of Leipzig ([2]). The zinks used for separating pairs are named by their catalogue number.

Figure 2 shows the result of the exploration of the two first basic concepts *straight zink* and *silent zink* (i.e., after Step 4 of the algorithm with $i = 2$). For instance, one can see in the diagram that *silent zink* is a subconcept of *straight zink*. The fact that not *everything* is a *straight zink* is asserted by the separating pair *Zink 1574* and *straight form*. The relation $\nearrow$ is indicated in the diagram by using the same symbol (e.g., *everything* $\nearrow$ *straight zink* by ⊖ and ⊕) Next we determine the largest lattice that is possibly generated by adding the next basic concept *curved zink* (Steps 5 & 6):

> "Is *Zink 1559* a *curved zink*?" — "No!" — "Has every *curved zink* the attribute *ground tone C*?" — "No!" — "Is *Zink 1558* a *curved zink*?" — "No!" — "Has each *curved zink* the attribute *recessed mouthpiece*?" — "No!" — "Is *Zink 1574* a *curved zink*?" — "No!" — "Has each *curved zink* the attribute *straight form*?" — "No!"

Figure 3 shows the context $\widetilde{\mathbb{K}}_3$ and the mappings $\widetilde{g}_3$ and $\widetilde{m}_3$. Steps 2 & 3 then determine the congruence relation on $\underline{\mathfrak{B}}(\widetilde{\mathbb{K}}_3)$ that reflects the dependencies between the concept *curved zink* and the concepts *straight zink* and *silent zink*.

> "Is the infimum of *straight zink*, *silent zink* and *curved zink* a subconcept of *nothing*?" — "Yes!" — "Is the infimum of *straight zink* and *curved zink* a subconcept of *silent zink*?" — "Yes!" — "Name a *curved zink* not having

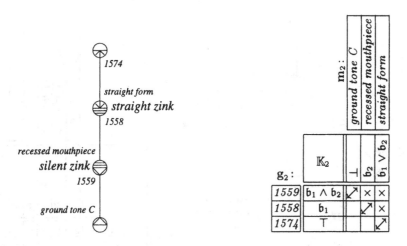

Fig. 2. The result of the exploration of the first two basic concepts

straight form!" — "*Zink 1563.*" — "Name an attribute of *curved zinks* that *Zink 1559* does not have!" — "*Attached mouthpiece.*" — "Name an attribute of the supremum of *silent zink* and *curved zink* that *Zink 1558* does not have!" — "*Recessed mouthpiece or curved form.*" — "Name an attribute of the supremum of *straight zink*, *silent zink* and *curved zink* that *Zink 1574* does not have!" — "*More than 6 finger holes.*"

Up to now (at Step 4 with $i = 3$), we have determined the complete lattice generated by the first three basic concepts *straight zink*, *silent zink*, and *curved zink*. It is shown in Figure 4. We continue the exploration in the same way with the remaining two basic concepts *cornetto* and *cornettino*. Finally, we get the context $\mathbb{K}_5$ as shown in Figure 5. Its line diagram shows all information about the hierarchical relationships between the five basic concepts. For example, we can deduce from it that there are no *silent zinks* that are also *cornettos*, because the infimum of *silent zink* and *cornetto* is *nothing*. We can further deduce that there are other zinks than those we chose for the exploration, because the supremum of all basic concepts is different from *everything*. The observation that the supremum of *cornetto* and *cornettino* is *curved zink* and their infimum is *nothing* reflects the fact that the *curved zinks* can be divided in two disjoint classes: *cornettos* and *cornettinos*.

Let us remark that, in the Fig. 5, *Zink 1558* is not laying below *attached mouthpiece*, even though Zink 1558 has an attached mouthpiece! *Zink 1558* and *attached mouthpiece* belong to different separating pairs, and so their relationship has not been asked from the expert.

If there are other subconcepts of *zink* we are interested in (for example *tenor zink*, *serpent* or *violoncel serpent*) we can continue the exploration by starting with the context $\mathbb{K}_5$ and adding the new basic concepts. This serial approach allows also to extend the acquired knowledge at a later time.

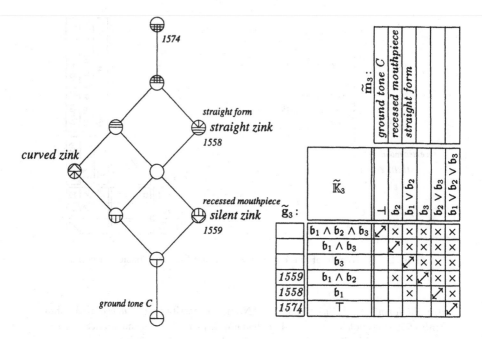

Fig. 3. The intermediate result $\widetilde{\mathbb{K}}_3$ and its concept lattice

5 Conclusion

The algorithm as described above is not able to treat incomplete knowledge. The user is assumed to reply to each question during the exploration either with "Yes" or "No". With a little change we can allow the answer "I don't know" to the question "Is the infimum of $\vec{x}$ a subconcept of the supremum of $\vec{y}$?": In this case the row $\vec{x}$ and the column $\vec{y}$ will not be deleted in $\widetilde{\mathbb{K}}_i$ and $\widetilde{g}_i(\vec{x})$ and $\widetilde{m}_i(\vec{y})$ will be set to the default value $?$. In Step 6 of the algorithm all $\widetilde{g}_{i+1}(\vec{x}, b_{i+1})$, $\widetilde{g}_{i+1}(\vec{x}, \top)$, $\widetilde{m}_{i+1}(\vec{y}, b_{i+1})$ and $\widetilde{m}_{i+1}(\vec{y}, \bot)$ will then automatically be set to $?$. These $?$ play the role of "possible separating pairs". During and after the exploration procedure the user can either replace them by a real separating pair or he can delete the corresponding row and column (if he is then sure that the inequality $\bigwedge \vec{x} \leq \bigvee \vec{y}$ holds). The result of the exploration can be shown by a list of line diagrams — one for each possibility of deleting corresponding rows and columns that are not confirmed by a concrete separating pair.

The algorithm generates in the worst case (i.e., the user denies all dependencies between the basic concepts) the free bounded distributive lattice $\mathrm{FBD}(b_1, \ldots, b_n)$, which is growing super-exponentially. However, the algorithm is working on the level of the formal contexts only, whose sizes are logarithmic in the sizes of the concept lattices. Hence, if the basic concepts are sufficiently related, then the exploration can be done in reasonable time. Its efficiency also depends on the ordering of the basic concepts: The stronger the first basic concepts are related, the smaller the contexts can be kept during the exploration.

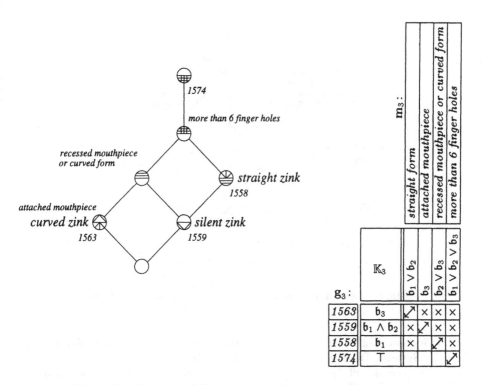

Fig. 4. Result of the exploration of the first three basic concepts

The final result, of course, is independent of this ordering. For basic concepts that are only weakly related, the whole lattice generated by them is often not requested. Then the basic concepts can be divided in stronger related classes which are explored separately (cf. [4]).

References

1. B. Ganter, R. Wille: Formale Begriffsanalyse: Mathematische Grundlagen. Springer, Heidelberg 1996
2. H. Heyde: Hörner und Zinken. Musikinstrumenten–Museum der Universität Leipzig. Katalog Bd. 5. VEB Deutscher Verlag für Musik, Leipzig 1982
3. U. Klotz, A. Mann: Begriffexploration. Diplomarbeit, TH Darmstadt 1988
4. G. Stumme: Exploration tools in formal concept analysis. In: *Ordinal and symbolic data analysis.* Studies in classification, data analysis, and knowledge organization **8**, Springer, Heidelberg 1996, 31–44
5. G. Stumme: The concept classification of a terminology extended by conjunction and disjunction. In: N. Foo, R. Goebel (eds.): PRICAI'96: Topics in artificial intelligence. LNAI **1114**, Springer, Heidelberg 1996, 121–131
6. G. Stumme: Concept Exploration – A Tool for Creating and Exploring Conceptual Hierarchies. In: D. Lukose, H. Delugach, M. Keeler, L. Searle, J. F. Sowa (eds.): *Conceptual Structures: Fulfilling Peirce's Dream.* LNAI **1257**, Springer, Berlin 1997, 318–331

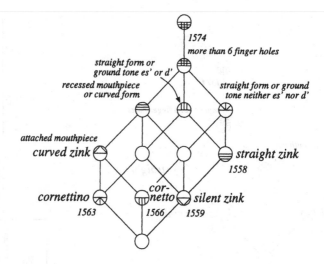

Fig. 5. Result of the Distributive Concept Exploration of zinks

7. G. Stumme: Concept Exploration – Knowledge Acquisition in Conceptual Knowledge Systems. Dissertation. Shaker, Aachen 1997
8. H. Wagner: Begriff. In: H. M. Baumgartner, C. Wild (eds.): *Handbuch philosophischer Grundbegriffe*. Kösel Verlag, München 1973, 191–209
9. R. Wille: Restructuring lattice theory: an approach based on hierarchies of concepts. In: I. Rival (ed.): *Ordered sets*. Reidel, Dordrecht–Boston 1982, 445–470
10. R. Wille: Tensorial decomposition of concept lattices. In: *Order* **2**, 1985, 81–95
11. R. Wille: Bedeutungen von Begriffsverbänden. In: B. Ganter, R. Wille, K. E. Wolff (eds.): *Beiträge zur Begriffsanalyse*. B. I.–Wissenschaftsverlag, Mannheim 1987, 161–211
12. R. Wille: Knowledge acquisition by methods of formal concept analysis. In: E. Diday (ed.): *Data analysis, learning symbolic and numeric knowledge*. Nova Science Publisher, New York, Budapest 1989, 365–380

Computing the Least Common Subsumer and the Most Specific Concept in the Presence of Cyclic $\mathcal{ALN}$- Concept Descriptions

Franz Baader and Ralf Küsters*

LuFG Theoretische Informatik, RWTH Aachen, Ahornstr. 55, 52074 Aachen, Germany
{baader,kuesters}@informatik.rwth-aachen.de

Abstract. Computing least common subsumers (lcs) and most specific concepts (msc) are inference tasks that can be used to support the "bottom up" construction of knowledge bases for KR systems based on description logic. For the description logic $\mathcal{ALN}$, the msc need not always exist if one restricts the attention to acyclic concept descriptions. In this paper, we extend the notions lcs and msc to cyclic descriptions, and show how they can be computed.

1 Introduction

Knowledge representation systems based on description logics (DL) can be used to describe the terminological knowledge of an application domain in a structured and formally well-understood way [3, 13]. Traditionally, the knowledge base of a DL system is built by first formalizing the relevant concepts of the domain (its terminology, stored in the so-called TBox) by *concept descriptions*, i.e., expressions that are built from atomic concepts (unary predicates) and atomic roles (binary predicates) using the concept constructors provided by the DL language. In a second step, the concept descriptions are used to specify properties of objects and individuals occurring in the domain (the world description, stored in the so-called ABox). DL systems provide their users with inference services that support both steps: classification of concepts and individuals and testing for consistency. Classification of concepts determines subconcept/superconcept relationships (called subsumption relationships) between the concepts of a given terminology, and thus allows one to structure the terminology in the form of a subsumption hierarchy. This hierarchy provides useful information on (implicit) connections between different concepts, and can thus be used to check (at least partially) whether the formal descriptions capture the intuitive meaning of the concepts. Classification of individuals (or objects) determines whether a given individual is always an instance of a certain concept (i.e., whether this instance relationship is implied by the descriptions of the individual and the concept). It thus provides useful information on the properties of an individual, and can

---

* Supported by "Studienstiftung des deutschen Volkes".

again be used for checking the adequacy of the knowledge base with respect to the application domain it is supposed to describe. Finally, if a knowledge base is inconsistent (i.e., self-contradictory), then it is clear that a modeling error has occurred, and the knowledge base must be changed.

This traditional "top down" approach for constructing a DL knowledge base is not always adequate, though. On the one hand, it need not be clear from the outset which are the relevant concepts in a particular application. On the other hand, even if it is clear which (intuitive) concepts should be introduced, it is in general not easy to come up with formal definitions of these concepts within the available description language. For example, in one of our applications in chemical process engineering [5], the process engineers prefer to construct the knowledge base (which consists of descriptions of standard building blocks of process models, such as reactors) in the following "bottom up" fashion: first, they introduce several "typical" examples of the standard building block as individuals in the ABox, and then they generalize (the descriptions of) these individuals into a concept description that (a) has all the individuals as instances, and (b) is the most specific description satisfying property (a).

The present paper is concerned with developing inference services that can support this "bottom up" approach of building knowledge bases. We split the task of computing descriptions satisfying (a) and (b) from above into two subtasks: computing the most specific concept of a single ABox individual, and computing the least common subsumer of two concepts. The *most specific concept* (msc) of an individual b (the *least common subsumer* (lcs) of two concept descriptions A, B) is the most specific concept description C (expressible in the given description language) that has b as an instance (that subsumes both A and B). For sub-languages of the DL used by the system CLASSIC [6], both tasks have already been considered in the literature [7, 9, 8]. However, the algorithms described in these papers only compute approximations of the msc of an individual. In fact, for ABoxes with cyclic dependencies between individuals, the msc of a given individual need not exist. Therefore we allow for *cyclic concept descriptions* (i.e., concepts defined by cyclic TBoxes) interpreted with greatest fixed-point semantics. The use of this semantics is motivated by the fact that (for the concept description language considered in this paper) it is the one best capturing the intuition underlying the msc. In particular, we will show that w.r.t. greatest fixed-point semantics the msc of an individual always exists. This is not the case for the least fixed-point semantics. The third possible semantics often employed for cyclic TBoxes, descriptive semantics, is not appropriate in this context since it does not provide for unique extensions of defined concepts [12].

Once one allows for cyclic concept descriptions, the algorithm for computing the lcs must also be able to deal with these descriptions. As a first solution to these problems, we consider cyclic concept descriptions in the language $\mathcal{ALN}$ (which allows for conjunctions, value restrictions, number restrictions, and atomic negations), and show how (1) the lcs of two such descriptions and (2) the msc of an ABox individual can be computed. In (2) we allow for cyclic de-

Table 1. Semantics of $\mathcal{ALN}$-concepts

syntax	semantics	name of construct
$\neg A$	$dom(I) \setminus A^I$	atomic negation
$C \sqcap D$	$C^I \cap D^I$	conjunction
$\forall R.C$	$\{d \in dom(I); R^I(d) \subseteq C^I\}$	value restriction
$(\geq m\,R)$	$\{d \in dom(I); |R^I(d)| \geq m\}$	at-least restriction
$(\leq n\,R)$	$\{d \in dom(I); |R^I(d)| \leq n\}$	at-most restriction

scriptions in the ABox, and the msc may also be a cyclic description. It should be noted that in languages allowing for disjunction (like $\mathcal{ALC}$), the lcs is just the disjunction of the given concepts, and thus computing it does not provide us with interesting information. The language $\mathcal{ALN}$ contains most of the constructors available in systems employing concept description languages that are not propositionally closed.

Our approach is based on the known automata-theoretic characterizations of subsumption w.r.t. cyclic terminologies with greatest fixed-point semantics [2, 11]. Because of the space limitation, we cannot give all the technical details. These details as well as complete proofs can be found in [4].

2 Definitions and notations

In this section, we introduce the description language $\mathcal{ALN}$ as well as the notions msc and lcs more formally, and show how they can be generalized to cyclic concept descriptions.

Definition 1 ($\mathcal{ALN}$-concept descriptions). $\mathcal{ALN}$-concept descriptions are formed from concept names and role names by means of the following syntax rules: $C, D \longrightarrow A \mid \neg A \mid C \sqcap D \mid \forall R.C \mid (\geq m\,R) \mid (\leq n\,R)$, where A denotes a concept name, R a role name, C, D concept descriptions, m a positive integer, and n a non-negative integer.

The semantics of $\mathcal{ALN}$-concept descriptions is defined by introducing the notion of an interpretation. An *interpretation* I consists of a domain $dom(I)$ and a mapping assigning a subset A^I of $dom(I)$ (the *extension of A*) to every concept name A, and a binary relation R^I over $dom(I)$ (the *extension of R*) to every role name R. This interpretation is extended to $\mathcal{ALN}$-concepts as defined in Table 1, where $R^I(d) := \{e \in dom(I) \mid (d, e) \in R^I\}$ denotes the set of *R-successors* of d in I.

In the following, we use $\perp$ to denote a concept description that is always interpreted by the empty set, such as $(\geq 2\,R) \sqcap (\leq 1\,R)$. In addition, we restrict our attention to the sub-language $\mathcal{FLN}$ of $\mathcal{ALN}$, which disallows atomic negation. In fact, as shown in [1], atomic negation can be simulated within $\mathcal{FLN}$, by using $(\leq 0\,R_A)$ in place of A and $(\geq 1\,R_A)$ in place of $\neg A$, where R_A is a new role name only used for this purpose.

Definition 2 (subsumption, lcs). *Let C, D, E be $\mathcal{FLN}$-concept descriptions.*

1. *C is subsumed by D $(C \sqsubseteq D)$ iff $C^I \subseteq D^I$ holds for all interpretations I.*
2. *E is a least common subsumer (lcs) of C, D iff it satisfies*
    - *$C \sqsubseteq E$ and $D \sqsubseteq E$, and*
    - *E is the least $\mathcal{FLN}$-concept description with this property, i.e., if E' is an $\mathcal{FLN}$-concept description satisfying $C \sqsubseteq E'$ and $D \sqsubseteq E'$, then $E \sqsubseteq E'$.*

As shown in [7], the lcs of two $\mathcal{FLN}$-concept descriptions always exists, and it can be computed in polynomial time. Things become less rosy, however, if we consider the most specific concept of ABox individuals.

Definition 3 ($\mathcal{FLN}$-ABoxes). *An $\mathcal{FLN}$-ABox is a finite set of assertions of the form $R(a, b)$ (role assertion) or $C(a)$ (concept assertion), where a, b are individual names, R is a role name, and C is an $\mathcal{FLN}$-concept description.*

In the presence of an ABox, an interpretation additionally assigns an element a^I of $dom(I)$ to each individual name a such that $a \neq b$ implies $a^I \neq b^I$ (unique name assumption). It is a *model* of the ABox $\mathcal{A}$ iff it satisfies $(a^I, b^I) \in R^I$ for all role assertions $R(a, b) \in \mathcal{A}$ and $a^I \in C^I$ for all concept assertions $C(a) \in \mathcal{A}$.

Definition 4 (instance, msc). *Let $\mathcal{A}$ be an $\mathcal{FLN}$-ABox, a an individual name in $\mathcal{A}$, and C an $\mathcal{FLN}$-concept description.*

1. *a is an instance of C w.r.t. $\mathcal{A}$ $(a \in_{\mathcal{A}} C)$ iff $a^I \in C^I$ for all models I of $\mathcal{A}$.*
2. *C is the most specific concept for a in $\mathcal{A}$ iff $a \in_{\mathcal{A}} C$ and C is the least concept with this property, i.e., if C' is an $\mathcal{FLN}$-concept description satisfying $a \in_{\mathcal{A}} C'$, then $C \sqsubseteq C'$.*

The following example demonstrates that the msc need not exist if the ABox contains cyclic role assertions: in the ABox $\mathcal{A} := \{R(a, a), (\leq 1 R)(a)\}$, the individual a does not have a most specific concept. In fact, it is easy to see that a is an instance of $\forall R. \cdots \forall R.((\leq 1 R) \sqcap (\geq 1 R))$ for chains of value restrictions of arbitrary length. Consequently, the msc cannot be expressed by a finite $\mathcal{FLN}$-concept description. However, the msc of a can be described by the recursively defined concept $A \doteq (\leq 1 R) \sqcap (\geq 1 R) \sqcap \forall R.A$, provided that this recursive definition is interpreted with greatest fixed-point semantics.

The example can also be used to illustrate why other semantics for cyclic definitions are not appropriate in this context. First, note that w.r.t. the least fixed-point semantics there is no msc for a. In fact, since a is an instance of $\forall R. \cdots \forall R.(\geq 1 R)$ for chains of value restrictions of arbitrary length, it follows that the msc of a is subsumed by all these concept descriptions. However, the characterization of inconsistency w.r.t. least fixed-point semantics [11] implies that a concept subsumed by these concept descriptions is inconsistent, and thus cannot have a as an instance. In particular, the concept A defined by $A \doteq (\leq 1 R) \sqcap (\geq 1 R) \sqcap \forall R.A$ is always interpreted by the empty set w.r.t. least fixed-point semantics. With respect to descriptive semantics, both the least fixed-point interpretation of A and the greatest fixed-point interpretation of A are allowed, which means that descriptive semantics does not uniquely determine an interpretation for a recursively defined concept.

Definition 5 (cyclic $\mathcal{FLN}$-TBoxes). *An $\mathcal{FLN}$-concept definition is of the form $A \doteq C$, where A is a concept name and C an $\mathcal{FLN}$-concept description. An $\mathcal{FLN}$-TBox is a finite set of $\mathcal{FLN}$-concept definitions such that every concept name occurs at most once as left-hand side of a definition.*[1]

The concept name A is a defined concept *in the TBox $\mathcal{T}$ iff it occurs on the left-hand side of a definition in $\mathcal{T}$. Otherwise, A is called* primitive concept.

The interpretation I is a model of the TBox $\mathcal{T}$ iff it satisfies $A^I = C^I$ for all concept definitions $A \doteq C \in \mathcal{T}$. It is well-known [12] that in the presence of cycles in the TBox, a given interpretation of the primitive concepts and roles (*primitive interpretation*) can have different extensions to a model of the TBox. The *gfp-semantics* chooses the greatest of these possible models as the gfp-model of the TBox. In the following we will employ this semantics to define the meaning of a TBox. As pointed out above, the other semantics for cyclic terminologies considered in the literature are not appropriate in this context.[2]

Because a gfp-model is uniquely determined by the primitive interpretation, the following definition of cyclic $\mathcal{FLN}$-concept descriptions and their semantics makes sense. Intuitively, a cyclic concept description is a cyclic TBox where one defined concept name is selected to represent the cyclic concept description defined by the TBox.

Definition 6 (cyclic $\mathcal{FLN}$-concept descriptions). *Assume that sets of primitive concept names N_P and of role names N_R are fixed. A cyclic $\mathcal{FLN}$-concept description $C = (A, \mathcal{T})$ is given by a defined concept A in a (possibly cyclic) $\mathcal{FLN}$-TBox $\mathcal{T}$ such that all the primitive concepts in $\mathcal{T}$ are elements of N_P and none of the defined concepts in $\mathcal{T}$ belongs to N_P.*

In this context, an *interpretation I* assigns subsets of $dom(I)$ to elements of N_P and binary relations on $dom(I)$ to elements of N_R. For a given cyclic concept description $C = (A, \mathcal{T})$, the interpretation C^I of C in I is the set assigned to A by the unique extension of I to a gfp-model of $\mathcal{T}$. This shows that, from a semantic point of view, cyclic concept descriptions C behave just like ordinary concept descriptions, i.e., a given interpretation I assigns a unique set $C^I \subseteq dom(I)$ to C. For this reason, the definition of subsumption and of the least common subsumer can be generalized to cyclic concept descriptions in the obvious way: just replace "$\mathcal{FLN}$-concept description" by "cyclic $\mathcal{FLN}$-concept description" in Definition 2. The same is true for the definitions of ABoxes, the instance relationship, and the most specific concept.

3 Computing the lcs of cyclic $\mathcal{FLN}$-concept descriptions

Both subsumption and the lcs of cyclic $\mathcal{FLN}$-concept descriptions can be computed using automata-theoretic characterizations of so-called value-restriction

---

[1] Note that we do not prohibit cyclic dependencies between definitions.
[2] See [12, 2] for a more formal definition of the semantics for cyclic terminologies.

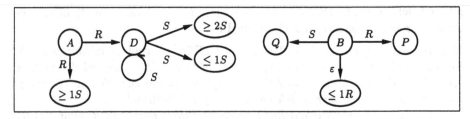

Fig. 1. The automata corresponding to $\mathcal{T}_A$ and $\mathcal{T}_B$.

sets. For convenience, we abbreviate the concept description $\forall R_1.\forall R_2 \cdots \forall R_n.C$ ($n \geq 0$) by $\forall R_1 \cdots R_n.C$, where $R_1 \ldots R_n$ is a word over the alphabet N_R of all role names (i.e., $R_1 \ldots R_n \in N_R^*$). For an interpretation I and a word $W = R_1 \ldots R_n$, we define $W^I := R_1^I \circ \cdots \circ R_n^I$, where $\circ$ denotes the composition of binary relations. The empty word ε is interpreted as the identical relation, and thus $\forall \varepsilon.C$ is equivalent to C.

Definition 7. *Let C be a cyclic $\mathcal{FLN}$-concept description and P a primitive concept name or a number restriction. Then the set $V_C(P) := \{W \in N_R^* \mid C \sqsubseteq \forall W.P\}$ is called the* value-restriction set *of C for P.*

Even for acyclic descriptions, these value-restriction sets may be infinite. For example, for the (acyclic) description $\bot := (\geq 2\,R) \sqcap (\leq 1\,R)$ and an arbitrary primitive concept name P we have $V_\bot(P) = N_R^*$. The value-restriction sets can, however, be represented by regular languages over the alphabet N_R. To obtain these languages, the TBox of a given cyclic $\mathcal{FLN}$-concept description C is translated into a finite automaton: the concept names and the number restrictions occurring in the TBox are the states of the automaton, and the transitions of the automaton are induced by the value restrictions in the TBox (see [2, 11] for details). For example, the TBoxes $\mathcal{T}_A$ and $\mathcal{T}_B$ defining the descriptions $C_A := (A, \mathcal{T}_A)$ and $C_B := (B, \mathcal{T}_B)$

$$\mathcal{T}_A: \quad A \doteq \forall R.D \sqcap \forall R.(\geq 1S) \qquad\qquad \mathcal{T}_B: \quad B \doteq (\leq 1R) \sqcap \forall R.P \sqcap \forall S.Q$$
$$D \doteq \forall S.D \sqcap \forall S.(\geq 2S) \sqcap \forall S.(\leq 1S)$$

give rise to the automata of Fig. 1. For a cyclic $\mathcal{FLN}$-concept description $C = (A, \mathcal{T})$ and a primitive concept or number restriction P, the language $L_C(P)$ is the set of all words labeling paths in the corresponding automaton from A to P. By definition, these languages are regular. In the example, we have, e.g., $L_{C_A}(\geq 2\,S) = RS^*S$ and $L_{C_B}(P) = \{R\}$.

It is easy to see that the inclusion $L_C(P) \subseteq V_C(P)$ always holds. However, since conflicting number restrictions can create inconsistencies (i.e., unsatisfiable sub-concepts), the inclusion in the other direction need not hold. Additionally, the set $V_C(P)$ may contain so-called C-excluding words:

Definition 8. *Let C be a cyclic $\mathcal{FLN}$-concept description. Then the set $E_C := \{W \in N_R^* \mid C \sqsubseteq \forall W.\bot\}$ is called the* set of C-excluding words.

Obviously, if $W \in L_C(\leq m\, R) \cap L_C(\geq n\, R)$ for $m < n$, then W must belong to E_C. Also, since $(\leq 0\, R)$ is equivalent to $\forall R.\bot$, we know that $W \in L_C(\leq 0\, R)$ implies $WR \in E_C$. In addition, if W belongs to E_C, then $WU \in E_C$ for all words U. Finally, for $W \in E_C$, at-least restrictions can also force prefixes of W to belong to E_C. In our example (see Fig. 1), the word R belongs to E_{C_A} since $RS \in E_{C_A}$ and $R \in L_{C_A}(\geq 1\, S)$. Consequently, $E_{C_A} = R\{R, S\}^*$ and it is easy to see that $E_{C_B} = \emptyset$

A more formal characterization of E_C, which also shows that E_C is a regular language, can be found in [11]. To be more precise, a finite automaton that accepts E_C and is exponential in the size of the automaton corresponding to C can be constructed. The following characterization of value-restriction sets is an easy consequence of the results in [11]:

Theorem 1. *Let C be a cyclic $\mathcal{FLN}$-concept description. Then*

1. *$V_C(P) = L_C(P) \cup E_C$ for all primitive concepts P;*
2. *$V_C(\geq m\, R) = \bigcup_{\ell \geq m} L_C(\geq \ell\, R) \cup E_C$ for all at-least restrictions $(\geq m\, R)$;*
3. *$V_C(\leq n\, R) = \bigcup_{\ell \leq n} L_C(\leq \ell\, R) \cup E_C R^{-1}$ for all at-most restrictions $(\leq n\, R)$.[3]*

Consequently, these sets are regular, and finite automata accepting them can be constructed in time exponential in the size of the automaton corresponding to C.

Using the notion of value-restriction sets, the automata-theoretic characterization of subsumption of cyclic $\mathcal{FLN}$-concept descriptions provided in [11] can be formulated as follows: $C \sqsubseteq D$ iff $L_D(P) \subseteq V_C(P)$ for all primitive concept names or number restrictions P. As an easy consequence, we obtain the following characterization of the lcs of such descriptions:

Corollary 1. *Let C, D be cyclic $\mathcal{FLN}$-concept descriptions. Then the cyclic $\mathcal{FLN}$-concept description E is the lcs of C and D if $L_E(P) = V_C(P) \cap V_D(P)$ for all primitive concept names or number restrictions P.*

Given automata for the (non-empty) value-restriction sets $V_C(P)$ and $V_D(P)$, it is easy to construct a cyclic $\mathcal{FLN}$-concept description E that satisfies this property (by simply translating the automata back into TBoxes). This shows that the lcs of two cyclic $\mathcal{FLN}$-concept descriptions can be computed in exponential time, and its size is at most exponential in the size of the input descriptions.

4 Computing the msc in $\mathcal{FLN}$-ABoxes with cyclic descriptions

In the following, we let $\mathcal{A}$ be an arbitrary but fixed $\mathcal{FLN}$-ABox with cyclic concept descriptions. In addition, we assume that $\mathcal{A}$ is consistent,[4] since for inconsistent ABoxes the msc is always the bottom concept $\bot$.

---

[3] For a language L and a letter R, we define $LR^{-1} := \{W \mid WR \in L\}$.

[4] An ABox is consistent iff it has a model. Note that testing $\mathcal{FLN}$-ABoxes with cyclic descriptions for consistency is a P-SPACE-complete problem [4].

In order to decide the instance problem and to compute the msc of an individual in $\mathcal{A}$, we again try to characterize value-restriction sets with the help of regular languages.

Definition 9. *Let a be an individual name in $\mathcal{A}$ and P a primitive concept name or a number restriction. Then the set $V_a(P) := \{W \in N_R^* \mid a \in_{\mathcal{A}} \forall W.P\}$ is called the* value-restriction set *of a for P.*

In addition to the automata corresponding to the cyclic concept descriptions in $\mathcal{A}$, we need an *automaton corresponding to $\mathcal{A}$*: the states of this automaton are the individual names occurring in $\mathcal{A}$, and the transitions are just the role assertions of $\mathcal{A}$, i.e., there is a transition with label R from a to b iff $R(a,b) \in \mathcal{A}$. For individual names a, b occurring in $\mathcal{A}$, the (regular) language $L_a(b)$ is the set of all words labeling paths from a to b in this automaton.

In the previous section, the value-restriction sets $V_C(P)$ for cyclic concept descriptions C could be characterized using the languages $L_C(P)$ and E_C. In order to characterize value-restriction sets for individuals, we first define a regular language whose rôle is similar to the one played by $L_C(P)$:

Definition 10. *Let a be an individual name in $\mathcal{A}$ and P a primitive concept name or a number restriction. Then the set*

$$L_a(P) := \{W \in N_R^* \mid \exists \text{ a concept assertion } C(b) \in \mathcal{A} \text{ and } U \in L_b(a) \\ \text{such that } UW \in L_C(P)\}$$

is called the predecessor restriction set *of a for P.*

In the situation described by the above definition, $C(b) \in \mathcal{A}$ implies that b^I belongs to C^I in any model I of $\mathcal{A}$. In addition, $U \in L_b(a)$ implies that a^I can be reached from b^I via (the interpretation of) the role chain U (i.e., b^I is a role predecessor of a^I). Thus, the value restriction $\forall UW.P$, which (because of $UW \in L_C(P)$) holds for all elements of C^I, and thus for b^I, propagates the value restriction $\forall W.P$ to a, i.e., $a^I \in (\forall W.P)^I$ holds for all models I of $\mathcal{A}$. This shows that $L_a(P) \subseteq V_a(P)$.

As for the corresponding inclusion stated in the previous section, this inclusion relationship may be strict, however. In a first attempt to overcome this problem, we introduce sets E_a corresponding to the sets E_C from the previous section. For this purpose, we adapt the syntactic definition of E_C (see the paragraph below Definition 8) by simply replacing the languages $L_C(\cdot)$ by $L_a(\cdot)$. Thus, if $W \in L_a(\leq m\, R) \cap L_a(\geq n\, R)$ for $m < n$, then W must belong to E_a; if $W \in L_a(\leq 0\, R)$, then $WR \in E_a$; etc. Unfortunately, this syntactic definition of E_a does not completely capture the semantic definition of the set of a-excluding words, i.e., the set of words E_a obtained this way may be smaller than $\{W \in N_R^* \mid a \in_{\mathcal{A}} \forall W.\bot\}$.

It turns out that this problem is a special case of the following more general problem: the definition of the languages $L_a(P)$ only takes into account value restrictions that come from predecessors of a. At-most restrictions in the ABox can, however, also require the propagation of value restrictions from successors of a back to a.

Let us first illustrate this phenomenon by a simple example. Assume that the ABox $\mathcal{A}$ consists of the following assertions: $R(a,b), (\leq 1\ R)(a), (\forall S.P)(b)$. It is easy to see that $RS \notin L_a(P) \cup E_a$. However, $(\leq 1\ R)(a)$ makes sure that, in any model I of $\mathcal{A}$, b^I is the only R^I-successor of a^I. Consequently, all $(RS)^I$-successors of a^I are S^I-successors of b^I, and thus $b^I \in (\forall S.P)^I$ implies $a^I \in (\forall RS.P)^I$. This shows that $RS \in V_a(P)$.

More generally, this problem occurs if concept assertions involving at-most restrictions in the ABox force role chains to use role assertions explicitly present in the ABox. In the example, we were forced to use the assertion $R(a,b)$ when going from a^I to an $(RS)^I$-successor of a^I. As a slightly more complex example, we assume that the ABox $\mathcal{A}$ contains the assertions

$$R(a,b), \quad R(a,c), \quad S(b,d), \quad (\leq 2\ R)(a), \quad (\forall R.(\leq 1\ S))(a),$$

and that $S \in L_c(P)$ and $\varepsilon \in L_d(P)$, where ε denotes the empty word. In a model I of $\mathcal{A}$, any $(RS)^I$-successor x of a^I is either equal to d^I or an S^I-successor of c^I. In the first case, $\varepsilon \in L_d(P)$ implies $x \in P^I$, and in the second case $S \in L_c(P)$ does the same. Consequently, we have $RS \in V_a(P)$, even though $RS \notin L_a(P) \cup E_a$. Here, we are forced to use either the assertions $R(a,b)$ and $R(b,d)$ or the assertion $R(a,c)$ when going from a^I to one of its $(RS)^I$-successors. Since in both cases the obtained successor must belong to P^I, a restriction on P must be propagated back to a from the successors of a.

Unfortunately, it is not yet clear how to give a *direct* characterization (as a regular language) of $V_a(P)$ that is based on an appropriate characterization of the set of words in $V_a(P) \backslash (L_a(P) \cup E_a)$ that come from this "backward propagation." Instead, we will first describe the complement of $V_a(P)$ as a regular language. Since the class of regular languages is closed under complement, this also shows that $V_a(P)$ is regular. In the following, we restrict our attention to the case where P is a primitive concept name. Number restrictions can be treated similarly.

Before we can give the characterization of $\overline{V_a(P)}$, we need to define one more set of words. Let $R_{\mathcal{A}}(a) := \{b \mid R(a,b) \in \mathcal{A}\}$ denote the set of explicit R-successors of a in $\mathcal{A}$, and let $|R_{\mathcal{A}}(a)|$ denote the cardinality of this set. In addition, let $c_a^{\leq R} := min\{n \mid \varepsilon \in L_a(\leq n\ R)\}$ denote the minimal number occurring in an at-most restriction that must hold for a. Then we define

$$N_a := \{\varepsilon\} \cup \bigcup \{R \cdot N_R^* \mid R \in N_R \text{ and } |R_{\mathcal{A}}(a)| < c_a^{\leq R}\}.$$

Intuitively, a word of the form RU belongs to N_a if at-most restrictions in the ABox do not force all R-successors of a to be reached using role assertions explicitly present in the ABox. The empty word is contained in N_a for technical reasons.

Using the language N_a as well as the languages $L_a(P)$, $L_b(a)$, and E_a, the complement $\overline{V_b(P)}$ of the value-restriction set of b for P can be described as follows:

$$\overline{V_b(P)} = \bigcup_{a \in I_{\mathcal{A}}} L_b(a) \cdot (N_a \cap \overline{L_a(P) \cup E_a}),$$

where I_A denotes the set of all individual names occurring in $\mathcal{A}$.

Intuitively, this identity can be explained as follows. Assume that the word W does not belong to $V_b(P)$. Then there exists a model I of $\mathcal{A}$ and an element x of $dom(I)$ such that $(b^I, x) \in W^I$ and $x \notin P^I$. A (possibly empty) initial segment V^I of the W^I-role path from b^I to x uses role assertions from $\mathcal{A}$. Let V be the maximal prefix of W for which this is the case, i.e., $W = VV'$ and there is an individual a in $\mathcal{A}$ such that $V \in L_b(a)$, $(b^I, a^I) \in V^I$, $(a^I, x) \in V'^I$, and (i) either $V' = \varepsilon$, (ii) or $V' = RV''$ and the transition from a^I to its R^I-successor on the V''-role path from a^I to x does not correspond to a role assertion in $\mathcal{A}$. In both cases, we can deduce that $V' \in N_a$. In addition, because $x \notin P^I$, the word V' cannot belong to $L_a(P) \cup E_a$.

For number restrictions P, the complement $\overline{V_b(P)}$ of the value-restriction sets can be characterized analogously. The only difference is that at-least restrictions require a slightly modified set N_a:

$$N_a(\geq m\,R) := \begin{cases} N_a \setminus \{\varepsilon\} & \text{if } |R_\mathcal{A}(a)| \geq m \\ N_a & \text{otherwise} \end{cases}$$

To sum up, we can give the following characterization of value restriction sets (see [4] for a formal proof of correctness):

Theorem 2 (value-restriction sets). *Let $\mathcal{A}$ be a consistent $\mathcal{FLN}$-ABox with cyclic concept descriptions, b be an individual name occurring in $\mathcal{A}$, P a primitive concept name, R a role name, m a positive integer, and n a non-negative integer.*

$$V_b(P) = \bigcup_{a \in I_A} L_b(a) \cdot \overline{(N_a \cap \overline{L_a(P) \cup E_a})},$$

$$V_b(\geq m\,R) = \bigcup_{a \in I_A} L_b(a) \cdot \overline{(N_a(\geq m\,R) \cap \overline{\bigcup_{\ell \geq m} L_a(\geq \ell R) \cup E_a})},$$

$$V_b(\leq n\,R) = \bigcup_{a \in I_A} L_b(a) \cdot \overline{(N_a \cap \overline{\bigcup_{\ell \leq n} L_a(\leq \ell R) \cup E_a R^{-1}})}.$$

Since the languages N_a, $L_a(P)$, $L_b(a)$, and E_a involved in this characterization are regular and finite automata accepting them can effectively be computed, the value-restriction sets are also regular and can effectively be computed. Using these sets, the instance problem can now be decided as follows:

Theorem 3 (instance). *Let $\mathcal{A}$ be a consistent $\mathcal{FLN}$-ABox with cyclic concept descriptions, C be a cyclic $\mathcal{FLN}$-concept description, and b an individual occurring in $\mathcal{A}$. Then $b \in_\mathcal{A} C$ iff for all primitive concept names or number restrictions P we have $L_C(P) \subseteq V_b(P)$.*

As an easy consequence of this theorem, we obtain the following characterization of the msc:

Corollary 2. *Let $\mathcal{A}$ be a consistent $\mathcal{FLN}$-ABox with cyclic concept descriptions, C be a cyclic $\mathcal{FLN}$-concept description, and b an individual occurring in*

$\mathcal{A}$. Then C is the msc of b in $\mathcal{A}$ if for all primitive concept names or number restrictions P we have $L_C(P) = V_b(P)$.

Given automata for the sets $V_b(P)$ it is again easy to construct a cyclic $\mathcal{FLN}$-concept description E that satisfies this property. This shows that the msc can effectively be computed.

5   Related and future work

An important topic for future work is to determine the exact worst-case complexities for computing the lcs and the msc, and for deciding the instance problem for $\mathcal{FLN}$-ABoxes with cyclic concept descriptions. Our algorithm for computing the lcs of two cyclic $\mathcal{FLN}$-concept descriptions is exponential, and we conjecture that this complexity cannot be avoided, i.e., there is no polynomial algorithm for computing the lcs in this case. One point supporting this conjecture is that subsumption for cyclic $\mathcal{FLN}$-concept descriptions is already PSPACE-complete (see [11]). It is, however, not clear how to reduce the subsumption problem (in polynomial time) to the problem of computing the lcs. In fact, if $C \sqsubseteq D$, then the lcs of C and D is equivalent to D, but testing for this equivalence may be as hard as testing for subsumption.

A naive analysis of the algorithms for deciding the instance problem and for computing the msc derived from our characterization of value-restriction sets would yield a triply exponential upper bound. In fact, the first exponential step is due to the fact that an automaton for E_a may already be exponential in the size of the input. The other two exponential steps are due to the two complements occurring in the characterization of the value-restriction sets.[5] We conjecture, however, that the instance problem can be decided in PSPACE, and that the msc can be computed in exponential time.

To the best of our knowledge, all the existing work on computing the lcs of description logic concepts [7,9,8] can only handle acyclic concept descriptions. In addition, the approach for computing the msc proposed by Cohen and Hirsh [9] yields only an approximation of the msc. In fact, since they allow for acyclic descriptions only, they cannot always derive an exact description for the msc. The pragmatic solution proposed in [9] is to restrict the length of value restriction chains occurring in the computed description by some arbitrary but fixed number. This way, one obtains an acyclic description, which may, however, be less specific than the real msc.

Kietz and Morik [10] consider the problem of inductively learning concept descriptions from ABoxes. On the one hand, this work is more restrictive than ours since it does not allow for complex descriptions (not even acyclic ones) in the ABoxes. On the other hand, it tries to solve a more ambitious problem since it tries to learn completely new descriptions from known ABox facts. To this purpose, several heuristic steps are employed. In contrast, computing the lcs

---

[5] since computing the complement of a regular language requires a powerset construction.

and the msc is a purely deductive problem that does not invent new descriptions: it just detects and collects commonalities of given descriptions in an appropriate way.

References

1. F. Baader. A formal definition for the expressive power of terminological knowledge representation languages. *J. of Logic and Computation*, 6(1):33–54, 1996.
2. F. Baader. Using automata theory for characterizing the semantics of terminological cycles. *Annals of Mathematics and Artificial Intelligence*, 18(2–4):175–219, 1996.
3. F. Baader and B. Hollunder. A terminological knowledge representation system with complete inference algorithms. In *Proceedings of the First International Workshop on Processing Declarative Knowledge*, volume 572 of *Lecture Notes in Computer Science*, pages 67–85, Kaiserslautern (Germany), 1991. Springer–Verlag.
4. F. Baader and R. Küsters. Computing the least common subsumer and the most specific concept in the presence of cyclic $\mathcal{ALN}$-concept descriptions. Technical Report LTCS-Report 98-06, LuFg Theoretical Computer Science, RWTH Aachen, Germany, 1998. See http://www-lti.informatik.rwth-aachen.de/Forschung/Papers.html.
5. F. Baader and U. Sattler. Knowledge representation in process engineering. In *Proceedings of the International Workshop on Description Logics*, Cambridge (Boston), MA, U.S.A., 1996. AAAI Press/The MIT Press.
6. A. Borgida, R. J. Brachman, D. L. McGuinness, and L. A. Resnick. CLASSIC: A structural data model for objects. In *Proceedings of the 1989 ACM SIGMOD International Conference on Management of Data*, pages 59–67, Portland, OR, 1989.
7. W. W. Cohen, A. Borgida, and H. Hirsh. Computing least common subsumers in description logics. In William Swartout, editor, *Proceedings of the 10th National Conference on Artificial Intelligence*, pages 754–760, San Jose, CA, July 1992. MIT Press.
8. W. W. Cohen and H. Hirsh. Learnability of description logics with equality constraints. *Machine Learning*, 17(2/3), 1994.
9. W. W. Cohen and H. Hirsh. Learning the classic description logic: Theoretical and experimental results. In *Proceedings of the Fourth International Conference on Principles of Knowledge Representation and Reasoning (KR'94)*, pages 121–133, San Francisco, Calif., 1994. Morgan Kaufmann.
10. J.-U. Kietz and K. Morik. A polynomial approach to the constructive induction of structural knowledge. *Machine Learning Journal*, 14(2):193–218, 1994.
11. R. Küsters. Characterizing the semantics of terminological cycles in $\mathcal{ALN}$ using finite automata. In *Proceedings of the Sixth International Conference on Principles of Knowledge Representation and Reasoning (KR'98)*, pages 499–510, Trento, Italy, 1998.
12. B. Nebel. Terminological cycles: Semantics and computational properties. In J. Sowa, editor, *Formal Aspects of Semantic Networks*, pages 331–361. Morgan Kaufmann, San Mateo, 1991.
13. W. A. Woods and J. G. Schmolze. The KL-ONE family. *Computers and Mathematics with Applications, special issue on knowledge representation*, 23(2-5):133–177, 1991.

Simultaneous Quantifier Elimination

Serge Autexier[1], Heiko Mantel[2], and Werner Stephan[2]

[1] Universität des Saarlandes, FB Informatik
Postfach 15 11 50, 66041 Saarbrücken, Germany
autexier@ags.uni-sb.de
[2] German Research Center for Artificial Intelligence (DFKI)
Stuhlsatzenhausweg 3, 66123 Saarbrücken, Germany
{mantel,stephan}@dfki.de

Abstract. We present a sequent calculus which allows the simultaneous elimination of multiple quantifiers. The approach is an improvement over the well-known skolemization in sequent calculus. It allows a lazy handling of instantiations and of the order of certain reductions. Simultaneous quantifier elimination is justified from a semantical as well as from a proof theoretical point of view.

1 Introduction

Sequent calculi are a very common search space representation. Originally developed by Gentzen [6] they have been applied in automated deduction, in logic programming, in formal program development, and other areas. During analytic proof search formulas in a sequent are decomposed into sub-formulas in a stepwise manner. The structure of sub-formulas and of formulas which are not decomposed is preserved. The preservation of structure is especially beneficial when user interaction is required. A user can recognize structures which e.g. in the context of formal methods [7] originate from a specification.

The relation between standard presentations of Hilbert type, natural deduction, and sequent calculi has been investigated by Avron [2] for the propositional case. The additional structure in sequent calculi usually provides advantages in proof search. In the presence of quantifiers additional differences between these type of calculi arise. Gentzen's rules for the elimination of quantifiers employ an eager handling of instantiations. This causes a high-degree of non-determinism in proof search which can be avoided by a lazy handling of instantiations with meta-variables together with a computation of instantiations by unification. *Skolemization* [13] is a well-known technique which guarantees that proofs constructed with a lazy handling of instantiations can be validated in general. In the context of sequent calculi, skolemization has been investigated for classical [4] as well as for non-classical logics [12, 9].

The technique for simultaneous quantifier elimination presented in this article is specific to sequent calculi. It provides an optimization over the usual approach for lazy handling of instantiations. The two justifications of its soundness yield different insights in the dependencies between formulas of a sequent in the presence of quantifiers.

After some fundamentals we present in section 3 a sequent calculus $\mathcal{K}$ with a rule for simultaneous quantifier elimination. We point out its advantages in comparison to usual handling of quantifiers in sequent calculus proof search. The soundness of $\mathcal{K}$ is demonstrated in section 4 using semantical and in section 5 using syntactical arguments. We conclude with some remarks on related work.

2 Fundamentals

Basing on [10], we define syntax and semantics of first-order logic. A *signature* Σ is a pair $(\mathcal{F}, \mathcal{P})$ consisting of a set $\mathcal{F}$ of operation symbols and a set $\mathcal{P}$ of predicate symbols. Each $f \in \mathcal{F}$ has an arity $n_f \in \mathbb{N}$ and each $p \in \mathcal{P}$ has an arity $n_p \in \mathbb{N}$. A Σ-*algebra* A has a *carrier set* S_A and assigns to each n_f-ary operation $f \in \mathcal{F}$ a total function $A(f) : (S_A)^{n_f} \to S_A$ and to each predicate $p \in \mathcal{P}$ a n_p-ary relation $A(p) \subseteq (S_A)^{n_p}$. *Constants* are 0-ary operations.

Syntax of First-Order Logic. The set $T_\Sigma(\mathcal{V})$ of *first-order terms* for a signature Σ and a set $\mathcal{V}$ of variables is defined recursively. For each $x \in \mathcal{V}$ holds $x \in T_\Sigma(\mathcal{V})$. If $t_1, \ldots, t_{n_f} \in T_\Sigma(\mathcal{V})$ then for any n_f-ary operation $f \in \mathcal{F}$ holds $f(t_1, \ldots, t_{n_f}) \in T_\Sigma(\mathcal{V})$. The set $wff(\Sigma, \mathcal{V})$ of *first-order formulas* for $\Sigma = (\mathcal{F}, \mathcal{P})$ and $\mathcal{V}$ is defined recursively. For $t_1, \ldots, t_{n_p} \in T_\Sigma(\mathcal{V})$ and $p \in \mathcal{P}$ with arity n_p the expression $p(t_1, \ldots, t_{n_p})$ is an *atomic formula* in $wff(\Sigma, \mathcal{V})$. If $\varphi, \psi \in wff(\Sigma, \mathcal{V})$ and $x \in \mathcal{V}$ then $\neg\varphi, \varphi \wedge \psi, \varphi \vee \psi, \forall x.\varphi, \exists x.\varphi \in wff(\Sigma, \mathcal{V})$ are formulas.

For a term t the function *Var* returns the variables and *Op* the operations which occur in t. The function *free* which returns the free variables of a formula is defined recursively over the structure of formulas, i.e. $free(p(t_1, \ldots, t_{n_p})) = \bigcup_{i=1}^{n_p} Var(t_i)$, $free(\neg\varphi) = free(\varphi)$, $free(\varphi \overset{\wedge}{\vee} \psi) = free(\varphi) \cup free(\psi)$, and $free(\overset{\forall}{\exists} x.\varphi) = free(\varphi) \setminus \{x\}$. *Op* returns for φ the operations which occur in φ.

Semantics of First-Order Logic. The *value* $A(\alpha)(t)$ of a term $t \in T_\Sigma(\mathcal{V})$ and the *value* $A(\alpha)(\varphi)$ of a formula $\varphi \in wff(\Sigma, \mathcal{V})$ for a Σ-algebra A and an assignment $\alpha : \mathcal{V} \to S_A$ where $free(\varphi) \subseteq \mathcal{V}$ is respectively an element of the carrier set S_A or a truth value (*true* or *false*).

- $A(\alpha)(x) = \alpha(x)$ for $x \in \mathcal{V}$,
- $A(\alpha)(f(t_1, \ldots, t_{n_f})) = A(f)(A(\alpha)(t_1), \ldots, A(\alpha)(t_{n_f}))$,
- $A(\alpha)(p(t_1, \ldots, t_{n_p})) = true$ iff $(A(\alpha)(t_1), \ldots, A(\alpha)(t_{n_p})) \in A(p)$,
- $A(\alpha)(\neg\varphi) = true$ iff $A(\alpha)(\varphi) = false$,
- $A(\alpha)(\varphi_1 \overset{\wedge}{\vee} \varphi_2) = true$ iff $A(\alpha)(\varphi_1) = true \overset{and}{or} A(\alpha)(\varphi_2) = true$,
- $A(\alpha)(\overset{\forall}{\exists} x.\varphi) = true$ iff $(A(\alpha[a/x])(\varphi) = true \underset{\text{for some}}{\text{for all}} a \in A(s))$.

where $\alpha[a/x]$ is the assignment: $\alpha[a/x](x) = a$ and $\alpha[a/x](y) = \alpha(y)$, if $y \neq x$. A formula φ is *valid in a Σ-algebra* A $(A \models_\Sigma \varphi)$ iff for any assignment α holds $A(\alpha)(\varphi) = true$. A formula φ is *valid* $(\models_\Sigma \varphi)$ iff it is valid in every Σ-algebra.

Substitutions. Let Σ be a signature and $\mathcal{V}$ be a set of variables for Σ. A function $\sigma : \mathcal{V} \to T_{\Sigma(\mathcal{V})}$ is called a *substitution*. The application of a substitution to a formula $\varphi \in wff(\Sigma, \mathcal{V})$ yields a formula $\sigma(\varphi)$, where all free occurrences of variables $x \in \mathcal{V}$ are replaced by $\sigma(x)$. If σ is the identity except for a finite number of variables $x_1, \ldots, x_n$, we denote σ by $[\sigma(x_1)/x_1, \ldots, \sigma(x_n)/x_n]$. $Dom(\sigma) = \{x_1, \ldots, x_n\}$ is called the *domain* of σ. A substitution σ is *admissible* for φ if for every sub-formula $Qx.\varphi'$ of φ holds $x \notin \sigma(y)$ for all $y \in free(Qx.\varphi')$. We require substitutions to be idempotent and admissible.

The following theorem states a fundamental relationship between substitutions and assignments. For a proof we refer the interested reader to [10].

Theorem 1 (Substitution Theorem). *Let V be a set of variables for a signature Σ, $\sigma : V \rightarrow T_{\Sigma(V)}$ a substitution, A a Σ-algebra, and $\beta : V \rightarrow S_A$ an assignment. Then for every $t \in T_{\Sigma(V)}$ holds $A(\beta)(\sigma(t)) = A(\alpha)(t)$, where $\alpha : V \rightarrow S_A$ is an assignment defined by $\alpha(x) := A(\beta)(\sigma(x))$ for every $x \in V$.*

We restrict ourselves throughout this article to formulas in *negation-normal form*, i.e. formulas where negation $\neg$ occurs only directly in front of atomic formulas. Using the de-Morgan laws any first-order formula can be transformed into an equivalent formula which is in negation normal form.

Sequents. A *(one-sided) sequent* s is a set Γ of formulas in negation-normal form denoted by $\longrightarrow \Gamma$. We define $free(\longrightarrow \Gamma) = \bigcup_{\varphi \in \Gamma} free(\varphi)$. Given an algebra A and an assignment $\alpha : V \rightarrow S_A$ with $free(s) \subseteq V$. The *value* $A(\alpha)(s)$ is *true* iff $A(\alpha)(\varphi) = true$ for some $\varphi \in \Gamma$. s is *valid in* an algebra A ($A \models_\Sigma s$) if for all assignments α $A(\alpha)(s) = true$. s is *valid* ($\models_\Sigma s$) if it is valid in all algebras.

A *sequent calculus* is a pair $\langle Ax, Inf \rangle$. Ax is a finite set of axiom schemes each of which is a decidable set of sequents. Inf is a finite set of inference rules. Each inference rule consists of a decidable set of pairs $(s_1, \ldots, s_n), s$ where $s_1, \ldots, s_n$ and s are sequents. s is called the *conclusion* and $s_1, \ldots, s_n$ the *premises* of the inference rule. A *principal formula* is a formula that occurs in the conclusion but not in any premise. Formulas which occur in a premise but not in the conclusion are called *side formulas*. All other formulas compose the *context*. Sequent rules can be represented graphically where the conclusion is written underneath the premises and separated from them by a horizontal line. A *derivation* of a sequent s from a set of sequents S is a finite sequence of sequents $s_1, \ldots, s_k$ with $k \geq 1$ and $s_k = s$ such that for each $i \leq k$ holds $s_i \in S$, s_i is an axiom in Ax, or there exist indices $i_1, \ldots, i_n$ such that there is an inference rule in Inf with conclusion s_i and premises $s_{i_1}, \ldots, s_{i_n}$. A sequent s is said to be *derivable* from a set of sequents S ($S \vdash s$) if there exists a derivation from S for it.

The one-sided sequent calculus $\mathcal{K}_c$ for formulas in negation normal form[1] is:

$$\frac{}{\longrightarrow \Gamma, \varphi, \neg\varphi} \; ax \qquad \frac{\longrightarrow \Gamma, \varphi_1 \quad \longrightarrow \Gamma, \varphi_2}{\longrightarrow \Gamma, \varphi_1 \wedge \varphi_2} \; \wedge \qquad \frac{\longrightarrow \Gamma, \varphi_1, \varphi_2}{\longrightarrow \Gamma, \varphi_1 \vee \varphi_2} \; \vee \qquad \frac{\longrightarrow \Gamma, \varphi[c/x]}{\longrightarrow \Gamma, \forall x.\varphi} \; \forall^* \qquad \frac{\longrightarrow \Gamma, \varphi[t/x]}{\longrightarrow \Gamma, \exists x.\varphi} \; \exists^{**}$$

$*$ c must not occur in $\longrightarrow \Gamma, \forall x.\varphi$ (*Eigenvariable condition*). $**$ t may be any term.

In *analytic proof search* with $\mathcal{K}_c$ one starts with the sequent to be proven and reduces it by application of rules until the *ax*-rule is applicable.

3 Simultaneous Quantifier Elimination

The quantifier rules of $\mathcal{K}_c$ cause problems in analytic proof search. Whenever the $\exists$-rule is applied a term t must be guessed immediately. To postpone the choice of t until more information about good choices of t are at hand is a superior approach. In order to do so the rule $\exists'$ depicted below inserts a free variable

---

[1] The restriction to formulas in negation-normal form and to one-sided sequents has only presentational purposes. The theory presented in this article could also be developed for arbitrary formulas and two-sided sequents.

X (sometimes also called *meta-variable*) which is implicitly existentially quantified. Thus, it may be instantiated later during proof search. However, precautions must be taken to guarantee the correctness of the resulting proofs because not all possible instantiations are admissible. *Skolemization* is used for this purpose. The rule *Skolem* inserts a *skolem-term* consisting of a new function symbol with all free variables of the sequent as arguments. Free variables may be instantiated during proof search. The instantiation of a variable affects all parts of a derivation where the variable occurs, i.e. *Inst* is a rewrite rule on derivations rather than an ordinary sequent rule. The *occur-check* ensures that a variable X can only be substituted by terms t which do not contain X.

$$\frac{\longrightarrow \Gamma, \varphi[X/x]}{\longrightarrow \Gamma, \exists x. \varphi} \, \exists' \qquad \frac{\longrightarrow \Gamma, \varphi[f(Z)/x]}{\longrightarrow \Gamma, \forall x. \varphi} \, Skolem^* \qquad \boxed{X} \rightsquigarrow \boxed{t} \quad Inst(X,t)^{**}$$

    * f must not occur in $s = \longrightarrow \Gamma, \forall x. \varphi$ and Z must contain all free variables of s.
   ** X must not occur in t and all variables and operations in t must also occur in the left-hand side proof-tree.

The calculus $\mathcal{K}_{sk}$ results from $\mathcal{K}_c$ by adding the rules $\exists'$, *Skolem*, and *Inst* while the rules $\exists$ and $\forall$ are removed.

The use of free variables and skolemization allows to postpone the instantiation until it can be computed, e.g. by unification. Nevertheless, if multiple quantified formulas occur in a sequent a principal formula must be determined. Although in some cases a principal formula can be chosen in a safe way, in general, the right order of reductions cannot be calculated from a sequent. This is demonstrated by the following example.

Example 2. Below a $\mathcal{K}_{sk}$-derivation with six rule applications is depicted.

$$\frac{\dfrac{\dfrac{\dfrac{\dfrac{\dfrac{\longrightarrow \varphi(X_1, f_1(X_1), Z_1), \neg\varphi(Z_2, X_2, f_2(X_1, X_2))}{\longrightarrow \varphi(X_1, f_1(X_1), Z_1), \exists z_2. \neg\varphi(z_2, X_2, f_2(X_1, X_2))} \, \exists'}{\longrightarrow \exists z_1. \varphi(X_1, f_1(X_1), z_1), \exists z_2. \neg\varphi(z_2, X_2, f_2(X_1, X_2))} \, \exists'}{\longrightarrow \exists z_1. \varphi(X_1, f_1(X_1), z_1), \forall y_2. \exists z_2. \neg\varphi(z_2, X_2, y_2)} \, Skolem}{\longrightarrow \exists z_1. \varphi(X_1, f_1(X_1), z_1), \exists x_2. \forall y_2. \exists z_2. \neg\varphi(z_2, x_2, y_2)} \, \exists'}{\longrightarrow \forall y_1. \exists z_1. \varphi(X_1, y_1, z_1), \exists x_2. \forall y_2. \exists z_2. \neg\varphi(z_2, x_2, y_2)} \, Skolem}{\longrightarrow \exists x_1. \forall y_1. \exists z_1. \varphi(x_1, y_1, z_1), \exists x_2. \forall y_2. \exists z_2. \neg\varphi(z_2, x_2, y_2)} \, \exists'$$

The proof attempt would have failed if we first had reduced the second formula.

A Rule for Simultaneous Quantifier Elimination. Simultaneous quantifier elimination is based on skolemization. However, it is superior since it allows a lazy handling of both instantiations and reduction orderings on quantified formulas.

We define *quantifier lists* ql recursively starting from the empty list ϵ and for a variable x by $\forall x. ql'$ and $\exists x. ql'$. In order to simplify the following definition we assume generators *vgen* and *fgen* which respectively generate new symbols for variables and operations on every call.

We define the *quantifier elimination function* QE which takes a quantifier list ql, a formula φ, and a set Z of variables as arguments and returns a formula. ql determines which quantifiers shall be eliminated from φ. Z is used in order to determine the arguments of skolem functions.

   – $\mathrm{QE}(\epsilon, \varphi, Z) := \varphi$,
   – $\mathrm{QE}(\forall x. ql, \varphi, Z) := \mathrm{QE}(ql, \varphi[f(Z)/x], Z)$, where $f := fgen$ is new.
   – $\mathrm{QE}(\exists x. ql, \varphi, Z) := \mathrm{QE}(ql, \varphi[X/x], Z \cup \{X\}$ where $X := vgen$ is new.

The rule *SQEl* for *simultaneous quantifier elimination* is depicted below.

$$\frac{\longrightarrow \Gamma, \psi_1, \ldots, \psi_n}{\longrightarrow \Gamma, \mathrm{ql}_1.\varphi_1, \ldots, \mathrm{ql}_n.\varphi_n} \ SQEl^*$$

* For each i $(1 \leq i \leq n)$ must hold $\psi_i = \mathrm{QE}(\mathrm{ql}_i, \varphi_i, \mathrm{free}(\longrightarrow \Gamma, \mathrm{ql}_1.\varphi_1, \ldots, \mathrm{ql}_n.\varphi_n))$.

The calculus $\mathcal{K}$ results from $\mathcal{K}_{sk}$ by replacing the rules $\exists'$ and *Skolem* by *SQEl*. $\mathcal{K}$ is complete with respect to $\mathcal{K}_{sk}$, i.e. for every sequent s which is $\mathcal{K}_{sk}$-derivable there is a $\mathcal{K}$-derivation, since $\exists'$ and *Skolem* can be simulated by *SQEl*. However, *SQEl* has advantages compared to these rules because one does not need to bother about the order of certain reductions.

Example 3. We reduce our example sequent by *SQEl*.

$$\frac{\longrightarrow \varphi(X_1, f_1(X_1), Z_1), \neg\varphi(Z_2, X_2, f_2(X_2))}{\longrightarrow \exists x_1.\forall y_1.\exists z_1.\varphi(x_1, y_1, z_1), \exists x_2.\forall y_2.\exists z_2.\neg\varphi(z_2, x_2, y_2)} \ SQEl$$

A comparison to example 2 shows the advantages of simultaneous quantifier elimination. First, one does not need to worry about the order of quantifier eliminations. Second, the skolem term in the second formula depends only on X_2 and not on both X_1 and X_2 as in example 2. This shows that the quantifier elimination of different formulas in a sequent do not depend on each other.

Remark 4. In the Isabelle system [11] for example a dual technique to skolemization is employed. According to this technique a universally quantified formula $\forall x.\varphi(x)$ is reduced to $\bigwedge x.\varphi(x)$ and an existentially quantified formula $\exists x.\varphi(x)$ to $\varphi(?x)$ where $\bigwedge$ is a meta-logic quantifier and $?x$ is a (higher-order) meta-variable. Due to lifting over quantifiers meta-variables receive arguments which essentially determine which constants may be used in instantiations. This causes close interdependencies between formulas in a sequent which are not present when skolemization is applied. Before a constant may be instantiated, i.e. appear as an argument of a meta-variable, the corresponding quantifier must have been reduced already. Therefore, it appears to be quite difficult to develop an optimized handling of quantifiers equivalent to *SQEl* for this technique. For details of the technique we refer the interested reader to [11].

4 Semantical Justification

In this section we present a correctness proof for $\mathcal{K}$ using semantical arguments. For this purpose an auxiliary calculus $\mathcal{K}_{aux}$ is defined which allows to reason about sequents with substitutions. The explicitly stated substitutions are used for meta-level arguments only. We prove the soundness of $\mathcal{K}_{aux}$ and then conclude the soundness of $\mathcal{K}$ from that. In the process we introduce orderings on constants and variables, an approach which is motivated by orderings on positions in the context of matrix characterizations.[3, 14]

Sequents with Substitutions. A *sequent with substitution s* is a pair $\longrightarrow \Gamma; \sigma$ consisting of a sequent $\longrightarrow \Gamma$ and a substitution σ. We define $\mathit{free}(s) = \bigcup_{\varphi \in \Gamma} \mathit{free}(\sigma(\varphi))$. The *value* $A(\alpha)(s)$ is *true* in an algebra A under an assignment $\alpha : \mathcal{V} \to S_A$ where $\mathit{free}(s) \subseteq \mathcal{V}$ iff $A(\alpha)(\longrightarrow \sigma(\Gamma)) = \mathit{true}$.

Below, we define the *auxiliary quantifier elimination function* QE_{aux} which takes a quantifier list ql, a formula φ, a set O of constants and variables, and a binary relation $\ll$ over O as arguments. ql determines which quantified variables shall be eliminated from φ. In O the set of all constants and variables introduced during the elimination are collected while a relation over these symbols is collected in $\ll$. QE_{aux} returns a triple consisting of a formula φ', a set O' of constants and variables, and an ordering $\ll'$ over O'.

- $QE_{aux}(\epsilon, \varphi, O, \ll) := \langle \varphi, O, \ll \rangle$,
- $QE_{aux}(\forall x.\text{ql}, \varphi, O, \ll) := QE_{aux}(\text{ql}, \varphi[c/x], O \cup \{c\}, \ll \cup \{(o,c) \mid \forall o \in O\})$,
  where $c := fgen$ is new.
- $QE_{aux}(\exists x.\text{ql}, \varphi, O, \ll) := QE_{aux}(\text{ql}, \varphi[X/x], O \cup \{X\}, \ll \cup \{(o,X) \mid \forall o \in O\})$
  where $X := vgen$ is new.

Example 5. With the appropriate symbols generated by *vgen* and *fgen* the value of $(\forall x_1 \exists y_1 \forall z_1, \varphi(x_1, y_1, z_1), \emptyset, \emptyset)$ under QE_{aux} is
$$\langle \varphi(X_1, c_1, Z_1), \{X_1, c_1, Z_1\}, \{(X_1, c_1), (X_1, Z_1), (c_1, Z_1)\}\rangle.$$

Orderings on Constants and Variables. QE_{aux} eliminates quantifiers in the order in which they occur in ql. This order is represented by the relation $\ll$ on the variables and constants introduced during elimination which is returned by QE_{aux}. Clearly, $\ll$ is an ordering, the *quantifier list ordering*.

For a set of variables $\mathcal{V}$, a set of constants $\mathcal{C}$, and a substitution σ we define two relations $\sim \subseteq \mathcal{V} \times \mathcal{V}$ and $\sqsubseteq \subseteq (\mathcal{V} \cup \mathcal{C}) \times \mathcal{V}$ as the minimal relations such that:

- for any $u, v \in \mathcal{V}$ if $\sigma(u) = v$ then $u \sim v$,
- for any $u \in \mathcal{V}$ and $v \in \mathcal{C} \cup \mathcal{V}$ if v occurs in $\sigma(u)$ and $\sigma(u) \neq v$ then $v \sqsubset u$,
- and for any $u, v \in \mathcal{V}$ if $v \sqsubset u$ and $u \sim u'$ then $v \sqsubset u'$.

We combine given orderings $\sqsubset$ and $\ll$ to a relation $\lhd \subseteq (\mathcal{C} \cup \mathcal{V})^2$, i.e. $\lhd = (\sqsubset \cup \ll)^+$ where $^+$ denotes the transitive closure. Indicating that $\lhd$ is intended to be usually irreflexive we call it a *reduction ordering*. If $\lhd$ is a reduction ordering over some set O of variables and constants and $O' \subseteq O$, then the *restriction* of $\lhd$ to O' is defined by $\lhd_{O'} := \{(o, o') \mid (o, o') \in \lhd \text{ and } o, o' \in O'\}$.

Calculus for Sequents with Substitutions. The auxiliary calculus $\mathcal{K}_{aux}$ is depicted below. Substitutions are explicitly stated and do not change in a $\mathcal{K}_{aux}$-proof. This is not problematic since we use the calculus only to reason about its soundness but not for proof search. Note, that in contrast to $\mathcal{K}$ in $\mathcal{K}_{aux}$ no skolem-terms are introduced during quantifier elimination.

$$\frac{}{\longrightarrow \Gamma, \varphi, \neg\varphi; \sigma} \, ax \qquad \frac{\longrightarrow \Gamma, \varphi_1; \sigma \quad \longrightarrow \Gamma, \varphi_2; \sigma}{\longrightarrow \Gamma, \varphi_1 \wedge \varphi_2; \sigma} \, \wedge \qquad \frac{\longrightarrow \Gamma, \psi_1, \ldots, \psi_n; \sigma}{\longrightarrow \Gamma, \text{ql}_1 \cdot \varphi_1, \ldots, \text{ql}_n \cdot \varphi_n; \sigma} \, SQEl_{aux}^{*} \qquad \frac{\longrightarrow \Gamma \sigma'; \sigma}{\longrightarrow \Gamma; \sigma} \, Subst^{**}$$

* For each $i \in \{1, \ldots, n\}$ holds $\langle \psi_i, O_i \ll_i \rangle = QE_{aux}(\text{ql}_i, \varphi_i, \text{free}(\longrightarrow \Gamma, \psi_1, \ldots, \psi_n), \emptyset)$, $\sqsubset$ the ordering from σ, $\ll = (\bigcup_{i=1}^{n} \ll_i)$, $\lhd = (\sqsubset \cup \ll)^+$, $O = \bigcup_{i=1}^{n} O_i$ the set of (free) variables and constants occurring in the premise and $\lhd_O$ is an irreflexive ordering.
** Where $\sigma \circ \sigma' = \sigma$ holds.

Example 6. The orderings $\ll$, $\sqsubset$, and $\lhd_O$ for the following rule application are depicted in the diagram to the right. $\ll$ is symbolized by solid arrows and $\sqsubset$ by dashed arrows.

$$\frac{\longrightarrow \varphi(X_1, c_1, Z_1), \neg\varphi(X_2, c_2, Z_2); \{Z_2/X_1, c_1/X_2, c_2/Z_1\}}{\longrightarrow \exists x_1.\forall y_1.\exists z_1.\varphi(x_1, y_1, z_1), \exists x_2.\forall y_2.\exists z_2.\neg\varphi(x_2, y_2, z_2); \{Z_2/X_1, c_1/X_2, c_2/Z_1\}} \, SQEl$$

$$\begin{pmatrix} Z_1 & Z_2 \\ | & \ddots & | \\ c_1 & & c_2 \\ | & \ddots & | \\ X_1 & & X_2 \end{pmatrix}$$

Theorem 7 (Soundness). *If there exists a $\mathcal{K}_{aux}$-proof $\mathcal{P}$ of a sequent with substitution s then s is valid.*

Proof. The proof is by induction on the structure of $\mathcal{P}$. The base case where $\mathcal{P}$ consists only of an application of ax is trivial. In the induction step a case distinction depending on the last rule application in $\mathcal{P}$ is made. We concentrate on the interesting cases where $\wedge$, *Subst*, or $SQEl_{aux}$ is applied. In each case we assume that all premises of the rule are valid and infer the validity of the conclusion. For a more detailed proof we refer the interested reader to [1].

- Let $\wedge$ be the last rule applied in $\mathcal{P}$. We assume that for every algebra A and every assignment α holds $A(\alpha)(\longrightarrow \Gamma, \varphi_1; \sigma) = true = A(\alpha)(\longrightarrow \Gamma, \varphi_2; \sigma)$. Let A be an arbitrary algebra and α be an arbitrary assignment. If there is a $F \in \Gamma$ such that $A(\alpha)(\sigma(F)) = true$, then $A(\alpha)(\longrightarrow \Gamma, \varphi_1 \wedge \varphi_2; \sigma) = true$ holds trivially. Otherwise, $A(\alpha)(\sigma(\varphi_1)) = true = A(\alpha)(\sigma(\varphi_2))$ must hold which implies $A(\alpha)(\longrightarrow \Gamma, \varphi_1 \wedge \varphi_2; \sigma) = true$.

- Let *Subst* be the last rule applied in $\mathcal{P}$. We assume that for every algebra A and every assignment α holds $A(\alpha)(\longrightarrow \sigma'(\Gamma); \sigma) = true$. According to the side condition of the rule holds $\sigma \circ \sigma' = \sigma$. Thus, $\longrightarrow \sigma(\Gamma) = \longrightarrow \sigma(\sigma'(\Gamma))$ and the validity of the conclusion follows.

- Let $SQEl_{aux}$ be the last rule applied in $\mathcal{P}$. The proof is done by induction over the number m of quantifiers eliminated, i.e. the sum of the lengths of the ql_i. The base case where $m = 0$ is trivial, since the premise and the conclusion are the same sequent. We first prove the case $m = 1$ with $s = \longrightarrow \Gamma, Qx.\varphi; \sigma$.

  • If $Q = \exists$, we assume that for every algebra A and every assignment α holds $A(\alpha)(\longrightarrow \Gamma, \varphi[X/x]; \sigma) = true$. Let A be an arbitrary algebra and α be an arbitrary assignment. The interesting case is where $A(\alpha)(\sigma(F)) = false$ for all $F \in \Gamma$ and $A(\alpha)(\sigma(\varphi[X/x])) = true$. Let σ' be the restriction of σ to $free(\Gamma \cup \{\exists x.\varphi\})$. Then
    $true = A(\alpha)(\sigma(\varphi[X/x])) = A(\alpha)(\sigma'(\varphi[X/x])) = A(\alpha)((\sigma'(\varphi))[\sigma'(X)/x])$
    $= A(\alpha[A(\alpha)(\sigma'(X))/x])(\sigma'(\varphi))$ by substitution theorem
    $= A(\alpha)(\exists x.\sigma'(\varphi))$ by definition of the semantics of $\exists$
    $= A(\alpha)(\sigma'(\exists x.\varphi)) = A(\alpha)(\sigma(\exists x.\varphi)) = A(\alpha)(\longrightarrow \Gamma, \exists x.\varphi; \sigma)$

  • If $Q = \forall$, we assume that for every algebra A and every assignment α holds $A(\alpha)(\longrightarrow \Gamma, \varphi[c/x]; \sigma) = true$. Let A be an arbitrary algebra and α be an arbitrary assignment. The interesting case is where $A(\alpha)(\sigma(F)) = false$ for all $F \in \Gamma$ and $A(\alpha)(\sigma(\varphi[c/x])) = true$. We consider all *variants* A_a of A, i.e. all algebras which differ from A only in the interpretation of c such that $A_a(c) = a$. The side-condition of $SQEl_{aux}$ and the definition of QE_{aux} ensure that $X \ll c$ holds for every $X \in free(\longrightarrow \Gamma, \forall x.\varphi; \sigma)$. Because $\lhd$ is required to be irreflexive for any $F \in \Gamma$, c does not occur in $\sigma(F)$ and thus, $A_a(\alpha)(\sigma(F)) = A(\alpha)(\sigma(F)) = false$. Let σ' be the restriction of σ to $free(\Gamma \cup \{\forall x.\varphi\})$. Then for all A_a holds
    $true = A_a(\alpha)(\sigma'(\varphi[c/x])) = A_a(\alpha)((\sigma'(\varphi))[c/x])$ since σ' is admissible
    $= A_a(\alpha[A_a(c)/x])(\sigma'(\varphi))$ by substitution theorem
    $= A_a(\alpha[a/x])(\sigma'(\varphi))$.
    For every $a \in S_A$ there is an A_a, thus $A(\alpha)(\longrightarrow \Gamma, \forall x.\varphi; \sigma) = true$.

In the induction step we assume the soundness of $SQEl_{aux}$ for the elimination of less than m quantifiers ($m > 1$) and show the soundness for m quantifiers. The irreflexivity of $\lhd$ ensures that there is a maximal element $o \in O$

with regard to $\lhd$. According to the definition of $\sqsubseteq$ o is not instantiated for any variable in O. Let o be introduced by the elimination of $Q_j x.\psi_j'$. We split the application of $SQEl_{aux}$ as follows into two applications of the rule where each of the applications reduces less than m quantifiers. Due to the choice of $Q_j x.\psi_j$ the side conditions for both rule applications are fulfilled.

$$\frac{\dfrac{\longrightarrow \Gamma,\psi_1,\ldots,\psi_j,\ldots,\psi_n\,;\sigma}{\longrightarrow \Gamma,\psi_1,\ldots,Q\textbf{\textit{x}}.\psi_j',\ldots,\psi_n\,;\sigma}\ SQEl_{aux}}{\longrightarrow \Gamma,\mathrm{ql}_1.\varphi_1,\ldots,\mathrm{ql}_j.Q\textbf{\textit{x}}.\varphi_j,\ldots,\mathrm{ql}_n.\varphi_n\,;\sigma}\ SQEl_{aux}}$$

1 quantifier elimination

$(m-1)$ quantifier eliminations

Remark 8. In the induction step of the above proof we show that it is always possible to focus on a single formula in a sequent. In the case where the rule $SQEl_{aux}$ is the last rule applied this is non-trivial because multiple formulas are reduced in a single rule application. Free variables in a sequent cause dependencies between formulas. Only the side condition of the rule $SQEl_{aux}$ allow us to single out a specific formula according to the reduction ordering and ensure in the case $\forall$ that this formula is valid in all variants of a specific algebra.

Theorem 9 (Soundness). *If there exists a $\mathcal{K}$-proof for a sequent then it is valid.*

Proof. There are three differences between $\mathcal{K}_{aux}$ and $\mathcal{K}$. In $\mathcal{K}_{aux}$ a substitution is explicitly stated in sequents, *Eigenvariables* have no arguments (i.e. are no skolem-terms), and the *Subst*-rule is a sequent rule while the *Inst*-rule of $\mathcal{K}$ is a rewrite rule on proof trees. Proof search in $\mathcal{K}_{aux}$ would require that an appropriate substitution is guessed before any rule may be applied. None of the rules in $\mathcal{K}_{aux}$ is capable to modify this substitution. This appears to be impractical, however, $\mathcal{K}_{aux}$ is only an auxiliary calculus. We argue that the skolemization based technique applied in $\mathcal{K}$ is a realization of the constraints imposed by $\mathcal{K}_{aux}$.

During proof search in $\mathcal{K}$ substitutions can only be applied globally to the proof tree using the *Inst*-rule. From all applications of *Inst* in a $\mathcal{K}$-proof $\mathcal{P}$ of a sequent s a substitution σ can be constructed such that a $\mathcal{K}_{aux}$-proof $\mathcal{P}_{aux}$ for $s;\sigma$ exists. $\mathcal{P}_{aux}$ can be constructed inductively from $\mathcal{P}$. An application of *Inst* in $\mathcal{P}$ results in an application of *Subst* on all open leaves of $\mathcal{P}_{aux}$. An application $SQEl$ results in an application of $SQEl_{aux}$. Skolemization ensures that the side-condition of $SQEl_{aux}$ holds, i.e. $\lhd_O$ is irreflexive. If $\lhd_O$ would not be irreflexive, then by construction of $\lhd_O$ the substitution were not idempotent – a contradiction. Any other $\mathcal{K}$-rule is mapped to the respective $\mathcal{K}_{aux}$-rule.

5 Syntactical Justification

Since the early seventies systems have emerged that use interactive proof strategies based on complex user defined proof rules. The soundness of these systems is guaranteed by explicitly performing a proof in the basic calculus for each (application of a) derived rule (or tactic). This *proof theoretic* approach is simple in the sense that no additional *formal* concepts are required. All we need is a system architecture that keeps up a consistent state of the overall proof generation process and forces us to expand all derived steps.

We present a generalization of this approach where in a formalized metalanguage we prove that a proof exists for all instances of a derived rule. As compared to tactical theorem proving here additional meta-logical concepts are required. However, the approach still is uniform in the sense that it relies on a fixed collection of formal concepts that are *syntactic* in nature. A main motivation of this paper is to compare this approach to a *semantic* justification which uses various concepts from model theory but which of course also could be formalized in a meta-level formalism.

The syntactic (or proof theoretic) approach seems to be particular useful for proof generation mechanisms that themselves use meta-level notions. For example, it provides a simple and clear semantics for meta-*variables* as placeholders for syntactic objects, like (object-level) variables, terms, and formulas. The approach is not limited to cases where the objects involved are first-class citizens with respect to (object-level) quantification nor is it restricted to meta-variables. In the context of the quantifier elimination rule also Skolem-functions are meta-level symbols.

The meta-level justification of quantifier elimination is *local* in the sense that we are able to guarantee a proof that replaces the derived step without any further proof transformation.

Basic Notions. We assume that the *abstract syntax* of the underlying object language is given as an abstract data type. Basic (static) types for this data structure include V for (object-level) variables, $TERM$ for (object-level) terms, and FOR for (object-level) formulas. The axiomatization uses *constructor symbols*, like $mk\text{-}and : [FOR, FOR \to FOR]$ and $mk\text{-}ex : [V, FOR \to FOR]$ for building up conjunctive and existentially quantified formulas, respectively. *Selectors* are used to decompose structured objects. As usual *predicates*, like Ex and All serve to detect the kind of formula we are dealing with.

In addition to the abstract syntax of the object language we rely on *auxiliary* data structures, like natural numbers (NAT), lists ($LIST(\ldots)$), and trees ($TREE(\ldots)$). For lists we use the following notation:

- $emptyl : LIST(\ldots)$ for the empty list
- $cons : [\ldots, LIST(\ldots) \to LIST(\ldots)]$ for adding an element in front of a list
- $\cdot\ : [LIST(\ldots), LIST(\ldots) \to LIST(\ldots)]$ for concatenating lists
- $.\ : [LIST(\ldots), NAT \to \ldots]$ for selecting elements
- $\downarrow\ : [LIST(\ldots), NAT \to LIST(\ldots))$ for computing the initial segment
- $||\ : [LIST(\ldots) \to NAT]$ for the length of a list
- $-\ : [LIST(\ldots), LIST(\ldots) \to LIST(\ldots)]$ for removing all occurrences of elements given by the second list from the first list.

Above the level of formula we have *sequents* and (proof) *trees* built up by $mk\text{-}seq : [LIST(FOR), LIST(FOR) \to SEQ]$ and $mk\text{-}tree : [SEQ, LIST(SEQ) \to TREE(SEQ)]$.

The function given by $fv_f : [FOR \to LIST(V)]$ computes a list containing all variables that have (free) occurrences in a formula. For terms we use fv_t. fv_f^* and fv_t^* are extensions to lists of formulas and terms, respectively. Substitutions are computed by $subst : [FOR, V, TERM \to FOR]$.

As our meta-language we use a higher-order language where all function symbols are interpreted as total functions.

Metalevel Representation of Simultaneous Quantifier Elimination. In a first step we define a set of trees given by a predicate Qe. Not all instances of this scheme represent valid proof steps. Those trees for which a proof in the basic calculus exists are filtered out by additional constraints later on.

$\forall t : TREE(SEQ).\forall fl : List(FOR).\forall l : LIST(LIST(TERM)).$

$\forall m : LIST(LIST([LIST(V) \rightarrow V])).\forall q : LIST(NAT).$

$\quad Qe(t, fl, l, m, q) \leftrightarrow (Fits(fl, l, m, q) \wedge$

$\quad\quad t \equiv mk\text{-}tree(mk\text{-}seq(emptyl, fl), cons(mk\text{-}seq(emptyl, elim^*(fl, l, m, q)), emptyl)))$

The succedent of the conclusion of the rule is given by fl the antecedent of both the conclusion and the premise being empty. The terms that are substituted for existential quantifiers are given by l. For each formula in fl there has to be a list in l of appropriate length. In the same way m contains lists of so-called Skolem-functions used to replace universally quantified variables. In the current stage of the development the functions in the lists of m are not constrained at all. All we know is their type: $[LIST(V) \rightarrow V]$. From this we already see that Skolem-functions compute (object-level) variables. Finally q determines the number of quantifiers that we want to remove from the quantifier prefix of each formula in fl. If there is no quantifier prefix for a member of fl then the corresponding number in q has to be zero. This as well as other (more or less obvious) *syntactic* constraints for the arguments are formalized by *Fits*.

We continue with the definition of $elim^*(fl, l, m, q)$ which computes the succedent of the premise of the rule:

$elim^*(fl, l, m, q) \equiv el^*(fl, l, m, q, 0) \qquad n \equiv |q| \rightarrow el^*(fl, l, m, q, n) \equiv emptyl$

$(n < |q| \rightarrow el^*(fl, l, m, q, n) \equiv$

$\quad\quad cons(elim(fl, fl.n, l.n, m.n, q.n, 0, 0), el^*(fl, l, m, q, n + 1))$

The function *elim* successively removes one quantifier after the other. Existentially quantified variables are replaced by terms given by the third argument. These terms correspond to the meta-variables used by the object-level proof procedure. The Skolem-functions given by the fourth argument are used to replace universally quantified variables. Skolem-functions are applied to a list of variables containing the free variables of fl and those variables occurring in the terms that have been substituted for existentially quantified variables before.

$(Ex(f) \wedge i \not\equiv 0) \rightarrow elim(fl, f, tl, sl, i, u, v) \equiv$

$\quad\quad elim(fl, subst(body(f), bvar(f), tl.u), tl, sl, i - 1, u + 1, v)$

$(All(f) \wedge i \not\equiv 0) \rightarrow elim(fl, f, tl, sl, i) \equiv$

$\quad\quad elim(fl, subst(body(f), bvar(f), sl.v(fv_f^*(fl) \cdot fv_i^*(tl \downarrow u))), tl, sl, i - 1, u, v + 1))$

$(\neg Ex(f) \vee \neg All(f) \vee i \not\equiv 0) \rightarrow elim(fl, f, tl, sl, i) \equiv f$

We are left with the problem of filtering out the valid instances of Qe. This is done by introducing an additional list of natural numbers e which defines a possible order of *sequential* quantifier elimination steps. If we have $e.n \equiv i$ this means that in the nth step the leading quantifier of the ith formula is removed. Of course e has to be constrained with respect to fl and q. For example the number of occurrences of i in e, denoted by $\sharp(e, i)$, has to be equal to the $q.i$. These additional constraints are formalized by $Adm(e, fl, q)$.

The main problem that has to be solved is to provide a suitable meaning for the Skolem-functions given by the lists in m. Note that $(m.i).j$ is the Skolem-function used to eliminate the jth universal quantifier in the ith formula. We define:

$$Skol(fl, l, m, q, e) \leftrightarrow \forall 0 \leq i < |m|.\forall 0 \leq j < |m.i|. \ (m.i).j \equiv$$
$$\lambda tl : LIST(TERM). \ s((fv^*(elim^*(fl, l, m, red(q, fl, e, i, j)))) - fv^*(fl)) \cdot tl),$$

where the reduced list $red(q, fl, e, i, j)$ is defined by

$$\forall 0 \leq k < |m|. \ red(q, fl, e, i, j).k \equiv \sharp(e \downarrow step(fl, e, i, j), k) \ .$$

s is a fixed function (the basic Skolem-function) that computes a variable which is not contained in the list of variables given as an argument and $step(fl, e, i, j)$ is the step in e in which the jth universal quantifier of $fl.i$ is removed.

Using this predicate we can clarify the nature of our syntactic Skolem-functions by proving the following basic theorem:

$$\forall t : TREE.\forall fl : LIST(FOR).\forall l : LIST(LIST(TERM)).$$
$$\forall m : LIST(LIST([LIST(V) \rightarrow V])).\forall q : LIST(NAT).\forall e : LIST(NAT)$$
$$((Adm(e, fl, q) \wedge Qe(t, fl, l, m, q) \wedge Skol(fl, l, m, q, e)) \rightarrow Prov(t))$$

Unfortunately this result is not yet satisfactory since during proof construction we allow *substitutions* involving Skolem-functions. To treat substitutions (for **metavariables denoting terms**) **we replace** fl **and** l by functions $\widetilde{fl} : [LIST(TERM) \rightarrow LIST(FOR)]$ and $\tilde{l} : [LIST(TERM) \rightarrow LIST(LIST(TERM))]$.
The function $gl : [LIST(LIST([LIST(V) \rightarrow V])) \rightarrow LIST(TERM)]$ provides the right hand sides of the substitutions.

Making the substituted terms depending on a structure m (of functions) allows to formalize substitutions that involve Skolem-functions. Every substitution occurring in the actual proof process can be represented as a list gl.

Again, $\widetilde{fl}, \tilde{l}, gl$, and q have to fit together which is expressed by the predicate $Fits_s$. Using these additional notations we are able to prove:

$$\forall gl.\forall \widetilde{fl}.\forall \tilde{l}.\forall q.(Fits_s(\widetilde{fl}, \tilde{l}, gl, q) \rightarrow \exists m.\exists e.(Fits(\widetilde{fl}(gl(m)), \tilde{l}(gl(m)), m, q) \wedge$$
$$Adm(e, \widetilde{fl}(gl(m)), q) \wedge \ Skol(\widetilde{fl}(gl(m)), \tilde{l}(gl(m)), m, q, e)))$$

Since the definition of gl allows the *nesting* of functions the choice of e (and therefore also of m) really depends on gl. In this way we have modelled the fact that the fullsemantics of the Skolem-functions can only determined a posteriori, that is after a substitution has been applied.

The meta-level formalization we have presented exactly models the usage of the quantifier elimination rule by separating the visible part, given by the argument list of the elements in m, from the hidden part, given by the additional arguments supplied to s. It is this hidden part that can only be determined after a substitution has been made.

6 Conclusion

We defined the sequent calculus $\mathcal{K}$ which incorporates a rule for simultaneous quantifier elimination. $\mathcal{K}$ is sound and complete. The more difficult proof of the soundness theorem has been carried out by semantical as well as by syntactical arguments. While the semantical perspective clarifies the interdependencies of formulas in a sequent the syntactical approach allows to translate $\mathcal{K}$-proofs into usual sequent proofs which do not contain any meta-level constructs. This translation preserves the structure of a proof. Subsequently, simultaneous quantifier elimination can be used in sequent calculi for non-classical logics as well. The simultaneous quantifier elimination rule presented in this article has been implemented in the VSE II system for formal software development which is currently under development at the DFKI as a successor of the VSE system [7].

Other systems handle quantifiers with different degrees of sophistication. Lazy handling of instantiations has been used in classical as well as in non-classical logics and in first-order as well as in higher-order formalisms. Except in sequent calculus and natural deduction calculi, Skolemization has been studied in the context of resolution, connection method and tableau calculi as well.

For instance in PVS [5] Gentzen-like quantifier elimination rules are used where instantiations must be guessed. Ketonen and Weyhrauch [8] present an approach where sequents are annotated by a substitution, like in the semantical part of this article, and used a technique similar to our quantifier list ordering. However, they have only classical quantifier rules with the corresponding non-determinism in proof search. In the Isabelle system [11] a technique dual to classical skolemization is used. In remark 4 we have pointed out that this technique causes close interdependencies between formulas in a sequent which make it quite difficult to develop an optimized handling of quantifiers equivalent to our simultaneous quantifier elimination rule.

References

1. S. Autexier and H. Mantel. *Semantical Investigation of Simultaneous Skolemization for First-Order Sequent Calculus*, Seki Report SR-98-05, 1998.
2. A. Avron. Simple Consequence Relations, In *Information and Computation 92*, p. 105–139, 1991.
3. W. Bibel. *Automated Theorem Proving*. Vieweg Verlag, 2nd edition, 1987.
4. K. A. Bowen. Programming with full first-order logic, In Hayes, Michie, Pao, Eds., *Machine Intelligence 10*, 1982.
5. J. Crow, S. Owre, J. Rushby, N. Shankar and M. Srivas. *A Tutorial Introduction to PVS*, Presented at WIFT'95, 1995.
6. G. Gentzen. *Untersuchungen über das logische Schließen*, Mathematische Zeitschrift. 39:179-210 and 405-431, 1935.
7. D. Hutter, B. Langenstein, C. Sengler, J. Siekmann, W. Stephan and A. Wolpers. Verification Support Environment (VSE), *High Integrity Systems*, p. 523-530, 1996.
8. J. Ketonen and R. Weyhrauch. A Decidable Fragment of Predicate Calculus, In *TCS, Volume 32-3*, 1984.
9. P. Lincoln and N. Shankar. Proof Search in First-Order Linear Logic and other Cut-Free Sequent Calculi, In *Proceedings of 9th LICS*, p. 282-291, 1994.
10. J. Loeckx, H.-D. Ehrich and M. Wolf. *Specification of Abstract Data Types*, Wiley-Teubner, 1996.
11. L.C. Paulson. *Isabelle, A Generic Theorem Prover*, Springer Verlag, 1994.
12. N. Shankar. Proof Search in the Intuitionistic Sequent Calculus, In D . Kapur, Ed., *Proceedings of CADE-11*, p. 522-536, 1992.
13. T. Skolem. Logisch-kombinatorische Untersuchungen über die Erfüllbarkeit oder Beweisbarkeit mathematischer Sätze, In *Skrifter utgit av Videnskapselskapet i Kristiania*, p. 4-36, 1920.
14. L. Wallen. *Automated Deduction in Non-Classical Logic*. MIT Press, 1990.

Deductive Verification of Invariants of State-Transition Systems

Dieter Hutter

German Research Center for Artificial Intelligence GmbH, Stuhlsatzenhausweg 3,
D-66123 Saarbrücken, Germany
hutter@dfki.uni-sb.de, Tel. -49-681-302-5317

Abstract. We present a modular technique to prove invariants of state-transition systems in a deductive framework. We show how the semantic knowledge of the given problem can be generically used to decompose the problem into modular tasks which can be successfully tackled with the help of techniques developed in the field of inductive theorem proving. As an example we present the mechanical verification of the invariant of a case study specifying a generic elevator.

1 Introduction

State-transition systems are commonly used to specify reactive systems. They are based on a view of a global state which can be manipulated by executing so-called transitions. Introducing special clock variable to model real time we obtain clocked transition systems for specifying real-time applications. Global properties of such a state-transition system are specified by invariants which have to be true in all reachable states. This forms a proof obligation when verifying the system. The application of state-transition systems in an industrial setting results in an increased complexity of the specification and also of the arising proof obligations. In the last years several industrial applications of state-transition systems have been performed using the *VSE*-system [VSE96] which is officially approved as a formal specification and verification tool wrt. the ITSEC-criteria (Information Technology Security Evaluation Criteria) by the German federal agency BSI (Bundesamt für Sicherheit in der Informationstechnik). Experience shows that the arising proof obligations usually cover several pages of first-order formulas which render a user guided proof search impossible.

Thus, there is a need for structuring the deduction process which decomposes large proof obligations into simpler tasks and synthesizes an overall proof from the arising partial solutions. This decomposition has to enable the use of specialized methods to solve specific problems and also to ease the speculation of lemmata needed to prove the theorem.

In this paper we present techniques to automate the proof of invariants of state-transition systems. While in practice such a proof obligation turns out to be a rather complex first-order formula, it has also an intrinsic syntactical structure which can be used to guide and automate the proof search. Proving the invariant of a state-transition system with respect to a specific transition T results in general in a proof obligation of the form

$$Req_T \wedge Ens_T \wedge Inv_{state} \rightarrow Inv_{state'}$$

where Inv_{state} and $Inv_{state'}$ denote the invariant of the system before and after performing a transition T. Req_T ("requires") denotes the precondition and Ens_T ("ensures") the specification of T. Basically we may think of this formula as a step case (wrt. the transition T) when applying induction on the reachable states of the system. We will adapt the rippling techniques developed in inductive theorem proving to show the invariants of state-based systems. Throughout this paper we will illustrate these techniques with the help of an example of a generic elevator.

2 Rippling and Annotated Formulas

Rippling [BSH+93,Hut97] is based on the notion of annotated terms where each occurrence of a symbol can be attached by additional information (encoded into the color of an occurrence) which is maintained during the deduction by the rippling calculus. E.g. $(a + b) \times (a - b)$ is an example of such an annotated term. The colors are used to represent the similarities explicitly. While the white parts denote the common parts of both sides of the equation to be proven, the grey symbols represent their differences. Thus, instead of describing differences by identifying minimal subterms which contain them (as in the RUE-approach), the notion of annotated terms allows one to represent the differences explicitly and therefore, seems to be a more adequate representation for implementing difference reduction techniques. Also, the explicit representation of differences is an important requirement in computing a measure of how far two terms or formulas differ which is a central aid in guiding (parts of) the proof search.

Using the rippling calculus the white parts of an annotated term stay — as a property of the calculus — invariant while the grey parts are subjects to change. In order to manipulate annotated terms correctly, the equations given as axioms are also colored such that the white parts on both sides coincide while the grey parts represent their differences. Examples of such annotated equations are given by:

$$(X + Y) \times Z = (X \times Z) + (Y \times Z) \tag{1}$$

$$X \times (Y - Z) = (X \times Y) - (X \times Z) \tag{2}$$

For example using (1) and (2) we are able to perform the following rewriting:[1]

$$(a + b) \times (a - b) \rightarrow (a \times (a - b)) + (b \times (a - b))$$

$$\rightarrow ((a \times a) - (a \times b)) + (b \times (a - b))$$

---

[1] For sake of simplicity we omit the details of matching and unification in the rippling calculus. The reader is referred to [Hut97] for details.

Notice that in all these annotated terms the white parts — namely $a \times a$ — stay fixed. These white parts are called the *skeleton skel(q)* of an annotated term q while the grey parts are called the *wave-fronts*. Precisely, the skeleton of such an annotated term q is a *set* of un-annotated terms which are obtained by successively replacing each subterm q' of q with a grey top-level symbol by some biggest subterm of q' with a white top-level symbol. We extend the notion of a skeleton to a equality by $skel(q = r) = \{q' = r' \mid q' \in skel(q) \text{ and } r' \in skel(r)\}$.

3 Specifications

The specification of state-transition systems in VSE [VSE96] consists of the description of system variables and a finite collection of transitions modifying these variables. Each system variable has a specific type which is related to some specified abstract datatype. A *state* is a (type-consistent) assignment of the system variables. A *transition* T maps each state into a set of *successor*-states and is denoted by a relation Ens_T which is formulated by a first-order formula. This formula refers to both, the unprimed system variables denoting the state *before* performing the transition, and the primed system variables representing the state *after* executing the transition. Transitions may also have a precondition Req_T which restricts the use of the transition to specific states.

3.1 States

In order to specify the elevator we will now define appropriate abstract datatypes used to declare the system variables. We use a slightly simplified version of the VSE input language.

First, the cabin door of the elevator may be either closed or open. In VSE enumeration datatypes are available to specify freely generated, finite datatypes:

```
TYPES : doorstates = ENUMERATED BY opened | closed
```

which results in a first-order formula $\forall X : doorstates\ X = opened \lor X = closed$.

In the same way we specify the different states of the cabin of the elevator inside the theory `cabadt`. A cabin is either moving or being halted:

```
TYPES : cabstates = ENUMERATED BY move | halt
```

The different directions in which the cabin can move are given in the theory `diradt` by the following datatype:

```
TYPES : dirstates = ENUMERATED BY up | down
```

For each floor there are buttons to request the elevator. The next datatype `buttonentry` is intended to store any request. Additionally each floor has an internal counter (encoded as an integer) which is used to count all stops of the cabin between the order and the arrival of the cabin at the denoted floor. Hence, proving that the value of this integer is always below a given value will guarantee some kind of *fairness* of the elevator.

```
TYPES : buttonstates = ENUMERATED BY req | noreq
        buttonentry =
            GENERATED BY mkbutton(state: buttonstates, count : int)
```

Now we have collected some prerequisites to specify the actual state of the elevator which consists in particular of an array of buttons[2] denoting the several floors, the position of the cabin door, the actual position of the cabin, whether the cabin is moving or not, and its direction. The specification of this state in VSE is sketched in the following figure:

```
OBJECT Elevator
  USING cabadt, diradt, ...
  DATA: buttons: ARRAY[INT]:buttonentry;
        door:    doorstates;
        pos:     int;
        cab:     cabstates;
        dir:     directions;
        ...
```

3.2 Transitions

A transition T is specified by a formula Ens_T relating the unprimed system variables, denoting the state before executing the transition, to the primed system variables, denoting the state after performing the transition. Transitions may be guarded by an additional formula Req_T preventing the execution of a transition in specific states.

For instance consider the transition **press** which specifies the press of some button in the elevator example:

```
PROC press
    MODIFIES buttons
    ENSURES
        EX i: minfloor <= i AND i <= maxfloor
            AND state(select(buttons', i)) = req
            AND ALL X: i = X
                        OR state(select(buttons', X))
                            = state(select(buttons, X));
        ALL X: count(select(buttons', X))
                = count(select(buttons, X))
```

The MODIFIES line specifies the set of system variables which are subject to changes while executing the transition. Thus **press** will only change the variable **buttons**. ENSURES describes the relation between the states before and after

---

[2] Actually ARRAY[INT]:buttonentry specifies an array of elements of type *buttonentry*. The array is not limited in its size, each integer may be used to index the array. Given an array *buttons* of that type, the term *select(buttons, i)* is used to refer to the value of its *i*-th cell.

executing **press**. The list of formulas is implicitly ∧-closed. Together with the
MODIFIES part we obtain the following first-order formula[3] Ens_{press} as a specification of **press**. To ease the description of the later proof procedure we assume
that this formula is given (or translated) in a skolemized normal form allowing
nested ∨,∧-formulas with negations occurring only in front of atomic formulas[4].

$$cab' = cab \wedge door' = door \wedge pos' = pos \wedge dir' = dir$$
$$\wedge \; minfloor \leq i \wedge i \leq maxfloor$$
$$\wedge \; state(select(buttons', i)) = req$$
$$\wedge \; (i = X \vee state(select(buttons', X)) = state(select(buttons, X)))$$
$$\wedge \; count(select(buttons', X)) = count(select(buttons, X))$$

As another example consider the transition **pass-down** denoting the move of
the cabin to the next lower floor:

```
PROC pass-down
    MODIFIES pos
    REQUIRES cab = moving;
             dir = down
             state(select(buttons, pos)) = noreq
    ENSURES
        pos' = p(pos)
```

In this case the transition decreases the system variable **pos** by one. Also **pos**
is the only system variable subject to modification. In contrast to the previous
example, **pass-down** is guarded by an additional requirement which demands
that the cabin is moving downwards and also that the button of the actual floor
is not pressed when the transition is performed.

3.3 Invariants

In order to specify properties of the overall state-transition system we formulate a
so-called *invariant* of the system. In VSE an invariant is encoded in a first-order
formula which represents overall safety properties which hold in all reachable
states. While the invariant Inv_{state} contains only unprimed system variables and
thus refers to the actual state, the corresponding $Inv_{state'}$, which we obtain by
replacing all unprimed system variables by their primed counterparts, refers to
the state after performing some transition T.

For example the invariant of the lift-example is a collection of formulas relevant to guarantee the safety of the system. In particular we demand that

- whenever the cabin is moving, the door is closed and by analogy, if the door
  is opened, the cabin is halted;

---

[3] We employ the Prolog convention of using capital letters to indicate (meta)variables
while e.g. i denotes a skolem constant.

[4] However, this is no restriction in principle, since using polarities of formulas it is
easy to lift our techniques also to non-normal forms.

- whenever the cabin is moving upwards (downwards), there is a request in some upper (lower) floor;
- each request is restricted to some existing floor;
- a fairness condition saying that there are at most twice as many stops between the request and arrival of the cabin at a specific floor; and
- the cabin operates only within existing floors.

Formally, we specify the invariant Inv_{state} of our elevator as follows:

$$(cab = move \rightarrow door = closed) \land (door = opened \rightarrow cab = halt) \qquad (3)$$

$$\land (cab = move \land dir = up) \qquad (4)$$

$$\rightarrow \exists \, floor_{req} : int \; floor_{req} \geq pos \land state(select(buttons, floor_{req})) = req$$

$$\land (cab = move \land dir = down) \qquad (5)$$

$$\rightarrow \exists \, floor_{req} : int \; floor_{req} \leq pos \land state(select(buttons, floor_{req})) = req$$

$$\land \forall X : int \; state(select(buttons, X)) = req \qquad (6)$$

$$\rightarrow (minfloor \leq X \land X \leq maxfloor)$$

$$\land \forall X : int \; count(select(buttons, X)) \leq (2 \times (maxfloor - minfloor)) \qquad (7)$$

$$\land \, minfloor \leq pos \land pos \leq maxfloor \qquad (8)$$

4 Proving the Invariants

To guarantee the system properties we have to verify that the specified invariant holds in all reachable states of the specified system. In order to prove such an invariant we can make use of an invariance rule for standard state-transition systems as it can be found for instance in [MP95] and reformulate the problem in a first-order setting. Then in particular, we have to prove that the invariant holds in any initial state and provided the invariant holds in some state, it holds also in all successor states accessible by some transition T. In this paper we focus on the latter case in which a given transition T has to preserve the specified invariant each time the transition is performed. The problem of proving invariants of state transition systems lies in the intrinsic complexity and size of these proof obligations. While the invariant has to include supporting lemmata and corollaries necessary to prove the desired properties, the specification of a transition usually consists of a large case analysis considering different states of the systems.

In order to tackle these proof obligations we propose a proof technique which is divided into two steps:

1. Appropriate rewrite rules are synthesized from the transition specification in order to manipulate terms or literals containing primed system variables. We are interested in rewrite rules the right hand sides of which do not contain any primed system variables. This step results in a set of *conditional* rewrite rules which give rise to a case analysis in a later proof.

2. The invariant to be proven is analyzed for occurrences of primed state variables which guides the selection of appropriate rewrite rules of the transition specification. This gives rise to an elaborated case analysis in order to deal with the conditionals of the rewrite rule. Proving the individual cases we distinguish between cases in which the selected rewrite rules contain non-primed system variables and so-called base cases in which no system variable is introduced by applying the rewrite rule. While in the first case we have to manipulate the invariant of the successor state in terms of the invariant of the previous state, in the latter case the proof of the invariant has to be done without this help.

4.1 Analysis of the Transition Description

The first step of our proof technique analyses the specification of a transition in order to generate appropriate rewrite-rules for a later invariant proof.

We call a term *primed* iff it contains at least one primed system variable. A primed term s in the specification is called a *head term* iff there is an unnegated equation $s = t$ in Ens_T. We call $s = t$ a primed equation and t the *body* of it iff t does not contain any primed system variable. However the equation is conditioned by a residuum $Cond(s = t)$. We obtain this formula denoting the negated condition of $s = t$ by replacing $s = t$ by false in Ens_T and simplifying the result with the help of standard boolean simplification rules (e.g. $A \land False \to False$ or $A \lor False \to A$). The formula $Cond(s = t) \lor s = t$ is called a *rewrite rule* of s in Ens_T if $Cond(s = t)$ does not contain any primed system variables. It is easy to show that each rewrite rule of s in Ens_T is a valid consequence of Ens_T. To ease the proof of the invariant we will shade the differences between the head term and the body of a rewrite rule in grey. As mentioned before, these grey parts constitute the wave-fronts of the rule while the other parts form the skeleton common to both sides.

For example consider the specification of **press**. Besides the head terms cab', $door'$, dir' and pos' with trivial rewrite rules

$$\boxed{cab'} = cab \quad (9) \qquad \boxed{dir'} = dir \quad (10) \qquad \boxed{door'} = door \quad (11) \qquad \boxed{pos'} = pos, \quad (12)$$

there are two head terms $count(select(buttons', X))$ and $state(select(buttons', X))$ with corresponding rewrite rules:

$$count(select(buttons', X)) = count(select(buttons, X)) \qquad (13)$$
$$state(select(buttons', i)) = req$$
$$i = X \lor state(select(buttons', X)) = state(select(buttons, X))$$

To generate suitable case analyses we normalize the obtained rewrite rules and group them into different classes. For normalizing these rules we use the concept of anti-unification: two head terms s_1 and s_2 are anti-unifiable iff there is a term s and two substitutions σ_1, σ_2 such that $\sigma_1(s) = s_1$, $\sigma_2(s) = s_2$, and for all $x \in DOM(\sigma_i)$, $\sigma_i(x)$ does not contain any primed system variable. We call two rewrite-rules *anti-unifiable* iff their head terms are anti-unifiable. Being anti-unifiable defines an equivalence relation which we use to factor the rewrite rules into classes. For each class we anti-unify the contained head terms $s_1, \ldots, s_n$ which results in a common term s and corresponding substitutions $\sigma_1, \ldots, \sigma_n$ with $\sigma_i(s) = s_i$. Without loss of generality we assume that $DOM(\sigma_i)$ (for all $1 \leq i \leq n$) does not share any variables with the original rewrite-rule. Then each rewrite rule $Cond(s_i = t_i) \vee s_i = t_i$ is normalized to

$$\left(\bigvee_{X \in DOM(\sigma_i)} \neg X = \sigma_i(X) \right) \vee Cond(s_i = t_i) \vee s = t_i.$$

Afterwards we eliminate literals of the form $\neg X = Y$ in the obtained rewrite rules of s by applying a substitution $\{X \leftarrow Y\}$ provided X does not occur in s.

In our example only $state(select(buttons', X))$ constitutes a class containing more than one normalized rewrite rule:

$$\neg X = i \vee state(select(buttons', X)) = req \tag{14}$$

$$X = i \vee state(select(buttons', X)) = state(select(buttons, X)) \tag{15}$$

while all other head terms constitute classes with exactly one (unchanged) rewrite rule (i.e. the rules (9) - (13)). The shadings of the rewrite rules indicate the differences (in terms of rippling) between head term and the body or the rule and will be used in the further process. In case of the transition **pass-down** we obtain (among others) the following shaded rewrite-rules:

$$\boxed{cab} = cab \quad (16) \qquad \boxed{dir} = dir \quad (17) \qquad \boxed{door} = door \quad (18) \qquad \boxed{pos} = \boxed{p(pos)} \quad (19)$$

Each rewrite rule constitutes its own class.

4.2 The Proof

While the generation of normalized rewrite rules of head terms is independent of the concrete invariant and can thus be done immediately after the specification of a transition, the next two steps of our proof procedure depend on the specific invariant to be proven.

As a first step of this phase we split the proof obligation $Ens_T \wedge Req_T \wedge Inv_{state} \rightarrow Inv_{state'}$ into a set of different obligations

$$\{Ens_T \wedge Req_T \wedge Inv_{state} \rightarrow Inv^1_{state'}, \ldots, Ens_T \wedge Req_T \wedge Inv_{state} \rightarrow Inv^n_{state'}\}$$

if $Inv_{state'}$ is a conjunction $Inv^1_{state'} \wedge \ldots \wedge Inv^n_{state'}$.

In a next step we will compute an appropriate case analysis for the proofs of the invariant parts. For this reason we analyze the contexts in which primed system variables occur. We say an occurrence π of a primed system variable in a formula Φ is *governed* by a head term s if there are occurrences π_1, π_2 with $\pi = \pi_1 \circ \pi_2$ such that s matches $\Phi|\pi_1$. Thus, each rewrite rule with head s can be used to manipulate the subterm containing this occurrence of the system variable.

Given a class of rewrite rules, like for instance $\{(14), (15)\}$ the conditions of the rewrite rule form a in general incomplete case analysis. Considering all classes the corresponding head terms govern some occurrences of a primed system variable, each class suggests some case analysis. Similarly to techniques in inductive theorem proving in order to formulate an appropriate case-analysis for induction[5], we use the suggested case analyses of these classes to impose a complete, common case analysis and attach those rewrite rules to a specific case, the conditions of which belong to this case.

Suppose, we have to prove the invariant of the transition **press**. Since **press** only modifies the system variable *buttons* the parts 3 and 8 are trivially proved. In case of part 7 the head term of (13) governs the only occurrence of a primed state variable and applying this rewrite rule finishes the proof. So we have a closer look at part 5 of the invariant. Thus we have to refute this part of $Inv_{state'}$:

$$cab' = move \wedge dir' = down \wedge (\neg Z \le pos \vee \neg state(select(buttons', Z)) = req) \tag{20}$$

assuming that the specification (9) - (15) of **press** and the invariant Inv_{state} of the state before executing **press** holds true.

Similarly to induction proofs the proof of the invariant is split into two parts. In the first part we are concerned with the removal of primed variables by using appropriate annotated rewrite rules. Thus, once we have eliminated all occurrences of primed variables, the wave-fronts of the manipulated theorem indicate the differences between the actual theorem and the invariant before performing the action. Hence, rippling techniques like rippling-out are used to minimize the differences by moving the wave-fronts towards top-level.

In our example the occurrences of cab' and dir' are governed by the trivial rewrite rules (9) and (10), thus the rewrite rules (9) and (10) governing the occurrences of cab' and dir' are used to rewrite (20):

$$cab = move \wedge dir = down \wedge (\neg Z \le pos \vee \neg state(select(buttons', Z)) = req) \tag{21}$$

The occurrence of the primed system variable *buttons'* in (21) is governed by the two rewrite rules (14) and (15) which suggests a case analysis on the property $Z = i$.

In the other case we use (14) to obtain a *non-recursive* case, thus we drop the annotations and apply (14) to (21) which results in:

$$cab = move \wedge dir = down \wedge (\neg Z = i \vee \neg Z \le pos \vee \neg req = req)$$

which simplifies to

$$cab = move \wedge dir = down \wedge i \le pos \tag{22}$$

---

[5] cf. for instance [Wal94] for a description of such a procedure.

In case of (15), (21) is rewritten to

$$\ldots \wedge \boxed{i = Z} \vee \neg Z \leq pos \vee \neg state(select(buttons, Z)) = req \tag{23}$$

Since the shaded differences occur now only on top-level we use the related part 5 of Inv_{state} and obtain:

$$i = floor_{req} \tag{24}$$

Finally (24) is used as a rewrite rule to reformulate (22) which yields

$$cab = move \wedge dir = down \wedge floor_{req} \leq pos$$

which is in contradiction to the other part of 5 demanding

$$\neg cab = move \vee \neg dir = down \vee \neg floor_{req} \leq pos$$

As another example consider the proof that the execution of the transition **pass-down** does not invalidate the invariant. Again we focus on part 5 of the invariant. By analogy to the previous example, trivial rewrite rules for cab', dir' and $buttons'$ are applied to simplify the goal to

$$cab = move \wedge dir = down \wedge (\neg Z \leq \boxed{pos'} \vee \neg state(select(buttons, Z)) = req \tag{25}$$

The occurrence of pos' is governed by the rewrite-rule (19). Applying it to (25) results in:

$$cab = move \wedge dir = down \wedge (\neg Z \leq \boxed{p(pos)} \vee \neg state(\ldots) = req \tag{26}$$

In order to reduce the differences of part 5 of Inv_{state} and $Inv_{state'}$, we use the rippling-out technique to manipulate the goal. Thus, we search for an appropriate rippling-out wave-rule, like

$$\neg X \leq \boxed{p(Y)} \rightarrow \boxed{X = Y \vee \neg X \leq Y}$$

in order to manipulate (26) to:

$$cab = move \wedge dir = down \wedge (\boxed{Z = pos} \vee \neg Z \leq pos) \vee \neg state(\ldots) = req \tag{27}$$

which enables the use of part 5 of Inv_{state}. Thus, we obtain as a remaining proof obligation:

$$floor_{req} = pos \tag{28}$$

which applied as a rewrite rule to (5) results in

$$\neg cab = move \vee \neg dir = down \vee state(select(buttons, pos)) = req$$

Further simplification and the application of the precondition of **pass-down** finally results in

$$noreq = req$$

which contradicts the specification of the abstract datatype **buttonstates**.

Summing up, we use the analysis of the transition description to compute an appropriate case-analysis for proving the individual components of the invariant while the form of the available rewrite rules determines the proof technique used to verify the single tasks. The computation of rewrite rules from the action specification is an easy task. We have to collect all occurrences of primed and non-primed state variables and sort these occurrences according to the specific contexts in which they occur. Based on these occurrences we compute a list of conditional equations or implications which have to be normalized in order to obtain identical left hand sides of the designated rules. The effort to do this is basically quadratic to the number of occurrences of state variables. This analysis is the basis to compute an appropriate case analysis for the intended verification of the invariant. Basically we collect all occurrences of state variables inside the invariant and compute the set of rules the left-hand side of which can be unified with some subterm of the invariant containing the state variables. Again this can be done without any search and results in a sophisticated case-analysis we use to split up the proof of the invariant. For each case of the proof we know about the rules we have to apply in order to get rid of the primed variables. Using coloring techniques we have an explicit representation of the syntactic differences between the invariant before and after performing the action. Rippling is used to remove these differences which usually is done without any search. Additionally the constraints introduced by rippling allow us also to speculate about inductive lemmata which have to be used in order to get the proof through.

5 Related Work and Conclusion

While in the past various frameworks have been developed to represent arising proof obligations of state-transition systems and to make them accessible for a mechanical verification, less work has been done in actually guiding the proof search. Within the STeP-system [BCC+96] verification diagrams [MP94] (generalized verification diagrams [BMS95]) are used to decompose the proof obligations while the arising subproofs are done without any special proof support. In the field of inductive theorem proving the rippling technique [BSH+93,Hut97] turned out to be a powerful method to guide inductive proof search which is documented in various papers.

We presented a technique to verify invariants of state-transition systems. Since our approach is based on logic we are not restricted to finite systems as it is the case when using model checking. We have implemented our techniques within the *INKA*-system [HS96] which is part of the *Verification Support Environment VSE* [VSE96]. Using this system we have successfully tested our techniques on several state-transition systems. For instance all the proof obligations arising from the verification of the invariant in our example of an elevator have been proven fully automatically within the system. The time spent to prove one case of such a proof obligation was typically less than a second.

References

[BCC+96] N.S. Bjørner, A. Browne, E. Chang, M. Colon, A. Kapur, Z. Manna, H.B. Sipma, T.E. Uribe: *STeP: Deductive-algorithmic verification of reactive and real-time systems*. 8th Computer Aided Verification CAV, Springer, LNCS 1102, 1996

[BMS95] A. Browne, Z. Manna, H.B. Sipma: *Generalized temporal verification diagrams*. 15th Conference on Foundations of Software Technology and Theoretical Computer Science, Springer, LNCS 1026, 1995

[BSH+93] A. Bundy, A. Stevens, F. v. Harmelen, A. Ireland, and A. Smaill: *Rippling: a heuristic for guiding inductive proofs*. Journal of Artificial Intelligence, pp. 185-253, No. 62, 1993

[HS96] D. Hutter, C. Sengler: *INKA - The Next Generation* 13th Int. Conference on Automated Deduction CADE, Springer, LNAI 1104, 1996

[Hut97] D. Hutter: *Colouring Terms to Control Equational Reasoning*. Journal of Automated Reasoning, Vol. 18, pp. 399-442, 1997

[MP94] Z. Manna, A. Pnueli: *Temporal verification diagrams* Int. Symp. on Theoretical Aspects of Computer Software, Springer, LNCS 789, 1994

[MP95] Z. Manna, A. Pnueli: *Temporal Verification of Reactive Systems: Safety*. Springer, New York, 1995

[Sha93] N. Shankar: *Verification of real time systems using PVS* 5th Computer Aided Verification CAV, Springer, LNCS 697, 1993

[VSE96] D. Hutter, B. Langenstein, C. Sengler, J. Siekmann, W. Stephan, and A. Wolpers: *Deduction in the Verification Support Environment (VSE)*. Formal Methods Europe 96, Oxford, Great Britain, 1996

[Wal94] C. Walther: *Mathematical Induction*. Handbook of Logic in AI and Logic Programming, Vol.2, Oxford Press, 1994

GOLEX — Bridging the Gap between Logic (GOLOG) and a Real Robot

Dirk Hähnel[†], Wolfram Burgard[†], and Gerhard Lakemeyer[‡]

[†] Universität Bonn, Institut für Informatik III, Römerstr. 164, D-53117 Bonn
{haehnel,wolfram}@cs.uni-bonn.de
[‡] RWTH Aachen, Lehrgebiet Informatik V, Ahornstr. 55, D-52056 Aachen
gerhard@cs.rwth-aachen.de

Abstract. The control of mobile robots acting autonomously in the real world is one of the long-term goals of the field of artificial intelligence. So far the field lacks methods bridging the gap between the sophisticated symbolic techniques to represent and reason about action and more and more reliable low-level robot control and navigation systems. In this paper we present GOLEX, an execution and monitoring system for the logic-based action language GOLOG and the complex and distributed RHINO control software which operates on RWI B21 and B14 mobile robots. GOLEX provides the following features: it maps abstract primitive actions into low-level commands of the robot control system, thus allowing the user to concentrate on the application rather than the inner workings of the robot; it monitors the execution of the primitive GOLOG actions, making it possible to detect simple execution failures and timeouts; and it includes means to deal with sensing and user input and to continue the operation appropriately. We present two different real-world applications in which GOLEX successfully operated a mobile robot in dynamic and even unstructured environments. These results suggest that the time is ripe for using symbolic action languages for mobile robot applications.

1 Introduction

To successfully perform their missions mobile robots must reliably fulfill and co-ordinate different kinds of subtasks like navigation, manipulation, perception, and interaction. Programming such robot applications using conventional programming languages is a very delicate and often frustrating enterprise, especially for people other than the designers of the robot. Partly as an answer to this dilemma the logic-based action language GOLOG [15] has been developed. It allows a user to specify at a very abstract level how primitive actions like *pickup(x)* change the world. More-over, such actions can be combined into high-level programs using familiar control structures such as loops or recursive procedures. GOLOG then verifies for a given description of the world whether a program is executable and, if successful, delivers a sequence of primitive actions which can then be handed to the robot for immediate execution.

Or so the theory goes. The problem is, of course, that there is still a big gap to bridge between a primitive action like *pickup(x)* and the actual (and hopefully correct) movements of the robot arm. This paper is about bridging this gap. At the moment there is no accepted theory of how to map abstract (logical) descriptions of actions into actual robot behavior, and this paper does not attempt to provide one either. In fact, we believe that experiments are needed first so that we can begin to understand what this mapping is about. Also, there is still widespread skepticism whether logic has a role to play at all in robotics, since previous attempts starting with SHAKEY [18] never left the laboratory and worked only in toy domains. Our work, perhaps for the first time, demonstrates that logic can be used successfully to control a robot in real world domains.

There are many issues that need to be addressed when implementing a high-level control language such as GOLOG. Here we focus on the following three, which cover both inherent problems when moving from the abstract to the concrete and problems due to current limitations of GOLOG.

Level of Abstraction: Primitive actions in GOLOG generally cannot be directly executed by the low-level control system.[1] For example, the action *pickup(letter)* has to be transformed in several control directives such as stop moving, initialize the gripper, move the gripper to the position of the letter, and close the gripper.

Execution monitoring: In GOLOG it is assumed that actions succeed provided their preconditions are met. This, however, is generally not the case in robotics. As an example, consider the situation in which the robot wants to go to a specific room, whose door it assumes to be open. However, it turns out that the door is in fact locked. Without monitoring the progress of the robot, the system would easily get stuck in front of the closed doorway.

Sensing and Interaction: GOLOG in its current form does not provide any means for incorporation sensing actions or interaction. Interaction with users, however, is a crucial aspect of a mobile robot operating, for example, as an interactive tour-guide in a museum. On the other hand, an office delivery robot has to detect the number of letters to be picked up in order to verify that none of them was lost during delivery.

To tackle these problems we developed GOLEX, a runtime and execution monitoring system for GOLOG that

- decomposes the primitive actions specified in GOLOG into a sequence of appropriate directives for the low-level robot control system, thus providing the necessary mapping from the abstract task level to the low level of the robot control software.
- permanently monitors the execution of the various and possibly parallel actions of the underlying robot control system. In case of a failure it chooses appropriate actions to recover from this situation and updates the logical representation of the state so that the system can restart from this situation.
- integrates simple forms of sensing and interaction into GOLOG. It permits the programmer to formulate actions that include interaction and sensing. To deal with situations in which the sensing or interaction has side-effects on the whole

---

[1] Although nothing prevents a user from specifying very low-level primitive actions in GOLOG, this would defeat the whole purpose of the language.

plan and not only on the currently executed action, it provides means for deriving a new plan by calling GOLOG using the description of the current state as the initial situation.

GOLEX has been implemented on top of the existing control software of the Bonn mobile robot RHINO [3,21], which consists of a number of asynchronous processes, loosely coupled through message passing. This software is being used by over 20 groups worldwide. GOLEX has been extensively tested in different applications and proved to be extremely robust in a real-world scenario, in which RHINO was deployed over several days as an interactive and autonomous tour-guide in the "Deutsches Museum Bonn" [4].

As for related work, issues such as execution monitoring certainly come up and need to be solved in any implementation of a robot control language. Most of these languages such as COLBERT [13] remain well below the level of abstraction of GOLOG and hence are hard to compare. Using logic to control a real robot was first attempted in the SHAKEY project [18]. It never made it beyond toy domains mainly because the robot hardware and low-level control software were neither reliable nor sophisticated enough in those days. In fact, between then and now most of the work in robotics has concentrated on fixing those shortcomings and issues of high-level control have regained interest only recently. The work closest to our own is perhaps [12]. There PRODIGY [6], a non-linear planning system, is coupled with a mobile robot. While the authors address issues similar to ours such as monitoring and failure recovery, their execution system ROGUE is tightly coupled with PRODIGY and thus cannot be readily used for GOLOG. Also, as far as we know, ROGUE has only been tested in controlled office environments.

The remainder of this paper is organized as follows. After a very brief description of GOLOG in Section 2 we present the architecture of the RHINO system in Section 3. The GOLEX system is described in Section 4. Finally, Section 5 describes two applications of GOLOG, a tour-guide robot and an office delivery task.

2 GOLOG — A Language for Specifying Actions

Since GOLEX only sees the output of a GOLOG program, which is a linear sequence of primitive actions, we will only hint at what GOLOG is about and refer the reader to [15] for details. GOLOG is based on the situation calculus [17], which itself is a dialect of the predicate calculus with three sorts: ordinary objects, actions, and situations. Situations are action histories constructed from an initial situation S_0 and a special two-place function do where $do(a, s)$ denotes the successor situation to s resulting from performing the action a. What is true at a situation is described in terms of *fluents*, which are predicates whose last argument is a situation.

Following [16], a situation calculus theory AX consists of a number of foundational axioms, precondition axioms for the actions, a specification of what is true after doing an action a in situation s,[2] and a description of what the world is like initially.

---

[2] This employs a solution to the frame problem by Reiter [19].

Given such an AX, GOLOG allows a user to write high-level programs where the primitive actions are those defined in AX and where complex actions can be formed using control structures known from conventional imperative languages. Here is an example of a simple procedure specifying coffee delivery:

proc *deliverCoffee*
   while ($\exists p$) *wantsCoffee(p)* $\wedge$ $\neg hasCoffee(p)$ **do**
     (πp).*goto(coffeeMachine); pickupCoffee; goto(p); giveCoffee(p)*
   endWhile
endProc

proc *goto(loc)*
   if *robotLocation(rloc)* $\wedge$ *rloc* $\neq$ *loc* **then** *drive(rloc, loc)* **endIf**
endProc

In this example, the operator πp non-deterministically chooses an action argument p for *goto(p)* that is a solution for the existentially quantified condition. The semantics of a GOLOG program is defined completely within the situation calculus. This is done using a special three-place macro *Do* which expands into a sentence of the situation calculus and where $Do(\rho, s, s')$ should be read as "the program ρ, when executed in situation s, leads to situation s'." The job of the GOLOG interpreter is then to find a sequence s' such that

$$AX \models Do(\rho, S_0, s').$$

If ρ = deliverCoffee, then s' could be

$$do(\ldots, do(giveCoffee(ray), do(drive(coffeMachine, ray), do(pickupCoffee, s0)))\ldots)$$

provided we specified in AX that Ray wants coffee and the robot starts at the coffee machine in situation S_0. It is s' which gets handed down to GOLEX for further processing.

3   The RHINO System Architecture

The RHINO system consists of more than 25 modules, each of which is designed to monitor or control dedicated aspects of the robot or its environment and to provide information to other modules. There is no centralized clock to synchronize the different components and the robot has to function even if major parts of its software fail or are temporarily unavailable (e.g., due to radio link failure).

The building blocks of this architecture are depicted in Figure 1. The on-board user interface consists of an on-board lap-top, a speech- and sound-board, and four colored buttons which allow users to interact with the robot. The task planner uses GOLOG to plan the activities of the robot and GOLEX to perform and monitor them. The navigation system or low-level control system of the robot consists of the collision avoidance routine [8], the map updating and path planning modules [21] and the localization system [5]. The task of the map building system is to update the information about the environment given new sensory input. The path planner computes cost-optimal paths from a starting position to a given target position given the current map of the environment. The localization module permanently estimates the position of the robot within its environment. Finally, the RHINO system contains various hardware control interfaces, for example, to a top-mounted pan-tilt-head carrying a stereo camera system or to the speech-board. All software modules communicate using TCX [7], a communication manager for point-to-point socket communication.

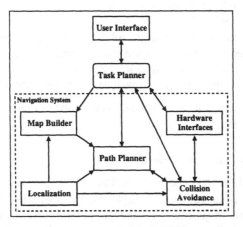

Figure 1: Major components of the RHINO control system

The RHINO navigation system has been proven robust and reliable in different applications [3,21]. The modularity provides a high flexibility with respect to new applications and supports the specialization of dedicated modules according to specific subtasks. The disadvantage of the decentralized architecture is that each module generally has to communicate with a variety of other modules. For example, the path planning system receives information from the localization system to estimate the current position of the robot, receives map updates from the map building module and transmits the next target point along the planned path to the collision avoidance system. Due to the asynchronous nature of the concurrently and independently running modules, the complexity of coordinating the various modules increases with the number of active modules. Moreover modules generally do not broadcast the successful completion of their tasks. For example, the collision avoidance simply stops the robot after reaching the target point obtained from the path planning module. Thus, the path planner has to monitor the progress of the robot and to transmit a new (intermediate) target points if the final destination has not yet been reached. Finally, modules may fail or abort and have to be re-initialized after restart. Thus, a high-level control system has to communicate with a series of different low-level control modules and has to permanently monitor the progress of the system to detect possible failures or the completion of the task.

4 GOLEX — The GOLOG Execution System

The GOLOG execution system GOLEX, which has been implemented in Prolog (together with a C-interface), is designed to support the control of a mobile robot equipped with the RHINO navigation system and to provide the programmer with the necessary level of abstraction on the Prolog level. During execution it handles user inputs and deals with possible timeouts of actions of the user or the robot. To summarize, the task of the GOLEX system is to

- refine primitive GOLOG actions into actions that can be carried out by the low-level controls system.
- permanently monitor the actions of the robot to verify that the primitive GOLOG actions have been successfully carried out, this way ensuring that the relevant state of the world is consistent with GOLOG's model.
- integrate simple forms of sensing as well as interaction with users.

How these different tasks are accomplished is described in more detail in the remainder of this section.

4.1 Refinement of Primitive Actions

Primitive actions in GOLOG have to be translated into a set of corresponding directives to the low-level control system accomplishing the desired task. For this purpose GOLEX includes a set of generic commands for possible actions carried out by the robot. These actions include primitives such as *robot_drive_path(L)* which successively transmits the list L of target points to the path planner so that the robot passes this sequence of points. Furthermore, it includes actions for turning the robot, for example, the predicate *robot_turn_to_point(P)* forces the robot to rotate so that it is heading towards P. It also contains commands for displaying images or texts on the on-board screen, to speak texts to play sounds, or to request user input. Finally, GOLEX provides primitives for receiving raw as well as abstract and preprocessed sensory input. For example, the primitive *free_space* is true, if there is no obstacle in front of the robot. This way, GOLEX allows to check, whether the path of the robot is blocked by a closed door.

Based on these primitives, the user can easily specify, how the primitive actions in GOLOG have to be translated into an appropriate sequence of navigation or display directives or user input requests. For example, in the tour-guide application the primitive *do(go(L), S)* is realized within GOLEX by the following Prolog clause:

```
exec(go(L)) :-
    position(L, (X, Y)),
    pan_tilt_set_track_point((X, Y)),
    target_message(L, M),
    speech_talk_text(["Please follow me to", L]),
    sound_play(horn),
    robot_drive_path([(X, Y)]),
    robot_turn_to_point((X, Y)).
```

4.2 Execution Monitoring

Because the other software components of the RHINO system generally do not report a failure, the GOLEX system has to constantly monitor the progress of the
robot and to detect whether the robot has accomplished the particular action. For
example, the primitive *robot_drive_path(L)* monitors, whether the robot has reached
the target point. The path planning module generally regards a target position as
reached if the robot is about 50cm away from it. To provide a higher accuracy at
the final destination, the *robot_drive_path(L)* primitive directly communicates with
the collision avoidance module to move the robot closer to the target and to achieve
the desired heading. Furthermore, it re-transmits the necessary information to each
connected module in case of transmission failures, resource conflicts between different modules or even in situations in which a module fails or is restarted again. For
example, the path planner stops the robot whenever it arrives at the target position.
If *robot_turn_to_point((X, Y))* starts to rotate the robot before this stop command is
received by the collision avoidance after the rotate command, the robot also stops
the final rotation and is facing the wrong direction. Thus, GOLEX monitors whether
this situation occurs and re-transmits the rotation command to the collision avoidance.

Several commands have additional arguments for timeouts. For example, *but-
ton_get_input(B, T)* waits the time T until a button is pressed. If no button was
pressed, it succeeds with B=0. Otherwise, B is bound to the number of the button
that was pressed. GOLEX also supports timeouts during the execution of actions.
For example the primitive *robot_go_path([P], T)* succeeds, if the robot reaches the
given P before the end of the time interval T and fails otherwise. This way the system
is able to consider time constraints while acting as a coffee delivery robot [20]:

```
exec_plan([startGo( Person, Place )| Other_actions], Done) :-
    wants_coffee(Person, Time_interval),
    ( robot_go_path([Place], Time_interval) ->
        execPlan(Other_actions, do(startGo(Person, Place), Done))
    ;
        write("Skipping "), write(Person), nl,
        retract(wants_coffee(Person, Time_interval)),
        ( do( deliver_coffee(Now), Done, New_actions) ->
            split(Done, New_actions, Remaining_actions),
            execPlan(Remaining_actions, Done)
        ;
            write("Aborting execution"),nl
        )
    ).
```

If GOLEX detects that the robot can no longer reach the destination before the
end of T it drops the user requests and re-plans using the current state as initial state.

4.3 Interaction

By providing primitives for user input, GOLEX adds the ability to interact with the
user. For example, the coffee delivery robot needs a confirmation that the user has
already taken his coffee. If the user does not respond after a certain amount of time,
the robot has to proceed with serving other people:

```
exec(serve_coffee_to(Person, Location)) :-
   robot_drive_path([Location]),
   robot_turn_to_point(Location),
   speech_talk_text(["Hi", Person,
                ". Please take your coffee and push a button"]),
   button_get_input(B, 10),
   ( B = 0 ->
       speech_talk_text(["Did you forget to push a button?"]),
       button_get_input(B1, 10),
       ( B1 = 0 ->
           speech_talk_text(["You seem to be very busy."])
       ;
           true
       )
   ;
       true
   ),
   speech_talk_text(["Thanks and good bye."]).
```

In both applications, GOLEX requires further information about the environment and the task. For example, in the tour-guide application it requires a map specifying the locations of the exhibits in the museum.

Furthermore, GOLEX supports two different types of user input that influences the currently executed plan of the robot. For example, in the museum tour-guide application visitors had the opportunity to request specific information about the currently visited exhibit, or even abort or change the current tour. The interaction with the users that want specific information about the current exhibit cannot be planned a priori in GOLOG, since it is unclear at the planning phase, which button will be pressed. The normal situation, however, is that the robot explains the exhibit to the visitors, reacts on the user input and after that continues with the currently planned sequence of exhibits. Thus, by providing a primitive action *explain(E)* to GOLOG, this type of interaction with the users can be achieved within GOLEX.

However, if the user requests to abort the tour or to be guided to another exhibit, GOLEX uses GOLOG to compute a new plan given the current state of the world as starting state. In such a situation it proceeds in a similar way as when a timeout occurs during a delivery job (see above).

5 Experimental Results

To evaluate the GOLEX system we performed two different experiments in different partially unstructured environments with the mobile robots RHINO (Figure 2a) from the University of Bonn and GOLEM from the University of Toronto (Figure 2b).

5.1 The Museum Tour-Guide Application

The first experiment has been carried out during the six day deployment of the mobile robot RHINO as an interactive personal tour-guide in the "Deutsches Museum Bonn", Germany [4]. The task of the robot was to guide visitors through the exhibition and to provide explanations about the exhibits (see Figure 3). During the 47 hours of operation, the actions of the robot were planned using GOLOG and the generated plans were executed by GOLEX.

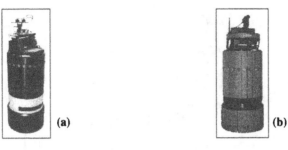

Figure 2: The mobile robots RHINO (a) and GOLEM (b) used for the experiments

Figure 3: RHINO giving a tour to visitors (a) and explaining an exhibit (b).

Over this period of time, the robot travelled approximately 18.6km. More than 2,000 real visitors and over 600 "virtual" Web-based visitors were guided by RHINO (see Figure 3). The robot fulfilled 2,400 tour requests by real and virtual visitors of the museum. Only six requests were not fulfilled which corresponds to an over-all success-rate of 99.75%. None of these failures were caused by the high-level planning system or by GOLEX. The key results are also summarized in Table 1. A typical path of the robot as well as the user interface are depicted in Figures 4 and 5.

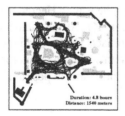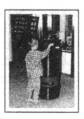

Hours of operation	47
Number of visitors	> 2000
Kilometers traveled	18.6
Maximal speed of travel	> 80
Average speed during motion	36.6
Number of requests	2400
Number of failures	6
Success rate	99.75%

Figure 4: Typical path of the robot.   Figure 5: RHINO's user interface.   Table 1: Some key results.

5.2 The Coffee Delivery Application

The second experiment is designed to demonstrate the applicability of GOLEX in a typical office delivery scenario. In this application the task of the robot GOLEM was to serve people with coffee [20]. Thereby it had to deal with time constraints given

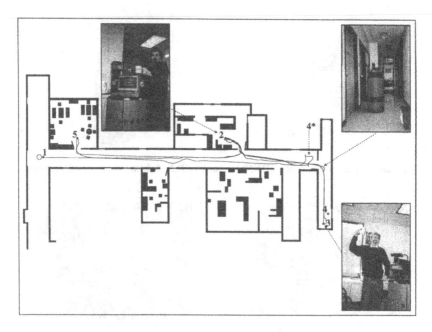

Figure 6: Path of the robot during the coffee delivery

by the time interval when the people had to be served. Whenever GOLEX detects, that the next customer cannot be served within the given amount of time, it skips this sub-plan from the current schedule and re-plans after removing this person from the list of persons to be served.

Figure 6 shows a typical run of GOLEM while serving three different people at the University of Toronto. It starts at position 1 and goes to the coffee machine at position 2. There GOLEM request for coffee which is uploaded by Mikhail and afterwards proceeds to Ray's office at position 3. After Ray took the coffee from the robot, GOLEM returns to the coffee machine to upload a further cup of coffee which has to be brought to Hector whose office is at position 4. On the way to Hector, the path of the robot is blocked by a crowd of people (position 4*). At the moment when the due time for serving Hector is expired, GOLEX retracts Hector's request and then computes a new plan using GOLOG. According to this plan, the visitor at position 5 is served next. After completing this task, the robot returns to position 2 and stops its delivery job.

6 Conclusions

In this paper we presented GOLEX, a runtime and execution monitoring system for GOLOG, that demonstrates, how mobile robot applications specified in a logical action language can be realized on top of existing low-level robot control software like that of the RWI B14 and B21 mobile robots [21]. GOLEX maps abstract primitive actions into low-level commands of the robot control system, thus allowing the user to concentrate on the application rather than the inner workings of the robot. Furthermore, it monitors the execution of the primitive GOLOG actions thus allowing to detect possible execution failures or timeouts. Finally, it incorporates user input and sensing and is able to continue the operation appropriately in such situations.

GOLEX has been implemented and tested extensively in different applications. In a long-term experiment GOLEX served as the execution monitoring system during a 47 hours lasting deployment of the mobile robot RHINO as an interactive tour-guide in the "Deutsches Museum Bonn". The robot fulfilled 99.75% of the user requests and none of the failures were caused by the high-level control system. It furthermore was applied in a typical office-delivery application where it controlled the mobile robot GOLEM to deliver coffee.

Although GOLEX has been proven to allow a robust execution of plans in these real world applications, there are many opportunities for future research:

- While there is a parallel version of GOLOG [9], GOLEX currently does not support parallel actions. For example, GOLEX is not able to react on user input while the robot travels to its destination. Supporting parallelism in general would require a resource management system since certain resources such as motors cannot be shared simultaneously.
- Specifying how to react to the outcome of a sensing action really should be handled at the abstract level of GOLOG. In fact, very recently there have been proposals to extend GOLOG with sensing actions [10,14]. Work is under way to adapt GOLEX to use these more expressive action languages.
- Similarly, it seems desirable to leave at least some part of execution monitoring under high-level user control. First results on how to specify such monitors in GOLOG have recently appeared [11], but they are still at a preliminary stage.
- Finally, when moving to more complex applications than the ones we reported on, the current techniques in GOLEX to deal with execution failures will probably not suffice. For example, rather than simply generating a new plan from scratch after a failure, plan transformation techniques as in [1] may be preferable.

While GOLEX was designed for the purpose of linking GOLOG to a real robot, GOLEX really only gets to see the output of GOLOG, that is, a sequence of primitive actions. Hence we expect it to be relatively easy to use GOLEX in conjunction with other action or planning languages such as TL [2] and RPL [1].

Finally, we strongly believe that both robotics and symbolic AI can benefit from each other. GOLEX is but one step in bringing the two fields closer together.

References

1. M. Beetz and D. McDermott. Improving robot plans during their execution. In Kris Hammond, editor, *Second International Conference on AI Planning Systems*, pages 3–12, Morgan Kaufmann, 1994.
2. W. Bibel. Let's plan it deductively. In *Proceedings of the Fifteenth International Joint Conference on Artificial Intelligence*, volume 2, pages 1549–1562, August 1997.

3. J. Buhmann, W. Burgard, A.B. Cremers, D. Fox, T. Hofmann, F. Schneider, J. Strikos, and S. Thrun. The mobile robot RHINO. *AI Magazine*, 16(2):31–38, Summer 1995.

4. W. Burgard, Armin B. Cremers, D. Fox, D. Hähnel, G. Lakemeyer, D. Schulz, W. Steiner, and S. Thrun. The interactive museum tour-guide robot. In *Proc. of the Sixteenth National Conference on Artificial Intelligence (AAAI-98)*, 1998. To appear.

5. W. Burgard, D. Fox, D. Hennig, and T. Schmidt. Estimating the absolute position of a mobile robot using position probability grids. In *Proc. of the Fourteenth National Conference on Artificial Intelligence*, pages 896–901, 1996.

6. J. G. Carbonell, C. A. Knoblock, and S. Minton. Prodigy: An integrated architecture for planning and learning. In K. Van Lehn, editor, *Architectures for Intelligence*. Erlbaum, 1990.

7. C. Fedor. *TCX. An interprocess communication system for building robotic architectures. Programmer's guide to version 10.xx.* Carnegie Mellon University, Pittsburgh, PA 15213, 12 1993.

8. D. Fox, W. Burgard, and S. Thrun. The dynamic window approach to collision avoidance. *IEEE Robotics and Automation Magazine*, 1997.

9. G. de Giacomo, Y. Lespérance, and H.J. Levesque. Reasoning about concurrent execution, prioritized interrupts, and exogenous actions in the situation calculus. In *Proceedings of the Fifteenth International Joint Conference on Artificial Intelligence*, volume 2, pages 1221–1226, 1997.

10. G. de Giacomo and H. J. Levesque. An incremental interpreter for high-level programs with sensing. Technical report, University of Toronto, 1998.

11. G. de Giacomo, R. Reiter, and M. M. Soutchanski. Execution monitoring of high-level robot programs. In *Proceedings of the Sixth International Conference on Knowledge Representation (KR 98)*, 1998. To appear.

12. K. Z. Haigh and M. M. Veloso. High-level planning and low-level execution: towards a complete robotic agent. In *Proceedings of the First International Conference on Autonomous Agents*, Marina del Rey, CA, February 1997.

13. K. Konolige. Colbert: A language for reactive control in saphira. In *KI-97: Advances in Artificial Intelligence*, pages 31–52. LNAI Series, Springer Verlag, 1997.

14. G. Lakemeyer. On sensing and off-line interpreting in golog. Technical report, RWTH Aachen, 1998.

15. H.J. Levesque, R. Reiter, Y. Lespérance, F. Lin, and R. Scherl. GOLOG: A logic programming language for dynamic domains. *Journal of Logic Programming*, 31:59–84, 1997.

16. F. Lin and R. Reiter. State constraints revisited. *Journal of Logic and Computation, special issue on actions and processes*, 4:665–678, 1994.

17. J. McCarthy. Situations, actions and causal laws. In *Semantic Information Processing*, pages 410–417. MIT Press, 1968.

18. Nils J. Nilsson. SHAKEY the robot. Technical report, SRI International, 1984.

19. R. Reiter. The frame problem in the situation calculus: A simple solution (sometimes) and a completeness result for goal regression. In V. Lifshitz, editor, *Artificial Intelligence and Mathematical Theory of Computation*, pages 359–380. Academic Press, 1991.

20. R. Reiter. Sequential, temporal golog. In *Proceedings of the Sixth International Conference on Knowledge Representation (KR 98)*, 1998. To appear.

21. S. Thrun, A. Bücken, W. Burgard, D. Fox, T. Fröhlinghaus, D. Hennig, T. Hofmann, M. Krell, and T. Schimdt. Map learning and high-speed navigation in RHINO. In D. Kortenkamp, R.P. Bonasso, and R. Murphy, editors, *AI-based Mobile Robots: Case studies of successful robot systems*. MIT Press, Cambridge, MA, 1998.

Structured Reactive Communication Plans –
Integrating Conversational Actions
into High-Level Robot Control Systems

Michael Beetz and Hanno Peters

University of Bonn, Dept. of Computer Science III, Roemerstr. 164,
D-53117 Bonn, Germany, beetz,peters2@cs.uni-bonn.de

Abstract. Specifying communication routines transparently and explicitly as part of robots' plans rather than hiding them in separate modules makes robots' communication behavior more effective, efficient, and robust. It enables robot control systems to generate, reason about and revise their communication behavior. The controllers can also synchronize the robots' conversations with other actions and use control structures to make the communication behavior flexible and robust. In this paper, we extend RPL, a reactive plan language, to allow for controlling conversational actions. The additional constructs constitute an interface between RPL and conversational actions that is identical to the interface between RPL and continuous control processes such as navigation. The uniformity of the two interfaces and the control structures provided by RPL enable a programmer to concisely specify a wide spectrum of communication behavior. This paper describes how these extensions are implemented and used by a robot office courier.

1 Introduction

The ability to perform natural language conversation significantly enhances robots' capabilities, augmenting both their abilities to perceive their environment and to effect changes within it. For instance, using natural language a robot can ask a person to open a door which it cannot open by itself. Being able to perform natural language communication also enables robots to both receive a wider range of job specifications and also to acquire information that cannot be sensed using their sensors.

Achieving the intended effects of speech acts often requires complex dialogs. For example, courier jobs given to a robot in natural language are sometimes ambiguous and have to be clarified. Thus, to equip a robot with reliable communication capabilities it is not sufficient to simply provide the necessary natural language understanding and generation capabilities. It is also necessary that the robot properly controls and synchronizes the execution of its speech acts, monitors their effects, and reacts properly to the speech acts performed by the people in its working environment.

In this paper we describe how we have equipped FAXBOT, an autonomous robot office courier, with natural language capabilities that satisfy the following requirements.

- **Communication as <u>action</u>.** Communication routines should be activated, controlled, and synchronized by the robot control system just like physical actions. Like other actions, speech acts have desired effects such as the acquisition of missing information.

- **Communication as Interaction.** The robot should always be able to process the speech acts it receives, interpret their content, and update its beliefs and course of action based on these speech acts. Taking into account the *inter*active rather than active character of communication requires adequate means for specifying reactive, robust, flexible, and efficient communication behavior.
- **Plans for Conversations.** Robots should reason about and replan their conversations based on its current state and tasks. They should also make use of different communication channels. Often it is better to point to objects than to describe the objects using natural language.

The idea of describing conversations in terms of speech acts that change the belief state of the listener is not new [Aus62,Sea69]. AI planning techniques for generating plans for communicating information can also be found in the literature (for instance, [CP79]). Nevertheless, the most widely used techniques for specifying flexible communication are dialog grammars [Rei81].

In this paper we propose the use of concurrent reactive plan languages for the specification of flexible and goal-directed dialog behavior. In general, concurrent reactive plans specify how an agent is to interact with its environment in order to accomplish its jobs. As a consequence, modern reactive plan languages provide appropriate control abstractions to specify concurrent action (with different priorities), reactive behavior, robust execution, exception handling, and context-specific execution of plan steps. These languages provide the appropriate means to specify the control and synchronization of different dialog threads because these are exactly the same problems that arise in the control of the robots' physical actions. Consider, for example, a sales talk where the sales representative has a plot of subgoals for convincing her client to buy a product. Besides leading the sales talk, the sales representative has to refute objections, which might require dialogs, and perhaps order lunch during the sales talk.

To the best of our knowledge, the idea of using concurrent reactive control language for the specification of flexible dialog behavior is new. In this paper we extend the planning language RPL [McD91] in such a way that it enables robots to lead restricted natural language dialogs and thereby carry out ambiguous commands and deal with situations that the robot cannot deal with by itself.

The remainder of this paper is organized as follows. The next section describes the robot control system and high-level plan language that the communication capabilities are integrated into. Next a brief explanation of the language interpretation (Section 3) and generation (Section 4) methods are given. Section 5 shows high-level plans of an autonomous robot office courier that applies communication actions. Section 6 discusses an electronic dialog between this robot and a person issueing a delivery command. We conclude with a brief review of related work and a discussion.

2 The FAXBOT Robot Controller

We carry out our research in the context of FAXBOT, an autonomous robot controller. It is designed for robust and efficient execution of a courier service on the autonomous mobile robot RHINO, an RWI B21 robot. FAXBOT operates in a part of an office building containing a large hallway, several offices, a library, and a classroom (see Figure 6).

FAXBOT operates over extended periods of time and carries out a schedule of multiple jobs, which can be changed at any time. Jobs are issued via electronic mail using strongly restricted natural language.

This section gives an overview of the FAXBOT's control modules, their roles, and their interaction. It also describes how these modules are controlled in a flexible and goal-directed way using a *structured reactive controller*.

2.1 Modules of the FAXBOT Controller

The FAXBOT control system runs modules which provide such capabilities as "collision avoidance," "localization," "motion planning," and "image processing." These modules run distributedly over the computer network and communicate asynchronously via message passing established by a communication management module (see Fig. 1). The modules run continuous control processes that can be activated and deactivated, and thereby provide a means for operating the robot.

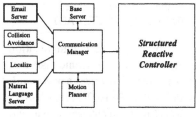

The module *structured reactive controller* [Bee96] combines the other modules so that they effect coherent goal-directed behavior. The main components of a structured reactive controller are the *process modules*, the *fluents*, the *structured reactive plan*, and the RPL *runtime system*. The elementary program units in the structured reactive controller are the process modules. Process modules constitute a uniform interface between RPL programs and the continuous control processes, such as collision avoidance and localization, run by other modules. Fluents, which are continuously updated according to the messages received by the structured reactive controller, provide information about the current state of the other modules of the control system. The structured reactive plan specifies how the robot is to respond to messages (from the navigation modules) and feedback (from the process modules) to accomplish its jobs (contained in the fluents). In summary, it is a collection of concurrent control routines that specify routine activities and can adapt themselves to nonstandard situations by executing planned responses [BM94].

Fig. 1: FAXBOT's Software architecture.

2.2 Extending FAXBOT to Perform Natural Language Communication

We have chosen "electronic mail" as the primary channel to communicate with people in its environment. Compared to spoken language, electronic mail allows for some important simplifications of the natural language communication task. The email is already a sequence of words. It is more reasonable to ask for writing correct English sentences. The identification of the dialog partner is simple: the name is contained in the *sender* line of the mail header. Finally, the real-time requirement for electronic mail is less challenging than in spoken language dialog.

To provide natural language communication capabilities the FAXBOT system (see figure 1) is extended by two additional modules: the "email server" and the "natural language server." The "email server" broadcasts each electronic mail sent to the computer account "RHINO" to the modules that have subscribed to "automatic" email update. It also provides the functions necessary for sending electronic mails. The "natural language server" provides the functions required for transforming electronic mails into an internal representation and analyzing the content of the email using the FAXBOT's world model.

To incorporate natural language capabilities into the structured reactive controller, we must specify the processes for natural language understanding and generation as process modules and store the information provided by them in global fluents.

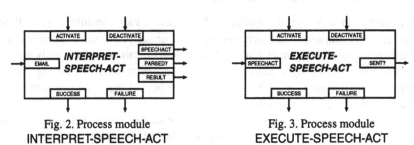

Fig. 2. Process module
INTERPRET-SPEECH-ACT

Fig. 3. Process module
EXECUTE-SPEECH-ACT

The interface between the structured reactive controller and the communication modules contains the fluents LAST-EMAIL, which contains the last electronic mail sent to the robot and NEW-EMAIL?, which is pulsed whenever FAXBOT receives a new email. The extension further contains the two process modules INTERPRET-SPEECH-ACT and EXECUTE-SPEECH-ACT. INTERPRET-SPEECH-ACT takes an electronic mail and translates it into a speech act with the content transformed into FAXBOT's internal representation. The fluent PARSED? signals the completion of the interpretation process and the fluent RESULT indicates whether the content of the email is inconsistent or ambiguous with respect to the robot's model of the world. EXECUTE-SPEECH-ACT takes an internally represented speech act, transforms it into an email, and sends it.

There are other means of communication that are available in the FAXBOT controller such as pointing, displaying graphics, the buttons mounted on the robot and so on. No further discussion of these facilities will be made in this paper.

3 Interpreting Electronic Mails

The interpretation of electronic mails proceeds in three steps: (1) transforming the electronic mail into an internal speech act representation; (2) parsing the content of the speech act; and (3) computing and analyzing the meaning of the speech act using the robot's world model.

3.1 Representing Emails in KQML

Emails are represented internally as KQML statements. KQML is a standardized language for the exchange of information between different knowledge-based systems [FLM95]. KQML messages communicate whether the content of a message is a request, order, etc [CL95]. FAXBOT can receive and perform requests, questions, acknowledgements, replies, and informative performatives.

The advantage of having representations of the purpose of electronic mails that abstract away from the contents of the mail is that this way the dialog behavior can be more concisely specified. In particular, at this level of abstraction we can specify which performatives are valid answers, whether responses are required, and so on.

From: peters2@cs.uni-bonn.de Date: Fri, 24 Oct 1997 12:03:57 To: rhino+tcx@cs.uni-bonn.de Subject: Library book Could you please bring the yellow book on the desk in room a-120 to the library before 12:30	(REQUEST 　:SENDER (THE PERSON 　　　　　(FIRST-NAME Hanno) 　　　　　(LAST-NAME Peters)) 　:RECEIVER (THE ROBOT (NAME RHINO)) 　:TIME (THE TIME-INSTANT 　　　　(DAY 24) (MONTH OCT) 　　　　(TIME 12:03)) 　:REPLY-WITH "Re: Library Book" 　:CONTENT content of the email 　:DEADLINE (A TIME-INSTANT 　　　　(BEFORE (DATE 12.30))))
Fig. 4. Typical electronic mail sent to FAXBOT	Fig. 5. KQML representation of the email from Fig. 4

Figure 4 shows a typical electronic mail sent to FAXBOT. Its internal representation using KQML is shown in figure 5. The algorithm for constructing KQML statements from emails determines the type of speech act, extracts the sender, the subject, and the time when the email was sent, transforms the pieces of information into the corresponding KQML statement.

3.2 Parsing the Content of Electronic Mails

After the KQML representation for an electronic mail is constructed, the content is parsed and transformed into the internal FAXBOT representation. This structured representation facilitates reasoning, retrieval, plan construction, etc. It provides logical connectives, is hierarchically structured and distinguishes between object descriptions, location descriptions, state descriptions, event specifications, and so on.

Input	Output
"Could you please bring the yellow book from Michael's desk in room A-120 to the desk in the library"	(ACHIEVE 　(LOC (THE BOOK 　　　(COLOR YELLOW) 　　　(ON (THE DESK 　　　　(OWNER (THE PERSON 　　　　　　(NAME MICHAEL))) 　　　　(IN (THE ROOM (NUMBER A-120)))))) 　(THE LOC (IN (THE ROOM 　　　　(FUNCTION LIBRARY)))))

We assume that the content of the electronic mail is written in correct English that satisfies the following additional restrictions. The body of the email is a single, self-contained sentence. Only a subset of correct english sentence constructions is accepted. Further the vocabulary is restricted to correctly spelled words from the office delivery domain. The parser signals an error if the sentences are not parsable. These failure signals can then be caught by control structures of the plan that make the plan tolerant against such failures. Recovery startegies might then ask the person sending the electronic mail for clarifications using examples of parsable sentences.

The content of electronic mails are parsed using a Definite Clause Grammar [PW80]. In particular we use an extension of the grammar described in [RN95] and [Nor92]. The grammar is extended by augmenting the vocabulary relevant for office delivery tasks (most notably rules for parsing temporal statements, room names, etc.). The second extension of the grammar enables the robot to parse the sentences it generates (see next section). Besides extending the expressiveness of the language we reduced the time required for grammatical processing using pattern matching techniques to filter out irrelevant grammar rules. Finally, we made the parser interruptable such that parsing processes can be terminated prematurely by deactivating them.

3.3 Interpreting the Content of Electronic Mails

The next step in the interpretation of emails is the identification of the objects the office courier has to pick up and the locations where they are to be picked up or delivered. FAXBOT operates in a part of an office building containing a large hallway, several offices, a library, and a classroom (see Figure 6). FAXBOT uses a symbolically annotated 3D world model of its environment that contains floor plan information for walls, doorways, and rooms and static pieces of furniture. This world model stores, among other information, the symbolic information that is used to interpret natural language commands and as domain knowledge for action planning.

To discuss how FAXBOT interprets an object description generated by the parsing step consider the following example:

```
(THE BOOK
    (COLOR YELLOW)
    (ON (THE DESK
        (OWNER (THE PERSON
            (NAME MICHAEL)))
```

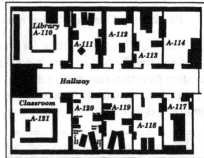

Fig. 6: Model of the office environment.

This object description contains a perceptual description of an object to be localized (LO), a description of a reference object (Michael's desk) and the spatial relation between them (cf. [Gap94,SGH+94]). Since in spatial descriptions reference objects are usually stationary objects with salient features FAXBOT requires reference objects to be contained in its environment model.

Thus, as a first step, the semantic interpretation component extracts the descriptions of reference objects and retrieves in the second step the set of objects in the environment model that satisfy these descriptions. If the query returns more than one map object, the job description is ambiguous. If the query returns no map object then the job specification is inconsistent with the robot's model of the environment. In both cases FAXBOT has to start a dialog to clarify the job specification.

4 Generating and Executing Speech Acts

For the generation of speech acts we use an extension of the language generation facilities of DUCK [McD85]. Essentially DUCK takes formulas written in predicate calculus and translates them into pseudo English sentences. To obtain more readable translations the programmer has to define skeletons for expressing predicates which are then compiled into rules. The rules for expressing logical connectors and handling the recursive structure of predicate calculus expressions are built into the system.

We have extended the facilities of the DUCK pseudo english generator to enable it to handle object and location descriptions and the different kinds of speech acts that the FAXBOT control system can generate. Thus, a typical object description like

```
(THE BOOK (COLOR YELLOW)
        (ON (THE DESK (SIZE BIG)
                (IN (THE ROOM (NUMBER A-120))))))
```

is translated into "the yellow book on the big desk in room A-120." Other examples of sentences that EXECUTE-SPEECH-ACT can produce are shown in section 6.

Since in electronic mail dialogs the content of an electronic mail is included in the answer, we have extended the parser so that it can parse the sentences that the pseudo english generator produces.

5 Communication Plans

Structured reactive plans are implemented in RPL (Reactive Plan Language) [McD91]. RPL provides conditionals, loops, program variables, processes, and subroutines. RPL also places high-level constructs (interrupts, monitors) and reactions (triggered by observed events) at the programmer's disposal. Interrupts and monitors are used to synchronize parallel actions and to make plans reactive and robust. The RPL constructs used to specify and synchronize conversation activity are the WITH-POLICY-, WHENEVER-, and WAIT-FOR-statements. See [McD91] for a complete description.

The RPL statement WITH-POLICY *P B* means "execute the primary activity *B* such that the execution satisfies the policy *P*." Policies are concurrent processes that run while the primary activity is active and interrupt the primary if necessary. Events that require FAXBOT to perform dialogs such as "receiving a command" are handled through fluents, program variables that signal changes of their values and thereby enable control threads to react to asynchronous events. The RPL statement WHENEVER *F B* is an endless loop that executes *B* whenever the fluent *F* gets the value "true." WAIT-FOR *F*, another control abstraction, blocks a thread of control until the fluent *F* becomes true.

The example on the right shows part of FAXBOT's high-level plan highlighting the plan steps for performing or processing speech acts. We see two global policies that ensure that incoming emails are processed immediately and ambiguous commands clarified. The other two conversational actions are part of the robot's primary activities, the ones intended to accomplish the robot's tasks.

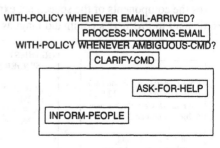

The robot generates conversation acts when it perceives situations that it cannot handle on its own. Below is a piece of a navigation plan that asks for help when the door of room A-120 that the robot intends to leave is closed.

```
WITH-POLICY PAR ESTIMATE-OPENING-ANGLE(EXIT(A-120))
          WHENEVER EXIT-OF-ROOM-A-120-CLOSED?
              LET SPEECH-ACT = MAKE-SPEECH-ACT
                              (FAXBOT,ALL,REQUEST,OPEN(EXIT(A-120)))
                  EXECUTE-SPEECH-ACT(SPEECH-ACT)
                  FAIL(CLOSED-EXIT A-120)
     LEAVE(A-120)
```

While leaving the room A-120 FAXBOT continously estimates the opening angle of the exit. Whenever the door angle estimator detects the door to be closed (the fluent EXIT-OF-ROOM-A-120-CLOSED? becomes true) FAXBOT generates a speech act as a request to all colleagues. This speech act has the content OPEN(EXIT(A-120)). Thus the body of the reaction sends an electronic mail that implements this speech act and signals a failure of the type CLOSED-EXIT that triggers replanning for the robot's overall course of action (see [BB98] for more details).

Another example that shows the advantages of tight integration of communication facilities into the robot control system is taken from an autonomous tour guide application. When the robot explains an exhibit and its distance sensors show that people are standing around the robot it points with its camera to the exhibit instead forming a natural language description of the exhibit. In this case the integration allows for the synchronized use of different modalities for communication purposes.

6   Conversations with FAXBOT

The following example demonstrates FAXBOT's communication behavior and how it is used to achieve competence in the robot's problem-solving behavior.

Wolfram: Could you please deliver the yellow book on the desk in room A-120 to the desk in the library before 12.30.
FAXBOT: Do you mean 'deliver the yellow book on Michael's desk in room A-120 to the desk in the library before 12.30' or 'deliver the yellow book on Dieter's desk in room A-120 to the desk in the library before 12.30' ?
Wolfram: Deliver the yellow book on Michael's desk in room A-120 to the desk in the library before 12.30.
FAXBOT: I will deliver the yellow book on Michael's desk in room A-120 to the desk in the library before 12:30.
Librarian: I will be out of the library for 45 minutes.
FAXBOT: OK. You will be back at 12:45.
FAXBOT: (sending an electronic mail to Wolfram) I can't accomplish the job "Deliver the yellow book on Michael's desk in room A-120 to the desk in the library before 12.30." The library is closed and the librarian won't be back until 12:50.

In more detail, this communication behavior is exhibited through the following problem solving steps. The first two steps show the electronic mail containing a command that is transformed into FAXBOT's internal representation. This representations makes the components of the speech act explicit and represents the content of the electronic mail in FAXBOT's command language.

```
From: peters@cs.uni-bonn.de)
Date: Fri, 24 Oct 1997 12:03:57
To: rhino+tcx@cs.uni-bonn.de
Subject: Command

Could you please bring
the yellow book on the desk
in room a-120
to the library before 12:30
```

```
(REQUEST
    :SENDER (THE PERSON (FIRST-NAME Hanno)
                        (LAST-NAME Peters))
    :RECEIVER (THE ROBOT (NAME RHINO))
    :TIME (THE TIME-INSTANT 10:24:12:03)
    :REPLY-WITH (YOUR COMMAND FROM 12.03)
    :CONTENT (ACHIEVE
                (LOC (THE BOOK
                        (COLOR YELLOW)
                        (ON (THE DESK
                                (IN (THE ROOM
                                        A-120)))))
                    (THE LOC (IN (THE ROOM LIBRARY))))
    :DEADLINE (A TIME-INSTANT (BEFORE (DATE 12.30))))
```

The conversation plans that the FAXBOT control system uses implement that the commands must be unambiguous with respect to the static aspects of the robot's world model and achievable. Thus if the interpretation process signals an ambiguity a control thread is triggered that leads the conversations necessary to make the command unambiguous.

After detecting the ambiguity in the command the FAXBOT controller generates a new speech act of the type query that contains as its content a disjunction of all instantiations of the original command that are consistent with the robot's model of the world (below right). This internal speech act representation is then transformed by the language generation process into pseudo English and the electronic mail is then sent to the person who issued the command (below right).

```
(QUERY
    :SENDER (THE ROBOT
                (NAME RHINO))
    :RECEIVER (THE PERSON
                (FIRST-NAME Hanno)
                (LAST-NAME Peters))
    :TIME (THE TIME-INSTANT
                (DAY 24) (MONTH OCT) (HOUR 12) (MINUTES 4))
    :REPLY-WITH (YOUR COMMAND FROM 12.03)
    :CONTENT (OR
                (ACHIEVE
                    (LOC (THE BOOK
                        (COLOR YELLOW)
                        (ON (THE DESK
                            (IN A-120)))
                            (OWNER DIETER))))))
                    (THE LOC (IN (THE ROOM LIBRARY)))))
                (ACHIEVE
                    (LOC (THE BOOK
                        (COLOR YELLOW)
                        (ON (THE DESK
                            (IN A-120)))
                            (OWNER MICHAEL))))))
                    (THE LOC (IN (THE ROOM LIBRARY)))))
    :DEADLINE (A TIME-INSTANT (BEFORE (DATE 12.30)))))
```

From: Rhino (rhino+tcx@cs.uni-bonn.de)
Date: Fri, 24 Oct 1997 12:04:35
To: peters2@cs.uni-bonn.de
Subject: Your Command from 12.03

Do You mean
  achieve that
    the yellow book on dieter 's desk
    in room a-120 is in the library
    before 12.30
  will be true
or
  achieve that
    the yellow book on michael 's desk
    in-room a-120 is in the library
    before 12.30
  will be true

Finally, the person issuing the command picks the intended instantiation of the original command and sends it back to FAXBOT. FAXBOT acknowledges the receipt of the command by repeating its interpretation of the command to be performed.

From: Hanno Peters (peters2@uran.informatik.uni-bonn.de)
Date: Fri, 24 Oct 1997 12:05:48 +0200 (MET DST)
To: rhino+tcx@uran.informatik.uni-bonn.de
Subject: Command-Revision

achieve that
  the yellow book on michael 's desk
  in-room a-120 is in the library before 12.30
will be true.

From: Rhino (rhino+tcx@cs.uni-bonn.de)
Date: Fri, 24 Oct 1997 12:08:35
To: peters2@cs.uni-bonn.de
Subject: Your Command from 12.05

I will achieve that
  the yellow book on michael 's desk
  in-room a-120 is in the library before 12.30
will be true.

7 Related Work

The problem of communicating with robots using natural language has been addressed in AI research from early on (cf. SHAKEY [Nil84] and SHRDLU [Win72]). More recent approaches comprise the work of Torrance and Stein [TS97] who studied the relation between natural language sentences and sensori-motor behavior for navigation tasks.

We have built our procedures for natural language interpretation and generation on top of implementations that were simple, well documented, and easily modifiable [RN95,Nor92]. As a result, neither the range of sentences that we can parse and interpret correctly nor the speed can compete with the "state of the art". Nevertheless, on average parsing takes less than three seconds which seems to be fast enough considering the time people require to read and answer their emails. [CMU$^+$97] gives an excellent and extensive review of current state of natural language processing techniques.

[CMU$^+$97] classifies approaches to modeling dialog behavior into dialog grammars (e.g. [Rei81]), plan-based models of dialog (e.g. [CP79]), and joint action theories of dialog (e.g. [LGS90]). Our work complements the research in this area in that it provides an appropriate implementation substrate for these approaches.

The TRAINS project is similar to our project in that it focusses on the integration of communication capabilities into a problem-solving agent. However, while the TRAINS project focusses on the reasoning aspects of building conversationally proficient problem-solving agent, we focus on the control and synchronization of conversational actions in a global problem solving context. The application of resource-adaptive computational methods to the generation and interpretation of conversational actions in dialogs [Wei97] is investigated within the READY project. FAXBOT also assigns time resources to threads of control. However, it does not yet apply automated reasoning techniques for determining adequate distributions of resources.

Other reactive robot control languages, such as RAP [Fir87] and ESL [Gat96], provide an expressiveness similar to RPL. So far, they neither have been extended to control conversational actions nor allow for sophisticated plan diagnosis and revision operations.

8   Conclusions

There are several motivations for equipping autonomous service robots with natural language capabilities. Being capable of receiving electronic mail and interpreting their contents provides the robot with an important means for acquiring symbolic information. In addition, being able to send requests helps the robot to overcome some of the restrictions of its effectors by asking for help. As we have pointed out earlier, an important aspect of a robot's communication capbility is the robustness of this capability. In this research we have aimed for one dimension of robustness: making the plans that employ communication actions failure tolerant. The language processing capabilities are rather simple and limited. As a consequence, experiments that measure the dialog success rate or skills for communicating are not appropriate for measuring the failure tolerance.

This research is part of a bigger research effort in which we try to develop *structured reactive controllers (SRCs)* as a uniform framework for the implementation of integrated control systems for autonomous robots acting in human working environments. In companion papers we have shown how image processing capabilities [BACM98] and planning capabilities [BM96] can be integrated into SRCs. The idea of having a single language for controlling and synchronizing the physical actions, image processing, planning, and communication capabilities of autonomous robots is a very powerful one. It allows the application of the same planning [BM94], execution, and learning techniques to all different modalities of robots and their combination.

Our research makes several contributions to the fields of robot control and natural language communication. One of the main contributions is a set of design principles for the integration of conversational actions into a robot control language. We have shown that control structures of modern robot control and planning languages can concisely and transparently specify flexible, reactive, and robust communication behavior. We have also argued that the protocol for interacting with conversational actions should be the same as the one for physical control routines: plans can start them and cause them to evaporate, but they run otherwise independently of the rest of the plan.

References

[Aus62]   J. L. Austin. *How To Do Things with Words*. Harvard University Press, Cambridge, Massachusetts, 1962.

[BACM98] M. Beetz, T. Arbuckle, A. Cremers, and M. Mann. Transparent, flexible, and resource-adaptive image processing for autonomous service robots. In H. Prade, editor, *Procs. of the 13th European Conference on Artificial Intelligence (ECAI-98)*, pages 632–636, 1998.

[BB98]   M. Beetz and M. Bennewitz. Planning, scheduling, and plan execution for autonomous robot office couriers. In R. Bergmann and A. Kott, editors, *Integrating Planning, Scheduling and Execution in Dynamic and Uncertain Environments*, volume Workshop Notes 98-02. AAAI Press, 1998.

[Bee96]   M. Beetz. *Anticipating and Forestalling Execution Failures in Structured Reactive Plans*. Technical report, yale/dcs/rr1097, Yale University, 1996.

[BM94]   M. Beetz and D. McDermott. Improving robot plans during their execution. In Kris Hammond, editor, *Second International Conference on AI Planning Systems*, pages 3–12, Morgan Kaufmann, 1994.

[BM96]   M. Beetz and D. McDermott. Local planning of ongoing activities. In Brian Drabble, editor, *Third International Conference on AI Planning Systems*, pages 19–26, Morgan Kaufmann, 1996.

[CL95]   P. Cohen and H. Levesque. Communicative actions for artificial agents. In *Proceedings of the International Conference on Multi-Agent Systems*, Cambridge, Ma, 1995. AAAI Press.

[CMU+97] R. Cole, J. Mariani, H. Uszkoreit, A. Zaenen, and V. Zue. *Survey of the State of the Art in Human Language Technology*. Cambridge University Press and Giardini, 1997. http://www.cse.ogi.edu/CSLU/HLTsurvey/HLTsurvey.html.

[CP79]   P. Cohen and C. Perrault. Elements of a plan-based theory of speech acts. *Cognitive Science*, 3(3):177–212, 1979.

[Fir87]   J. Firby. An investigation into reactive planning in complex domains. In *Proc. of AAAI-87*, pages 202–206, Seattle, WA, 1987.

[FLM95]   Tim Finin, Yannis Labrou, and James Mayfield. *Software Agents*, chapter KQML as an agent communication language. MIT Press, Cambridge, Ma, 1995.

[Gap94]   K.-P. Gapp. Basic meanings of spatial relations: Computation and evaluation in 3d space. In *Proc. of the Thirteenth National Conference on Artificial Intelligence*, pages 1393–1398, 1994.

[Gat96]   E. Gat. Esl: A language for supporting robust plan execution in embedded autonomous agents. In *AAAI Fall Symposium: Issues in Plan Execution*, Cambridge, MA, 1996.

[LGS90] K. E. Lochbaum, B. J. Grosz, and C. L. Sidner. Models of plans to support communication: An initial report. In *Proc. of AAAI-90*, pages 485–490, Boston, MA, 1990.

[McD85] D. McDermott. The duck manual. Research Report YALEU/DCS/RR-399, Yale University, 1985.

[McD91] D. McDermott. A reactive plan language. Research Report YALEU/DCS/RR-864, Yale University, 1991.

[Nil84] Nils J. Nilsson. Shakey the robot. Technical Note 323, SRI International, Menlo Park, California, 1984.

[Nor92] P. Norvig. *Paradigms of Artificial Intelligence Programming: Case Studies in Common Lisp*. Morgan Kaufmann, San Mateo, CA, 1992.

[PW80] F. Pereira and D. Warren. Definite clause grammars for language analysis. In *Artificial Intelligence*, pages 231–278, 1980.

[Rei81] R. Reichman. *Plain-speaking: A theory and grammar of spontaneous discourse*. PhD thesis, Harvard University, Cambridge, Massachusetts, 1981.

[RN95] S. J. Russell and P. Norvig. *Artificial Intelligence: A Modern Approach*. Prentice-Hall, Englewood Cliffs, NJ, 1995.

[Sea69] John R. Searle. *Speech Acts: An Essay in the Philosophy of Language*. Cambridge University Press, Cambridge, 1969.

[SGH⁺94] E. Stopp, K. Gapp, G. Herzog, T. Lngle, and T. Lth. Utilizing spatial relations for natural language access to an autonomous mobile robot. In B. Nebel and L. Dreschler-Fischer, editors, *KI-94: Advances in Artificial Intelligence.*, pages 39–50, Berlin, Heidelberg, 1994. Springer.

[TS97] Mark C. Torrance and Lynn Andrea Stein. Communicating with martians (and robots). Technical report, MIT Artificial Intelligence Laboratory, 1997.

[Wei97] T. Weis. Resource-adaptive action planning in a dialogue system for repair support. In B. Nebel, editor, *Proceedings der 21. Deutschen Jahrestagung fr Knstliche Intelligenz*, Berlin, New Yor, 1997. Springer.

[Win72] Terry Winograd. Understanding natural language. *Cognitive Psychology*, 3(1), 1972. Reprinted as a book by Academic Press.

Towards a Methodology for Developing Application-Oriented Report Generation*

Helmut Horacek[1] and Stephan Busemann[2]

[1] Universität des Saarlandes, FB 14, Informatik
Postfach 1150, D-66041 Saarbrücken
horacek@cs.uni-sb.de

[2] DFKI GmbH
Stuhlsatzenhausweg 3, D-66123 Saarbrücken
busemann@dfki.de

Abstract. Although research in natural language generation has led to the development of numerous methods and reusable software tools, we feel that building comparably simple application systems still involves more hand-crafted skills than systematic methodology. In our view, this is due to the fact that most available tools are oriented towards contributing to a general purpose generation system rather than supporting the economic development of dedicated applications. In order to improve this situation, we present a methodology for developing application-oriented report generation with limited effort, emphasizing domain- and user-specific preferences over general-purpose communicative principles. Key parts in our approach comprise building an ontologically minimal initial representation on the basis of user parameters and associated domain data, the successive refinement of this initial representation by making implicit information explicit enough for fleshing out selected text and sentence patterns, and the opportunistic combination of linguistically motivated methods with template-based generation. This methodology should enable system developers to build application-oriented report generators more systematically and with reduced effort.

1 Introduction

Although research in natural language generation (NLG) has led to the development of numerous methods and reusable software tools, we feel that building comparably simple application systems today still involves more hand-crafted skills than systematic methodology. In our view, this is due to the fact that most available tools (e.g. SURGE [Elhadad and Robin, 1996], KPML [Bateman, 1997]) are based on *in-depth* approaches to NLG contributing to a general purpose generation system rather than supporting the economic development of dedicated applications. They require, for instance, detailed input specifications,

---

* This work has been supported by a grant from the European Union to the project TEMSIS (Telematics Applications Programme, Sector C9, contract no. 2945).

some of them being irrelevant for the application in hand. Even more importantly, today's tools rarely help in organizing application conventions systematically and efficiently, and in relating non-linguistic to linguistic specifications at whatever level of description, ranging from deep semantic representations to surface forms.

While in-depth approaches to NLG are indispensable for scientific progress in the field, we suggest that certain types of applications can, at present, be built more successfully by systematically adopting more *shallow* techniques, which emphasize domain- and user-specific preferences over general-purpose communicative principles (cf. [Busemann and Horacek, 1998] for a more extensive argumentation). Motivated by the application-related deficits of general tools, we have developed a methodology for shallow multi-lingual report generation. Key parts in our approach comprise building an ontologically minimal initial representation on the basis of user parameters and associated domain data, the successive refinement of this initial representation by making implicit information explicit enough for fleshing out selected text and sentence patterns, and the opportunistic combination of linguistically motivated methods with template-based generation. Our shallow methodology was put to the test within the multi-lingual report generator developed for the TEMSIS project.

The paper is organized as follows. The TEMSIS application environment is outlined in Section 2. Section 3 describes and motivates the methods for building a report generator in a systematic and efficient manner. Based on the experience gained, we discuss the process of developing systems of a similar kind in Section 4. Finally, Section 5 characterizes the applicability conditions and the limitations of our approach.

2   The TEMSIS NL Generation Application Environment

In this section, we illustrate the goals pursued in TEMSIS from an application-oriented perspective. With TEMSIS, a Transnational Environmental Management Support and Information System was created as part of a transnational cooperation between the communities in the French-German urban agglomeration, Moselle Est and Stadtverband Saarbrücken. Networked information kiosks are being installed in a number of communities to provide public and expert environmental information.

The timely availability of relevant environmental information will improve the planning and reactive capabilities of the administration considerably. Current measurement data are made available on the TEMSIS web server. The data include the measurement values of several pollutants, the location and the time the measurements were taken, and a variety of thresholds. Besides such data, the server provides metadata that allow for descriptions of the measuring locations, of the pollutants measured and of regulations or laws according to which a comparison between measurements and thresholds can be performed.

This information can be accessed via the internet through a hyperlink navigation interface.[3]

The verbalization of NL air quality information in French and German is an additional service to the environmental administrations reducing the need to look up multiple heterogeneous data. Reports contain statements about the average and maximum values of the concentration of air pollutants over certain periods of time, about relations to threshold values, about comparisons with values from preceeding time periods, canned text descriptions of measuring locations and pollutants, and diagrams showing long-term developments. The generated texts can be edited and further processed by the administrations to fit additional needs.

The structures of the texts originated from discussions with the TEMSIS user group. The reports were classified into seventeen types. The user group also provided a set of sample texts, which we categorized into nine assertion types. This categorization helped us to accomodate the wordings in the reports to the demands of the domain.

In order to obtain a report, a user specifies his demands by choosing from a hierarchy of options presented to him within the hyperlink navigation interface. The user has to specify a pollutant, a measuring location, a time interval, and in some cases comparison parameters, which leads to the instantiation of one of the seventeen report types. In addition, descriptions of pollutants and measurement stations can be requested. These are stored as canned texts in the TEMSIS database. In (1) a sample user request is shown followed by an excerpt of the resulting text translated into English. Altogether, the system can generate 384 report structures that differ in at least one linguistic aspect.

```
(1)  :LANGUAGE GERMAN
     :POLLUTANT SO2
     :MEASURING STATION "Carling"
     :REPORT-TYPE AVERAGE
     :TIME January/98
```

The concentration of sulfur dioxyde in the air at the measurement station "Carling" in January 1998 was 20 µg/m³, so that the threshold value I1 of 140 µg/m³ for a 30 minute interval according to TA-Luft has not been exceeded (an annual threshold value is related to a daily measurement value here). In December 1997, the value was 25 µg/m³, so that the threshold value has not been exceeded either.

The development of the TEMSIS report generator had to be carried out under rather tight resource constraints. With an investigation of eight person months, the system had to be built from scratch in large parts. We decided to reuse the TG/2 production system for shallow linguistic verbalization [Busemann, 1996] as well as some of its subgrammars including e.g. rules for temporal expressions. We looked for simple and application-oriented solutions, at the same time envisioning systematicity and a methodological development process.

---

[3] The URL is http://www-temsis.dfki.uni-sb.de/.

We refrained from reusing large in-depth NLG resources such as SURGE [Elhadad and Robin, 1996] or KPML [Bateman, 1997], because their adaptation to the needs of TEMSIS would have required considerable effort for developing interfaces to the feeding components. Moreover, the use of such resources within relatively small applications like the present one means a certain overshot.

Altogether, we believe that both the kind of functional requirements and the need of keeping the develoment effort very small are by far not unique for the TEMSIS report generation scenario. Our aim is thus to elaborate a methodology for developing systems of this kind efficiently.

3 Report Generation in TEMSIS

In this section, we illustrate the techniques used within the TEMSIS report generator. We first introduce some terms that are central for our methods:

- *User specifications* or *parameters* are the input data which trigger the composition of a report.
- These specifications play the role of *influence factors* in individual report parts, and they may be interpreted differently according to the specific assertion types. For instance, while the expression "sulfur dioxyde" used for confirming the user's choice of pollutant is interpreted as the type of pollutant, that same expression refers to the concentration of the pollutant in the air if it occurs within an assertion about threshold passing.
- *Variations* in the reports and their statements break down into two sorts. Linguistically motivated variations mainly originate from aggregation operations and depend on the target language chosen, with some of the aggregations made possible due to peculiar data constellations (e.g., identical value comparison outcomes). Variations in content have their source purely in data-specific constellations. For instance, if a measured value does not exceed some threshold, an otherwise conveyed comparison with a higher threshold is skipped.

We have partitioned the generation process into three phases (disregarding the access to the database according to the user parameters, which yields actual measurement data):

1. Organizing the material to convey in terms of single statements on the basis of user parameters.
2. Recasting the domain-oriented specifications in language-adequate, but language-neutral, terms by successively refining the specifications obtained so far.
3. Transducing the resulting intermediate structure into French or German texts, by an opportunistic combination of linguistically motivated methods with template generation.

With major simplifications, these tasks correspond to the classical phases of text planning, lexicalization, and realization, organized in a traditional pipe-line architecture. However, some of our techniques and the interfaces involved deviate from usual standards. Due to the conventionalized nature of our reports, using linguistically motivated methods, such as RST-based text planners, would be an overshot. Moreover, in-depth lexicalization methods are only an option in our approach, but we are using more surface oriented processes due to the limited functional requirements and available resources. While content realization does not encode meaning by itself, the template-based verbalization in TG/2 uses rules depending on the domain and the task at hand. Such dependencies render a simple pipe-lined architecture feasible.

In the following, we elaborate the main concepts in each phase and illustrate them with sample representations in English for the reader's convenience.

3.1 Phase 1: Text organization

Organizing the material that goes into a report is supported by two sorts of data structures:

- *Report skeletons* describe the application conditions of report types and provide a basic text structure to be filled with single statements.
- *Assertion structures* capture data-driven options and variations in single statements and bind relevant user parameters and domain data – the influence factors – to these statements.

Report skeletons consist of lists of assertion structures. In a report skeleton, the application conditions serve to match user specifications for selecting a unique report type, to access domain data according to these specifications, and to activate further specifications implicitly associated with a report type, such as suitable threshold specifications. Selecting a report skeleton causes the associated assertion structures to be instantiated.

```
(2)   (AVERAGE POLLUTANT
              MEASUREMENT-STATION
              TIME
              (#'DESCRIBE-VALUE VALUE)
              (#'DESCRIBE-THRESHOLD THRESHOLD)
              (#'DESCRIBE-COMPARISON COMPARISON))
```

Assertion structures consist of a small number of condition-action pairs evaluated like a case statement. Example (2) is an assertion structure for a statement about an average value including a threshold comparison, such as the sample text following (1). It is referred to from report skeletons representing average value reports, and is picked up in case a suitable threshold for the selected pollutant is available in view of the user's time specification. The elements of this assertion structure are interpreted in three different ways (see the instantiated structure in (3)):

- The first predicate, in (2) AVERAGE, becomes the value of the PRED feature of the assertion to be built.

- Atomic elements, in (2) POLLUTANT, MEASUREMENT-STATION, and TIME, indicate that the referred elements of the user specification are to be copied into the assertion, where they appear as attribute-value pairs.
- List elements are evaluated as procedure calls. Their parameters denote database access results for the selected report. These procedures yield descriptions of the relevant data, either as a simple attribute-value pair for atomic values (VALUE 20), or as an attribute with a list of attribute-value pairs as its value (the values of the attributes THRESHOLD and EXCEEDS).

Example (3) shows the instantiated assertion structure, originating from (2), for the central statement of the sample text in (1).

```
(3) ((PRED AVERAGE)
     (POLLUTANT SO2)
     (MEASUREMENT-STATION "Carling")
     (TIME ((YEAR 1998) (MONTH 1)))
     (VALUE 20)
     (THRESHOLD ((AMOUNT 140)
                 (THRESHOLD-TIME YEARS)
                 (LAW-NAME TA-LUFT)
                 (THRESHOLD-NAME I1)
                 (MEASUREMENT-DURATION 30-MINUTES)))
     (EXCEEDS ((TIMES 0))))
```

Altogether, organizing the material to convey results in filling these data structures by interpreting user parameters accordingly. The interpretation of user parameters yields at least a partial order of statements out of an unordered set of specifications. Ontologically, the semantically condensed predicates in the user specifications are split into operationally interpretable predicates, with context-sensitive and conventionally motivated details added according to statement types. Restrictions in this interpretation process include the absence of recursion in statement expansions, and a lack of convenience in expressing data dependencies across statements – identical expressions need to be included in several assertion structures referred to by some report skeleton.

The internal organization of statement specifications is encoded in a condensed form: a top level predicate represents the type of each assertion and encapsulates the entire meaning of the associated assertion with the exception of the attached influence factors. Each of the influence factors is represented as an attribute value pair, linked to the top level predicate by an unambiguous attribute. The value itself may be one of the following:

- An atomic value, such as an option, or a name; an example is the pollutant identifier (see (3)).
- A list of values, such as a data vector; an example is a list of measurement values.
- An attribute value structure, for structured influence factors with internal dependencies; an example is a time specification (see (3)).

Altogether, this categorization imposes some sort of minimal ontology on the initial proposition representation to encapsulate 'domain communication knowledge' [Kittredge *et al.*, 1991], and it makes local parameter and data dependencies explicit.

3.2   Phase 2: Recasting information

The second processing phase, recasting the information, manipulates initial representations of assertion structures like (3). It takes care of augmenting, restructuring, and aggregating them, to meet the properties of the TG/2 verbalizer. In particular, no linguistic facts are made explicit since this is left to TG/2.

Augmenting statement specifications means making information implicitly entailed or available elsewhere explicit at the place it is needed. This concerns reestablishing report-wide information, as well as making locally entailed information accessible. An example for the latter is the unit in which the value of a measurement is expressed (see (4)). Examples for the former are the choice of the target language, and more interestingly, the number of diagrams depicted, copied into the introductory statement to these diagrams. This treatment is much simpler than using a reference generation algorithm, but it relies on a fixed number of diagrams for a given report skeleton.

Example (4) shows the result obtained for (3) except to aggregation, with changes in bold face.

```
(4)  ((PRED AVERAGE)
     (POLLUTANT SO2)
     (LANGUAGE GERMAN)
     (MEASUREMENT-STATION "Carling")
     (TIME ((YEAR 1998) (MONTH 1)))
     (VALUE ((AMOUNT 20) (UNIT mg/m3)))
     (THRESHOLD ((AMOUNT 140) (UNIT mg/m3)))
     (SOURCE ((LAW-NAME TA-LUFT)
              (THRESHOLD-NAME I1)
              (PERIOD ((MEASUREMENT-TIME DAYS)
                       (THRESHOLD-TIME YEARS)))))
     (MEASUREMENT-DURATION 30-MINUTES)
     (EXCEEDS ((TIMES 0))))
```

TG/2-oriented recasting ranges from renaming an attribute over reifying it as a structured value, such as (AMOUNT 20) in (4), raising an embedded partial description by one level, such as (MEASUREMENT-DURATION 30-MINUTES) in (4), to complex operations such as building lists of attribute value pairs from data vectors. Most of these operations are data-driven utilizing schemata as they were elaborated for linguistically motivated lexicalization [Horacek, 1996]. In contrast to that work, some of our schemata are purely application-oriented, and they are 'heavier' in terms of the number of schema parameters and the size of the structures covered. In TEMSIS, we use twelve schema classes and about hundred instantiations.

In other approaches, the lexicalization process and the structural mappings involved are determined by the lexemes and the grammatical structures in the target language. In contrast, our approach breaks down the composition through mapping schemata only as far as distinctions between phrasings are required. In particular, the treatment of language specificity is handed over to TG/2. This design, which results in a much smaller number of mapping schemata, has two important consequences:

- The search control is eased significantly, because a single mapping schema is available only in most cases.
- The coarse-grained partitioning makes writing the schemata much easier, so that problems of expressibility are unlikely to occur.

As a last part of information recasting, some sorts of aggregation are performed. Operations that remove partial descriptions or add simple structures are invoked, driven by a small set of declaratively represented rules, operating on a discourse memory. Most of the rules aim at avoiding repetitions of optional constituents (e.g., temporal and locative information) over adjacent statements. The rules are formulated to meet application particularities, such as impacts of certain combinations of a value and a threshold comparison outcome, rather than to capture linguistic principles. Before aggregation, the internal representations of the two sentences in the text following (1) are identical except to the value and the month. After aggregation, the representation of the second sentence is reduced to (5), the newly added REPEAT slot giving raise to the use of *either* in TG/2. Several parts have been elided, as a comparison with (4) reveals.

```
(5) ((PRED AVERAGE) (LANGUAGE GERMAN)
     (TIME ((YEAR 1997) (MONTH 12)))
     (VALUE ((AMOUNT 25) (UNIT mg/m3)))
     (EXCEEDS ((TIMES 0))) (REPEAT YES))
```

3.3 Phase 3: Linguistic verbalization

Finally, our dedicated verbalization component, TG/2, selects appropriate production rules for the sorts of statements and some key parameters. The productions consist of conditioned rewrite rules with a context-free backbone. Their right-hand side consists of canned text elements, lexemes, or non-terminal symbols corresponding to recursive rule activation. This way, canned texts, template techniques and context-free grammars are integrated into a single formalism [Busemann, 1996].

The string of template elements in (6)[4] corresponds to the right-hand side of a rule verbalizing average values. The applicability conditions for this rule include the requirement that the TG/2 input contain the specification (PRED AVERAGE).

---

[4] Capitalized words within brackets are place holders; a question mark following an opening bracket indicates an optional constituent.

```
(6)  "the concentration of " <POLLUTANT> "in the air "
     <? "at" MEASUREMENT-STATION> <? "on" DATE> "was "
     <VALUE> "(" <T1> "is related to " <T2> "here)."
```

TG/2 improves over existing tools that provide comparably poor support for both complex phrasings and for sychronising their functionality across several languages. Phrasal composition comprises fine-grained parts, such as time and value descriptions, as well as rather coarse-grained ones, such as the example above, where the expression in parentheses is triggered by the difference of the attribute values of (MEASUREMENT-TIME <T1>) and (THRESHOLD-TIME <T2>) (e.g. *an annual threshold is related to monthly values here*).

This organisation works in a comparably simple way without the need to model the associated linguistic features and their cross-language differences in full detail. More precisely, TG/2 allows us to model exactly at the level of granularity dictated by the domain, meeting our resource constraints well.

4 Developing an Application-Oriented Report Generator

In this section, we illustrate the development process of an application-oriented report generator. We abstract away from particularities of the TEMSIS scenario in order to obtain a development methodology for applications with similar properties. The development process can be divided into three major activities:

- Organizing the material to convey by structuring it in terms of proposition sequences, and making influence factors on individual propositions explicit.
- Designing an intermediate representation structure mediating between statement specifications and a suitable verbalization component.
- Fleshing out data structures that support manipulations of the intermediate representation structure: mapping schemata, aggregation and grammar rules.

The first activity, organizing the material to convey, is based on user specifications. Report specifications and a corpus of sample texts, which are the two central building blocks that formally untrained users can and should provide to system builders, must be examined in terms of their cross-dependencies (cf. [Reiter *et al.*, 1997]). Sentence patterns must be abstracted from these examples, and they must be categorized and related to report specifications. This analysis should lead to definitions of report skeletons, assertion specifications, and influence factors, composed in a systematic way, as described in the previous section. There is a certain choice involved between having a larger number of report types, or assertion propositions with more conditionals.

The contribution of the process model underlying this activity lies in providing a specific approach to build initial representations with a widely free vocabulary that can be accomodated to elements in an associated knowledge base. Building such a draft specification is based on human pre-analysis to build schemata that bear some similarities to McKeown's [McKeown, 1985]. Our schemata can also represent conditionals, but they are flat structures without recursion, and their instantiation is geared by user-based specifications rather than by linguistically motivated concepts such as focus constraints.

The second activity, designing an intermediate representation structure, is influenced by two factors imposing different demands on this structure: (1) the distinctions necessary in the output texts must be represented explicitly and as economically as possible; (2) an available verbalization component should be made exploitable. Several divergent attitudes towards resolving the ontological differences between domain-oriented perspectives (which manifest themselves in initial representations) and language-oriented perspectives (which manifest themselves in – in-depth – intermediate representations) may result:

- For a canned text verbalization component, that difference is essentially ignored; necessary distinctions are made explicit, and resulting structures are directly converted into text templates.
- For a shallow verbalization component such as TG/2 (also some of the so-called intermediate techniques in IDAS [Reiter *et al.*, 1995] fall under this type), bridging that difference is transferred to the verbalization component's grammar rules;
- For an in-depth realization component such as SURGE, structure-changing rules should take care of bridging that ontological difference.

Depending on which approach is chosen, there is some sort of compensative effect between minimal development effort, as in the first alternative, and optimum extendability, as in the third alternative.

Finally, the third activity, fleshing out the various sorts of production rules involved, depends on choices made for the intermediate representation structure. For a shallow approach, building a small set of schemata that map complete substructures is frequently adequate. For more in-depth approaches, a much larger set of elementary schemata is required. In the former case, a certain amount of effort is certainly needed to enhance the set of schemata available for a new application. In the latter case, more effort is needed to analyze the differences between initial and intermediate representations in terms of their decomposition into schemata that are elementary enough for the ontological level of the intermediate representation structure. Similar trade-offs concern aggregation and grammar rules.

5 Applicability and Limitations

Our methodology is applicable to reports in which the organization principles underlying the information conveyed and the associated wordings reflect more the domain conventions and the user preferences than the linguistic concepts. These reports can exhibit only limited degrees of variations, their structure and content is widely determined by parameters, and reasoning about contents of a knowledge base should be restricted to subtasks with a local impact. All conventions and preferences are interpreted much more directly and concretely than typical rhetorical parameters for experimental systems, such as "colloquial", "verbose" etc., so that reasoning about them is not required.

Our methodology covers reports of a complexity comparable to those produced by Ana [Kukich, 1983], FOG [Boubeau et al., 1990], IDAS [Reiter et al., 1995], and it may in large parts be extendible to those produced by PLANDOC [McKeown et al., 1994]. Ana is the first natural language report generator, and the kind of texts it produces can still be considered valuable today. However, Ana is implemented as a widely unstructured rule-based system, which does not seem to be easily extendable and portable. In comparison to that, we gain over Ana through several motivated representation levels with well-defined structures and vocabulary. Moreover, our generator is widely driven by easily readable and interpretable data structures rather than by collections of production rules for each of three processing phases in Ana. Hence, we assess our main contribution in comparison to Ana as an increase of systematicity, which rather similarly holds for FOG. In comparison to IDAS, we are lacking a component for referring expressions, but we gain in terms of multi-linguality. In comparison to PLANDOC, we also gain in terms of multi-linguality, and our approach requires significantly less development effort. However, PLANDOC has a number of more powerful components, such as the sorts of aggregation it can deal with, and it has available to it the generality of SURGE.

In this context, the limitations and prospects of our approach can be assessed as follows (cf. [Busemann and Horacek, 1998] for more details):

- Aggregation techniques can easily be extended, although their formulation would require rather accessing properties of domain parameters than evaluating in-depth linguistic features.
- Extending the approach by a reference mechanism is possible, but this would require major enhancements to the report structure and statement representation schema, and to the associated interpretation processes.
- Modeling the language structures explicitly in more detail is definitely an option that can and should be pursued. However, the more the flexibility is increased this way, the bigger become the problems of search control and mastering expressibility in the lexicalization phase.

6 Conclusion

In this paper, we have presented a methodology for developing application-oriented shallow report generators with comparably low development effort. We have described the TEMSIS generator as an instance for the domain of air-quality reports. The development process comprises building an ontologically minimal initial representation on the basis of user parameters and associated domain data, the successive refinement of this initial representation by making implicit information explicit enough for fleshing out selected text and sentence patterns, and the opportunistic combination of linguistically motivated methods with template-based generation. We have discussed a number of options in the development process, with divergent costs and benefits. While this methodology allows one to develop systems that can only produce reports of limited complexity, the comparably low effort associated makes our approach competitive.

References

[Bateman, 1997] John Bateman. KPML delvelopment environment: multilingual linguistic resource development and sentence generation. Report, German National Center for Information Technology (GMD), Institute for integrated publication and information systems (IPSI), Darmstadt, Germany, January 1997. Release 1.1.

[Boubeau et al., 1990] L. Boubeau, D. Carcagno, E. Goldberg, R. Kittredge, and A. Polguere. Bilingual generation of weather forecasts in an operations environment. In *Proceedings of the 13 th International Conference on Computational Linguistics (COLING-90), Volume 1*, pages 90–92, Helsinki, 1990.

[Busemann and Horacek, 1998] Stephan Busemann and Helmut Horacek. A flexible shallow approach to text generation. In Eduard Hovy, editor, *Nineth International Natural Language Generation Workshop. Proceedings*, Niagara-on-the-Lake, Canada, 1998.

[Busemann, 1996] Stephan Busemann. Best-first surface realization. In Donia Scott, editor, *Eighth International Natural Language Generation Workshop. Proceedings*, pages 101–110, Herstmonceux, Univ. of Brighton, England, 1996. Also available at the Computation and Language Archive at http://xxx.lanl.gov/abs/cmp-lg/9605010.

[Elhadad and Robin, 1996] Michael Elhadad and Jacques Robin. An overview of SURGE: a reusable comprehensive syntactic realization component. In Donia Scott, editor, *Eighth International Natural Language Generation Workshop. Demonstrations and Posters*, pages 1–4, Herstmonceux, Univ. of Brighton, England, 1996.

[Horacek, 1996] Helmut Horacek. Lexical choice in expressing metonymic relations in multiple language. *Machine Translation*, 11:109–158, 1996.

[Kittredge et al., 1991] Richard Kittredge, Tanya Korelsky, and Owen Rambow. On the need of domain communication knowledge. *Computational Intelligence*, 7:305–314, 1991.

[Kukich, 1983] Karen Kukich. Design and implementation of a knowledge-based report generator. In *Proceedings of the 21st Annual Meeting of the Association for Computational Linguistics*, pages 145–150, Cambridge, MA, 1983.

[McKeown et al., 1994] Kathleen McKeown, Karen Kukich, and James Shaw. Practical issues in automatic documentation generation. In *Proceedings of the 4 th Conference on Applied Natural Language Processing (ANLP)*, pages 7–14, Stuttgart, 1994. Morgan Kaufmann.

[McKeown, 1985] Kathleen McKeown. Discourse strategies for generating natural language texts. *Artificial Intelligence*, 27:1–41, 1985.

[Reiter et al., 1995] Ehud Reiter, Chris Mellish, and John Levine. Automatic generation of technical documentation. *Applied Artificial Intelligence*, 9, 1995.

[Reiter et al., 1997] Ehud Reiter, Alison Cawsey, Liesl Osman, and Yvonne Roff. Knowledge acquisition for content selection. In *Proceedings of the 6th European Workshop on Natural Language Generation (ENLGWS-97)*, pages 117–126, Duisburg, 1997.

Concepts for a Diagnostic Critiquing System in Vague Domains[1]

Ulrike Rhein-Desel, Frank Puppe
Institute for Artificial Intelligence and Applied Informatics,
Würzburg University, Am Hubland, D-97074 Würzburg

Abstract. Since the seminal work of Perry Miller about medical critiquing systems in the eighties, there has been remarkable little further research. We present a knowledge level analysis of the types of knowledge and reasoning strategies necessary for an diagnostic critiquing system in vague domains. Instead of building a critiquing system from scratch, we investigate how to enrich a knowledge-based diagnostic system with additional knowledge for critiquing. There are three kinds of additional knowledge: 1. Knowledge for the analysis of the reliability of a diagnostic conclusion for a given case taking into account reliability and completeness of data, reliability of the diagnostic knowledge and the explanation of the diagnostic conclusion. 2. Knowledge about the importance of a diagnosis (e.g. treatibility, danger, urgency), and 3. Multiple diagnostic models including partial knowledge like explicit critiquing rules or guidelines.

1. Introduction

Since the late sixties a large number of researchers have worked on concepts and prototypes for intelligent systems which assist physicians in diagnosis and treatment. Decision support systems such as expert systems usually receive facts and information about a patient's symptoms as input data and suggest possible diagnoses, optionally together with explanations. However, at least in medical domains, decision support systems cannot take the responsibility for their solutions, which still remains with the physician. Therefore it seems plausible that they should be able to comment the solutions derived by the user. Only if the user's solutions are not reasonable, they should criticize recognized weaknesses, otherwise they should provide no output. In the eighties, Perry Miller [Miller 86] proposed critiquing systems as a new type of system with the aim to enhance the acceptance of conventional medical expert systems by physicians.

In the late eighties, some critiquing systems were developed for small medical or technical applications [Silverman 92]. Most systems remained a prototype. Although in the last few years the term *critiquing system* became a common term particularly in medical informatics [Bemmel & Musen 97], hardly any new projects or systems came up. One reason for the missing breakthrough despite broad acceptance might be the complexity of critiquing knowledge in vague domains. In [Bemmel & Musen 97], a critiquing system is defined as a "decision support system that allows the user to make the decision first; the system then gives its advice when the user requests it or when the user's decision is out of the system's permissible range." Critiquing systems observe the inputs and decisions of the user and try to verify the decisions. They only attract attention in critical situations.

The input/output behavior of critiquing systems in comparison to expert systems is shown in figure 1. Systems of both types receive symptoms as input and output explanations for

[1] This work has been supported by the Deutsche Forschungsgemeinschaft (DFG) under the grant Pu 129/2-1.

the solution and the decision making process on demand (dashed line). The difference is that critiquing system have the diagnoses as a second input whereas diagnoses are the output of an expert system. The main output of a critiquing system is the critique.

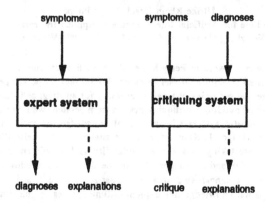

Figure 1: Input and output of expert systems and critiquing systems

Two straightforward architectures of critiquing systems are:
- Formalization of explicit knowledge on when to criticize a solution. This approach was followed in particular in the early critiquing systems. While it works in well defined domains (e.g. for checking whether mandatory constraints are fulfilled by a proposed solution) it is not very promising for vague and complex diagnostic domains.
- Comparing the solution derived by an expert system with the solution of the user and criticizing major differences. This approach is quite popular for knowledge based training systems (e.g. [Puppe & Reinhardt 95]) but it assumes that the expert system's expertise is superior to the user. The last assumption might be fulfilled for students and preselected well-known cases but not for experts and arbitrary cases.

In the following analysis, we present concepts to combine both approaches and to add additional knowledge and reasoning strategies. In the next chapter we start with tasks and some requirements for critiquing systems and describe how a critiquing system works in general. Chapter 3 is the core of this paper. There we describe the concepts for the critiquing knowledge and how this critiquing knowledge can be integrated in a decision support system. An illustrative example from the field of simple pediatrics is given in chapter 4. Finally, chapter 5 presents conclusions and future work.

2. Tasks and Requirements for the Critiquing System

While in some domains, critiquing solutions is easier than inferring them, in vague and complex domains like medical diagnosis, it is often impossible to find out the correct solution with acceptable costs and risks. If many equally acceptable solutions and various tradeoffs must be considered, critiquing solutions is quite a complex task.

The critiquing system uses some guiding questions which are important for checking the quality and the appropriateness of the user's solution:

1. Is there knowledge against this solution?
2. Is the solution reliable?
3. Is the solution complete?
4. Are there better solutions?

The first question concerns knowledge on undesired or forbidden situations. If there is a rule which makes explicit that in the given situation the chosen solution is not correct, the critiquing system must give a corresponding message to the user. Reliability of a solution depends on the reliability of both the data and the knowledge to infer that solution. It also includes, that there is sufficient input data available for assessing the solution. A solution is complete, if it covers (explains) all the major symptoms. Even if a solution passes all these questions, there might be other even more plausible solutions.

In addition to these questions, it is useful to perform a sensitivity analysis: If slight modification of values of symptoms change the diagnosis or the scoring of the diagnosis, the solution is perhaps not reliable. One possible reaction of the critiquing system is the request that the user should check the symptoms in question whether he is sure about the corresponding values.

Some critiquing systems (e.g. HYPERCRITIC [Mosseveld & van der Lei 90], systems of the ATTENDING-family [Miller 86], critiquing system of ONCOCIN [Silverman 92], ship damage control system [Ramachandran & Wilkins 96] or CASSY [Gerlach & Onken 94]) have a component which represents an ideal expert as yardstick for the correctness of the user's decision. A disadvantage of such an architecture is its lack of flexibility. The decisions of a user might be not optimal, but still acceptable. In such a situation, a system with an ideal-expert-component reports a warning. However too many low level warnings impair the acceptance of a critiquing system. Moreover, the concept of an ideal expert hinders considering different possible alternatives of treatment or diagnostic decisions. Users in technical fields with only few possible alternatives in each situation might accept such rigorous systems. In medical applications the situation is different; in many situations the possible alternatives can not be judged right or wrong.

Besides medical knowledge which is necessary for any medical decision support system, critiquing systems need additional special knowledge. A basic requirement for our critiquing system is that it has to cope with different aspects of uncertainty:
- uncertainty about the quality of the basic knowledge base,
- uncertainty about the completeness of the data,
- uncertainty about the correctness of the data,
- and even uncertainty about the quality of the critiquing knowledge.

Critiquing knowledge from different sources with different granularity and with different views can provide more redundancy and allows critiques and comments with higher certainty. The critiquing knowledge necessary for judging these uncertainties comes from various knowledge sources.

To be practically useful, the critiquing system should be able to help the user in situations with only partial available information. In such situations, a conventional decision support system cannot work. A critiquing system may help in such situations because it tries to infer solutions using only the information at hand, tries to judge the reliability of the data and the solutions and thus helps the user not to overlook facts or to remind him of rare but relevant hypotheses.

In medical decision making it is often necessary to consider the development of the symptoms, the momentary situation gives not enough information. For example, in the medical field of pediatrics a lot of diagnoses can only be found taking into account the development of the disease. Many children's diseases begin with unspecific fever. The characteristic symptoms such as exanthemas appear one or even several days later. So in the beginning a correct diagnosis is very difficult if it is possible at all. Therefore, the representation of time is often of crucial importance.

Besides the use of the development schemes for diagnostic purposes, critiquing systems are also very useful for monitoring the development of a disease. Knowing the normal development they check from the input data and the history of the current case if a complication is likely to appear or if there are other problems with the current interpretation of the case. However, this aspect will not be dealt with in this paper.

3. The Critiquing Knowledge

Critiquing knowledge divides into direct and indirect knowledge. Direct critiquing knowledge is an explicit representation of specific situations and constellations which require critique or comments from the system. Indirect critiquing knowledge is knowledge from which the critiquing system infers these situations and constellations. Indirect knowledge is modeled not only for critiquing purposes; it can be used by other components of a decision support system as well.

Existing critiquing systems mostly use direct critiquing knowledge. An example is the critiquing system based on the expert system ONCOCIN [Silverman 92]. In the critiquing process the expert system solution is suppressed. Instead, it is compared with the user's solution. The comparison uses a set of pre-programmed rules for the allowable discrepancies pairwise for diagnoses and prescribed drugs. This approach is very exhaustive and not reusable in other applications. Other critiquing systems or prototypes of critiquing systems have similar concepts.

The difficulties with direct knowledge can be summarized as follows:
• direct knowledge is impracticable for bigger applications,
• direct knowledge hinders flexible judgement of suboptimal but correct solutions,
• the approaches are not easy to adopt to other applications.

Nevertheless, direct critiquing knowledge is useful for identifying frequent mistakes and dangerous situations. For all other situations and decisions, indirect critiquing knowledge has advantages. In this contribution, we suggest to employ the knowledge of an expert system[2]

[2] The basic items of the knowledge representation are diagnoses, therapeutic actions, investigations, symptoms and rules expressing the relations. Using the rules, the diagnoses and actions

as the base for the indirect knowledge of a critiquing system. It is necessary to augment and modify the knowledge representation before it can be used by the critiquing system. In the following parts of this chapter we describe the necessary concepts for the knowledge representation of the critiquing knowledge.

3.1 Reasons for Unreliability of Conclusions

The reliability of the conclusions of a critiquing system depend on
- the reliability of the data,
- the completeness of the data,
- the reliability of the knowledge, and
- the degree of conflicting evidence.

The input data of a critiquing system can be unreliable or incomplete. The reliability of data depends on the reliability of its source. If the physician is not sure about some symptoms because the symptom has not manifested yet or because he lacks experience, then the corresponding input data has low reliability. Generally, data from examinations or laboratory tests are more reliable than anamnestic data. According to these categories, all symptoms automatically get an a-priori reliability mark which can be overwritten by the user. The completeness of data depends on the number of available symptoms in relation to the number and importance of symptoms necessary for a diagnosis.

The reliability of the knowledge depends on the certainty of the expert who has modeled the knowledge. If the expert is not certain about some details or if some parts of the modeled knowledge are not yet well understood, the knowledge is less reliable. Conflicting evidence is given in situations with evidence both in favor of and against a solution or if there are several high rated competing solutions, where only one of them can be correct.

If a conclusion is unreliable, the system has two possibilities: Either it critiques this situation with a corresponding hint to the user or it tries to increase the reliability. In the latter case, it is necessary to ask the user whether he is certain about the input and whether it is possible to get more data. The situations in which the system might ask the user for data are the following:
- The unreliability of the conclusion depends on the incompleteness of the data. Additional data could increase the reliability.
- The symptoms which are of particular importance for the diagnosis are unreliable (e.g. anamnestic data). Then the user is asked if he is really sure about the data which he should confirm by a reliability mark. Changed data or changed reliability marks could increase the reliability.
- In case of conflicting evidence, additional or changed data or changed reliability marks could help to increase or decrease the evidence of the conclusion. This could lead to a situation with lower conflicting evidence.

---

are concluded from the symptoms. The solutions are ordered according to the rating of their probability.

In a situation in which the unreliability of the diagnosis depends on the unreliability of the knowledge itself, the only possibility for the critiquing system is to inform the user about the unreliability and its reason.

3.2 Knowledge for Focusing the Critique

The critiquing system should not ask for additional information too often, otherwise the system disturbs the user more than it helps. It is important to focus on important questions with answers having high relevance. For example if competitor diagnoses with conflicting evidence lead to the same actions then asking for additional data is superfluous.

For focusing on critical situations, additional knowledge is necessary. So the knowledge representation must be extended with some additional parameters:
- **treatibility**: The term *treatibility* means that treatment is possible. This parameter gives the grade of treatibility for the diagnoses. In this parameter the utility of a treatment is already subsumed.
- **danger**: For all diagnoses their degree of *danger* must be specified. This parameter indicates that the respective diagnoses are dangerous or critical for the patient without treatment.
- **urgency**: This parameter marks diagnoses which have to be treated immediately.

Possible actions (e.g. treatments, technical investigations) of the user are augmented with two parameters:
- **risk**, indicates actions that are risky for the patients, and
- **usefulness**, indicates how useful actions with respect to what diagnoses are.

If the diagnosis is sufficiently clear and there are different treatments without clear preferences, but with quantifiable benefits and risks, then decision theory (see e.g. [Russell & Norvig 95]) is a powerful tool to find out the best action.

All these parameters and combinations thereof provide knowledge for focusing the critique. The parameter *treatibility* firms as a leading parameter. If the diagnosis is not treatable, further consideration of other parameters is not necessary. In particular, no risky actions should be considered in such a case. Any violation must lead to a critique from the system.

The concrete use of the other parameters is summarized in the following list. For all items of the list, treatibility of the diagnoses is assumed.
- If a diagnosis is dangerous, this diagnosis must be handled with high priority.
- The parameter *urgency* of a diagnosis means that the necessary therapeutic action must be chosen, otherwise the user should get a critique. However, if the diagnosis is unreliable and the treatment is risky, it is difficult to decide. As already mentioned, decision theory - if the necessary numbers are available - should be the first choice.
- The parameter *risk* is also important in the following situations:
  - If the diagnosis for therapeutic action is unreliable, the action should be delayed until the reliability is increased with additional data.
  - If the action is a risky investigation and there are other means to increase the reliability of the diagnosis, the user should be informed.

- The parameter *usefulness* helps judging the appropriateness of an action, if the corresponding diagnosis is not specified by the user. If the system cannot find a sufficient reason for an action, or its cost/benefits analysis is bad, the system should question the action.

3.3 Critiquing Knowledge from Different Knowledge Bases

In practice, a critiquing system employs knowledge bases of different quality and different functions for the critiquing process:

- **direct vs. indirect knowledge** The distinguishing aspect of these types of knowledge is whether an explicit description of the critiquing situations is given (direct) or whether these situations have to be inferred (indirect).
- **systematic vs. partial knowledge** This functional aspect of the knowledge means that only systematic knowledge can be used to infer solutions for a new whereas partial knowledge helps judging other knowledge or deals with special aspects.

We distinguish four types of knowledge assisting in critiquing systems which can be characterized with the help of the above concepts:

	direct	indirect
systematic	–	(enriched) conventional knowledge bases
partial	fault knowledge	partial formalized knowledge

- **systematic direct critiquing knowledge**
  Since it is usually impossible to enumerate all possible faults a diagnostician can do, we left this cell empty.
- **fault knowledge**
  Fault knowledge contains explicit descriptions of e.g. typical mistakes or critical situations.
- **(enriched) conventional knowledge base**
  The conventional knowledge base of a decision support system (e.g. categorical, heuristic, set-covering, functional, statistical, case-based etc. including combinations thereof) is complete enough to be used for inferring solutions to a previously unknown case. The knowledge base should be enriched with knowledge for focusing the critique as stated in section 3.2.
- **partial formalized knowledge**
  Partial formalized knowledge may be represented with the same or different representations as conventional knowledge bases, but is limited in its scope so that it does not cover the whole domain. Examples are constraints, suggestions, regulations, guidelines etc.

Often, partial knowledge contains rules or constraints without consideration of special cases or exceptions, where it might give no advice at all. In the context of a critiquing system, partial knowledge can often be viewed more reliable than conventional knowledge bases if applicable. If a decision or a planned therapeutic action is not in agreement with the partial knowledge, a corresponding critique from the system is often appropriate.

As a typical example of partial knowledge, medical guidelines gain importance in the discussion about quality management in medicine. They can be defined as a "systematically developed report, which has the aim to support physicians and patients with the decision about useful actions of medical care under the specific clinical circumstances." [Ohmann 97]. Integrating guidelines in the critiquing system defines a „lower bound" for the critique. Decisions which are not in agreement with a guideline should trigger critique.

The consistency of different types of knowledge for the same application is an issue of special interest. The minimal requirement is, that inferences from the partial and the covering knowledge should not contradict inferences from the complete knowledge. However, even this is difficult to guarantee in complex domains. A way to circumvent this problem is to assess the reliability of different knowledge packages in advance and to prefer the critique of the most reliable knowledge package in the case of contradictions.

4. Example[3]

The algorithms underlying the critiquing process are illustrated with a small example and not presented technically. The disease of the example is whooping cough, which is very contagious with a contagion index of 80%. Particularly for small children whooping cough is very dangerous, up to 5% of small babies die. There exists a vaccination against whooping cough, but this vaccination is only possible for children which are elder than 3 month. The disease is interesting for a critiquing system because it manifests itself quite late after at least one week and is not easy to diagnose.

In medical literature, for example in [Pschyrembel 98], the development of diseases is described verbally using clinical stages or phases and also graphically. Typical examples are given in Figure 2 and Figure 3. They show the developments of whooping cough and measles. The horizontal lines indicate the existence of the corresponding symptom, named at the right side of the figure. The gradients of the lines represent an increase or a decrease of the corresponding symptom

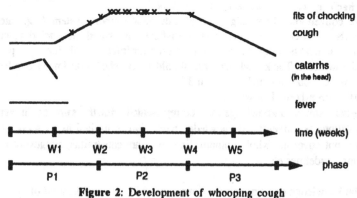

Figure 2: Development of whooping cough

In figure 2 the normal development of whooping cough is presented. In [Pschyrembel 98] the duration of the phases are given with their minimum and maximum. The duration in figure 2 are for ease of this graphic the minimal duration. The disease consists of three

---

[3] The example serves mainly for illustration and is therefore strongly simplified.

phases. The first phase looks like a cold with fever and a little coughing. In the second phase the cough becomes worse, even with fits of chocking particularly during night time. In the third phase everything gets better, the cough normally lasts for some days but without the fits of chocking.

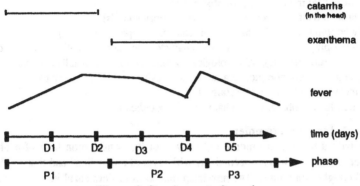

Figure 3: Development of measles

Measles has three phases as well (figure 3). The main symptom, the characteristic exanthema, appears in the 2nd phase. The 1st phase reminds of the 1st phase of whooping cough. With both diseases the patients have fever and some catarrhs in the head. This means that they have a rhinitis, an otitis or a conjunctivitis. In the 1st phase the diseases can not be distinguished, a correct diagnosis is not possible without technical investigations.

For the other diagnoses of our example, influenzal infect, bronchitis and pseudo-croups, we do not present such a diagram because in the example the development of these diseases is not important. We first sketch the knowledge necessary for the example critiquing system. All diagnoses of the example are treatable. This parameter is not explicitly listed in the description of the knowledge. The parameters being normal are not mentioned. Then we present the situation with a verbal description of the case. The physician's conclusions and the system's inferences are shown in a more formal, but also verbal form.

Knowledge of the system:
- fault knowledge
  - if not antibiotics for whooping cough 2nd phase, then critique
  - if fever without observable symptoms and no examination of urine, then critique
- partial formalized knowledge
  - if febrile seizures (Fieberkrämpfe), keep fever lower 38.5
- conventional knowledge base
  - pedriatic knowledge base containing infectious diseases
  - *(a) Knowledge for focusing the critique*
  - (whooping cough 1st phase: dangerous)
  - (whooping cough 2nd phase: dangerous, urgent)
  - (pseudo-croup: dangerous)
  - (prescription of nose drops:
    - usefulness (influenzal infect, bronchitis, whooping cough 1st phase))
  - (prescription of antipyretics:
    - usefulness (measles 2nd phase, bronchitis, influenzal infect)

(prescription of antibiotics:
        usefulness (whooping cough 2nd phase, bronchitis, influenzal infect)
        risky (patient is allergic))
(b) set-covering knowledge base
(influenzal infect: fever, rhinitis, otitis)
(bronchitis: fever, cough, rhinitis, respiratory sounds)
(whooping cough 1st phase: fever, catarrhs, unspecified cough)
(whooping cough 2nd phase: characteristic cough with fits of chocking (Erstickungsanfälle), bacteriological examination for Bordetella pertussis)
(pseudo-croup (allergic): characteristic cough with fits of chocking)
(measles 1st phase: fever, catarrhs)
(measles 2nd phase: fever, characteristic exanthema)

Situation 1 for the example:

A mother with a nearly three month old baby is in the consultation hour of a physician. The mother reports that it is the second day with fever of about 38.5° and that the baby has a cold and coughs sometimes. The physician diagnoses an influenzal infect and prescribes some nose drops and some antipyretics which can be given if the baby becomes nervous from the fever. At the moment the physician has no hints on something else. The physician wants to see the baby again if the symptoms last for the next two days.

Conclusions from situation 1:

- doctor's diagnosis: influenzal infect
- doctor's action: prescription of nose drops and antipyretics
- system's diagnosis: influenzal infect (favorite),
        bronchitis (suspicious),
        whooping cough 1st phase (suspicious)
        measles 1st phase (suspicious)

System's results:
The diagnosis of the system and the doctor differ, the system has on its list of suspicious diagnosis a dangerous diagnosis which needs special attention. This diagnosis is dangerous but not urgent. The actions of the doctor are also reasonable for this diagnosis. The system gives no critique but marks the case as having perhaps a wrong doctor's diagnosis. This mark allows to reconsider the diagnosis more easily.

Situation 2 for the example:
In the second week after the first consultation the mother comes to the physician with her baby early in the morning, because the baby had some coughing attacks, one with a fit of chocking during the last night. The baby has no fever and the cold has disappeared. The physician had some cases of pseudo-croup in the last week and so he thinks of this diagnosis in the case of the baby. The mother's description of the cough fits to this disease. The physician prescribes nothing, he recommends to appease the baby in such situations. Sometimes fresh, moist air, that is opening the window, may help during an attack.

Conclusions from situation 2:
- doctor's diagnosis: pseudo-croup
- doctor's action: recommendations (mentioned above) for the mother
- system's diagnosis: whooping cough 2nd phase (favorite)
  (development of the disease causes this favorite, although bacteriological examination is missing),
  pseudo-croup (suspicious)

System's inferences:
- check fault knowledge
  result: nothing applies to this situation, no critique
- check reliability of the diagnosis and the data
  method: calculate from the reliability of the symptoms
  result: main symptom (cough) from anamnesis,
  symptom value (fit of chocking) is reliable (overwritten),
  diagnosis is reliable
- check completeness of doctor's diagnosis
  result: doctor's diagnosis is o.k.
- check partial formalized knowledge
  result: nothing applies to this situation, no critique
- check system's diagnoses
  doctor's diagnosis is suspicious for the system
  system has different favorite diagnosis
  result: checking of favorite diagnosis,
  one symptom is missing
- check the relevant critiquing parameters
  result: whooping cough is dangerous, 2nd phase is dangerous and urgent,
  associated action (antibiotics) is missing (negative knowledge),
  action (antibiotics) critique is necessary

System's results:

The physician gets the critique that he should check for whooping cough (bacteriological examination) immediately. If this is not possible fast enough, the critiquing system recommends to prescribe antibiotics.

For the last consultation situation the system favorites whooping cough 2nd phase as a diagnosis, because input data matches the developments. Whooping cough 2nd phase is dangerous and urgent. Therefore the system informs the user about the symptom's favorite diagnosis and tries to increase the evidence of this disease. Since it is dangerous and urgent, the system reminds the user of the missing result of the bacteriological examination and the need to start an antibiotics therapy soon. Nevertheless, the physician decides if the critique of the system is qualified and how he reacts on the suggestions.

5. Conclusion

Critiquing systems help the physician with the decision making process indirectly, commenting the user's decisions only in critical situations. For reuse of knowledge, critiquing systems might be based on the knowledge base of an diagnostic expert system, but requires additional knowledge as outlined in this paper. Our next step we are currently working on is to implement these concepts in a shell kit and to evaluate them with real world domains and cases, especially in comparison to training systems [Puppe et al. 98].

6. References

[Bemmel & Musen 97] van Bemmel, J. and Musen, M. (1997): Handbook of Medical Informatics, Springer.

[Gerlach & Onken 94] M. Gerlach, M. and Onken, R. (1994): CASSY - The Electronic Part of a Human-Electronic Crew, In: 3rd International Workshop on Human-Computer-Teamwork, Cambridge, UK.

[Miller 86] Miller, P. (1986): Expert Critiquing Systems - Practise-Based Consultation by Computer, Springer.

[Mosseveld & van der Lei 90] Mosseveld, B. and van der Lei, J. (1990): HYPERCRITIC: A Critiquing System for Hypertension. In: O'Moore et al: Medical Informatics, Europe '90, Lecture Notes in Medical Informatics, Springer.

[Ohmann 97] Ohmann, C. (1997): Was ist Qualitätsmanagement? in: Scheibe (Hrsg.): Qualitätsmanagement in der Medizin - Handbuch für Klinik und Praxis, ecomed.

[Puppe & Reinhardt 95] Puppe, F., Reinhardt, B. (1995): Generating Case-Oriented Training from Diagnostic Expert Systems, Machine Mediated Learning, Vol 5, Nr. 3&4.

[Puppe et al. 98] Puppe, F., Puppe, B., Reinhardt B., Schewe S. und Buscher, H.P. (1998).: Evaluation medizinischer Diagnostik-Expertensysteme zur Wissensvermittlung., in: Informatik, Biometrie und Epidemiologie in Medizin und Biologie 29, Nr. 1.

[Pschyrembel 98] Pschyrembel (1998): Klinisches Wörterbuch, de Gruyter.

[Ramachandran & Wilkins 96] Ramachandran, S. and Wilkins, D. (1996): Temporal Control Structures in Expert Critiquing Systems, In: TIME-96, Workshop of the FLAIRS 96, Florida.

[Russell & Norvig 95] Russell, S., Norvig, P. (1995): Artificial Intelligence - A Modern Approach, Chapter 16 "Making Simple Decisions", Prentice Hall.

[Silverman 92] Silverman, B. (1992): Survey of Expert Critiquing Systems; Practical and Theoretical Frontiers, CACM, Vol.35, No.4.

The Treatment of Time in a Case–Based Analysis of Experimental Medical Studies

Alexander Seitz and Adelinde M. Uhrmacher *

University of Ulm, D–89069 Ulm, Germany,
seitz@ki.informatik.uni--ulm.de,
WWW home page: http://www.informatik.uni--ulm.de/ki/seitz.html

Abstract. Case–based approaches are employed within a multitude of application areas one of which is the prediction of dynamic behaviour. Given a situation the possible development after a time span shall be determined. If only a small set of heterogenously structured cases describing observations at a variety of time points is given to start with, as it is the case when experimental medical studies shall be analysed, it becomes necessary to analyse and evaluate the temporal horizon from case to case differently, and treat time as a first class variable. This is the strategy OASES (Our Approach to Simulation based on Experimental Studies) employs. For this purpose, OASES utilises knowledge implicit in cases for matching and adaptation. Whether different time points do match in the current situation or how different time points of observation might effect the development, is decided based on cases which time is an explicit part of. *Keywords*: Case–Based Reasoning; Case–Based Similarity Ranking; Case–Based Adaptation; Prediction; Experimental Studies

1 Introduction

Time is a variable hardly addressed in case–based reasoning systems. However, if the behaviour of a dynamic system is the subject of the reasoning process, information about time has to be processed. We are interested in analysing and predicting the effect of certain settings in medical experimental studies. The knowledge that is available shows itself not as an explicit model about the objects, interrelations and causal forces of the domain [9], but as a set of observations which are temporally interrelated. If all observations occur based on a fixed set of variables with a fixed frequency, they form a traditional time series, whose homogeneous structure, given a sufficient number, supports an inductive analysis. In this case an a priori time window can be determined to define the temporal range within which interrelations between observations are likely. Based on the time window the original temporal relation can be flattened into cases whose variables are indexed with time [11, 12, 16]. Other approaches abstract time

* The research was sponsored by the Forschungsschwerpunktprogramm Baden Wuerttemberg. We would like to thank the Department of Orthopaedic Research and Biomechanics at the University of Ulm for their cooperation.

into several general trends [14]. In the case of experimental studies a variety of rather short time series based on different situations and time spans reflect different aspects of the underlying behavioural pattern. No inductive methodology can decide whether current observations should be explained with respect to observations a few hours or a few days before nor seems any abstraction of time useful. In analysing experimental medical studies time seems only interpretable with respect to the single observation, same as interpolation procedures between different time points suggest themselves based on the specifics of the observation. Rather than keeping time as a separate dimension, time becomes an intrinsic part of the experimental setting. Therefore, OASES [4] encodes time as just another experimental parameter and utilises intensively the knowledge inherent in cases to determine whether different time points do match in the current situation or how different time points of observation might effect the development.

2   The Application Domain

OASES has been put firstly to test in the area of bone healing. Despite the large number of experimental studies the significance and importance of single factors in general are still unknown in this area. Factors that influence fracture healing are both local (degree of local trauma, vascular injury, infection, etc.) and systemic (age, hormones, etc.). Besides biological interventions (osteogenic, osteoconductive and osteoinductive methods), mechanical and physical interventions (mechanical, electrical and ultrasound stimulation) and their effect on bone formation are analysed [6]. The experimental setting is typically expressed by a set of experimental parameters, for example 'species' or 'osteotomy', whereas the results are measured by result parameters, for example the 'torsional stiffness' of the fixed bone. Sometimes, the data are described quantitatively, often only qualitatively. As experimental studies typically analyse the effect of single factors in a given experimental setting, often comparative statements can be found, e.g. "more proliferate callus formation was seen in the less–rigidly fixed groups [7]". The influence of parameter changes on the healing process is expressed by mathematical factors, differences or just nominal changes. In publications, isolated or absolute results for each group can be found as well as comparative assessments between groups. Although the 650 cases which encode around 50 experimental studies are very different with respect to the set of variables, their scaling niveau and the observation frequency, they all describe or assess a healing situation by referring to certain time points of observation, capturing snapshots of the underlying system (Fig. 1). These time points indicate situations relative to the beginning of the experiment neglecting the influence of time at a larger scale, e.g. the influence of seasons on the healing process. Thus, each experiment can be interpreted as a short time series, between 1 to 10 observations with a frequency which varies between hours and weeks.

Since time has a different meaning for different species and different experiments, each experiment defines its own temporal horizon, which determines how temporal differences are interpreted. The time chosen for observation belongs to the experimental design, as do osteosynthesis, gap width and other experimental parameters and, therefore, is treated as such.

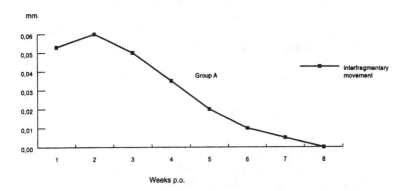

Fig. 1. Experimental Studies as "Time Series" — snapshots of the interfragmentary movement at different time points [3].

3 Case–Based Prediction

Case–based prediction implies that at least part of the model the prediction is based upon, is encoded as cases. OASES utilises intensively the knowledge inherent in cases and avoid widely the necessity to define or derive general knowledge [4]. Even if a general and closed domain model can not be induced nor validated, more about existing studies and their interrelation will be learned. The single steps in OASES are summarised in Fig. 2, some of which will be explained in detail within the following sections.

3.1 Matching Cases

First, the system has to find experiments that help in predicting the outcome of a given healing situation at a certain time. Since parameters are identified by their name, an apparently simple method of matching is checking parameters for equal values. Weighted Euclidean distances assess differences [5, 12] by assuming an explicit weighting of features which requires the possibility to determine the relevance of parameters in general. Often, however, the invariance of feature weightings over the case space proves to be inadequate [17]. What effect a different time of observation will have depends on the species and other experimental parameters, and can therefore not be determined in general.

In a first selection process we search for cases in the form of experiments that are sufficiently similar to the given situation and thus might be useful candidates for the prediction process. We compare the inquiry with cases by comparing values of all experimental parameters, including the time of observation. We

1. Input of inquiry I
2. For all results R in database ;; Select cases sufficient similar.
   (a) *Diff* = Number of not exchangeable parameter values in R and I
   (b) If *Diff* $\leq$ Diff$_{max}$;; Diff$_{max}$ is specified by the user.
      – Store R for further inspection
3. For all stored results R ;; Order cases according to their usability.
   (a) Given parameter names $p_1, \ldots, p_n$ for parameters in R or I, according values $v_{1,1}, \ldots, v_{n,1}$ and $v_{1,2}, \ldots, v_{n,2}$ in R and I, compute usability U of R for processing I by

$$U = \frac{1}{n} \sum_{i=1}^{n} \mathrm{PAd}(p_i, v_{i,1}, v_{i,2}, R, I) \ .$$

   (b) if $U \geq$ U$_{min}$;; U$_{min}$ specified by user.
      – Store R for adaptation and final presentation
4. For all stored usable results R ;; Adapt Cases.
   (a) Combine adaptation rules for R
   (b) Adapt R according to combined rule
5. Present stored results in descending order of usability

Fig. 2. The Case–Based Algorithm in Pseudo–Code.

refer to the inquiry as a case, too, and calculate the *similarity* between two cases:

- Two cases are *similar*, if the number of parameters whose values are not exchangeable does not exceed a threshold specified by the user.
- Two parameter values are *not exchangeable*, if they do not lie within a given tolerance region nor does an experimental study, i.e. a comparative result, exist which states that the values can be exchanged in the given situation.

Apart from the de facto equality of parameter values, different metrical values can be matched if they lie within a specified tolerance span. Often, experiments, i.e. cases, can be found whose comparative results support the exchangeability of parameter values by varying the corresponding parameter and declaring no effect on the inspected result parameter.

An experiment contradicts the exchangeability of two values of a parameter, if it claims an influence on the result. In that case the values are assumed to be dissimilar. Its claim is also valued by its similarity. The most similar experiment decides the issue. If the values are considered dissimilar, according to the stored cases, and the experiment that argues an influence is sufficient similar, it will be used within the adaptation process. Because the most "similar" case is not necessarily the one observed at the same time point, interpolations between different time points are a frequent form of adaptation.

When valuing the experiments supporting or opposing the exchangeability of values, the concept of similarity is again employed. This results in a recursive definition of similarity. The user specifies how many stages of similarity computation at most are reached. At the lowest level of recursion values are checked for identity.

Not each case which is found sufficient similar to the given inquiry is necessarily useful for forecasting the expected behaviour. It must be possible to adapt parameter value differences and modify the result of the found study accordingly. Therefore a second selection process complements the first. Based on the set of selected cases which have been found to be sufficient similar those are preferable whose differences can be explained away by cases in the case base. Those cases are used to produce adaptation hypotheses. The adaptability PAd of parameter values is quantified by a number ranging from 0 to 1. The value of 0 means, that no adaptation is possible whereas 1 documents full adaptability. Let I be the given inquiry, R a result to be compared with I. Furthermore, assume that v_1 and v_2 are the corresponding values of a parameter p that has to be adapted. Then $\text{PAd}(p, v_1, v_2, I, R)$ is computed as follows:

- If $v_1 = v_2$ then $\text{PAd} = 1$.
- If the exchangeability of v_1 and v_2 is documented by a comparative experiment, its similarity is used as the adaptability of the values (see above).
- If values can be adapted by the adaptation methods described below, the adaptability equals to the quality score of the applied adaptation method. Applicability and quality score of an adaptation method depends on similarity of the adaptation hypotheses, and, in the case of interpolation, the value difference that has to be bridged. For that purpose, let v_l and v_r be the parameter values between which the interpolation has to be done; v_{min} and v_{max} describe the value span of the parameter. Furthermore, let IS_{min} designate a minimum interpolation specificity. The specificity IS for the interpolation between v_l and v_r is computed as

$$IS = \text{IS}_{min} + \left(1 - \left|\frac{v_r - v_l}{v_{max} - v_{min}}\right|\right)(1 - \text{IS}_{min}) \ .$$

IS lies in the interval $[0, 1]$. The lower the minimum IS_{min}, the worse interpolations over wide ranges are assessed, lowering the quality score of the adaptation rule. IS is multiplied with the usability of the adaptation hypothesis.

- If v_1 and v_2 are metrically scaled and can not be adapted, the *adaptability* of parameter values is determined depending on their difference. In the whole, three minor deviations between two experiments might more easily be tolerated than one major one. A ratio between their metric distance and the overall value span of the regarded parameter in the case base is computed. If the distance equals to the span, the adaptability gets the value 0. With the distance becoming smaller the adaptability converges to a maximum value specified by the user that must be less than or equal to 1. Let MA_{max} be the specified maximum and v_{min} and v_{max} specify the value span of parameter p, the adaptability PAd of the parameter values is computed as

$$\text{PAd} = \left|\frac{v_2 - v_1}{v_{max} - v_{min}}\right| \text{MA}_{max} \ .$$

Given parameter names $p_1, \ldots, p_n$ for parameters in a result R or the inquiry I with according values $v_{1,1}, \ldots, v_{n,1}$ and $v_{1,2}, \ldots, v_{n,2}$ in R and I, the usability U of R for computing the outcome of a given inquiry I is computed as the arithmetic mean of the parameter adaptabilities, expressed in the formula

$$U = \frac{1}{n} \sum_{i=1}^{n} \text{PAd}(p_i, v_{i,1}, v_{i,2}, R, I) \ .$$

If the found case is identical with the inquiry, i.e. all parameter values are exchangeable, or the found case is sufficient similar and no adaptation rules can be applied the case results are presented as the answer to the user inquiry. Typically, however, the result of cases has to be adapted. Cases that support the usability are used to produce adaptation rules to answer the inquiry and forecast the likely result of the experimental setting. Since different adaptation methods are available which might result in different adaptation hypotheses with different quality scores, only the adaptation method which offers the highest quality score enters the calculation of the usability and will be applied during adaptation.

3.2 Adaptation methods

Adaptation methods are used to modify the original result of an experiment that is different to the inquiry in some parameters. Using adaptation methods results in corresponding adaptation rules, which have to be combined. See also Sect. 3.4.

Exact adaptation Exact adaptation requires an experiment that exactly describes the difference of two parameter values. For example, the user asks OASES to predict the effect of a certain experimental setting on the periosteal callus. OASES finds an experiment result in the literature (O'Sullivan et al, 1994 [13]) that matches to a certain degree the parameter settings given by the user but differs in weight and experiment duration. The value '12 weeks' for the latter has to be adapted to a value '6 weeks' stated by the user. Another experiment (Aro et Chao, 1993 [1]) is found which exactly varies these two values and states as a comparative result the periosteal callus is decreasing from 6 weeks to 12 weeks. The described change can be used as an adaptation rule. The similarities between the experiment and the cases to be adapted, are combined to a quality score for the adaptability of the parameter values.

Interpolation between absolute results When an experiment differs from the inquiry in some metrically scaled experimental parameter and its result parameter is metrically scaled, interpolation between absolute results may be applied. Time is one of the few parameters typically metrically scaled, and lends itself for an "interpolation between absolute results".

If multiple metrical scaled parameters have to be adapted, the system tries to employ a modified Shepard–Interpolation [15], which uses relative instead of absolute distances between vectors, bypassing the problem of different ranges of variation for different parameters. If such a joint interpolation is not possible, single interpolations are combined.

In Fig. 3, a joint interpolation is done over the parameters 'interfragmentary movement' and 'experiment duration'. The inquiry specifies the vector (0.15 mm, 3.5 weeks) while the absolute experiments use vectors (0.0 mm, 2.0 weeks) and (0.2 mm, 4 weeks), respectively. The result of the originally found experiment is adapted accordingly. Interpolation is done linear and weighted by the ratio between the footholds and the general value range. The quality score of the resulting adaptation rule is the usability score of the adjoined absolute experiment which supports the interpolation multiplied with the weight mentioned above.

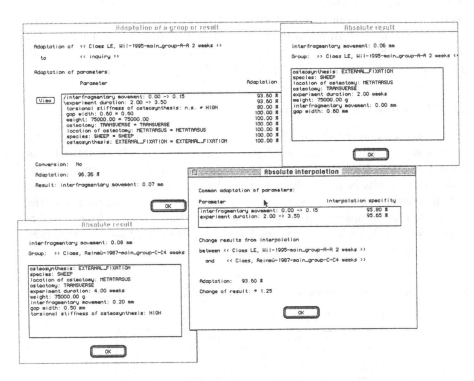

Fig. 3. Interpolation over multiple parameters

3.3   Interpolation using comparative results

Even comparative results can be used for interpolation on condition that the experiment parameter variation comprises the metrically scaled values that have to be adapted. As an example, the user wants to know the result of applying a certain healing method after 6 weeks and a study is found in the case base documenting results after 4 weeks. In this case, a comparative study might help that describes the change of the result parameter between 4 weeks and 8 weeks by a factor of, say 2.0. Proceeding from 4 to 6 weeks instead of 8 weeks means that the doubling of the original result value has to be adapted to an increasing of 50 %, resulting in a factor of 1.5.

The modified comparative result is used as an adaptation rule. To get a quality score of the adaptation rule, the usability between the single components of the comparative experiment with the cases to be adapted is determined. Afterwards the usability values are multiplied.

Using mean values for adaptation If a parameter value v_1 has to be adapted to a value v_2, the method of using mean values collects cases that treat the result parameter and either value v_1 or value v_2. It calculates the mean values of the result parameters within these two groups. The ratio of the second mean value to the first is used as an adaptation rule. Cases used for computing the mean values are weighted according to their similarity. The average similarity of both groups defines the quality score for the adaptation rule.

3.4 Combining adaptation rules

Adaptation rules describe value changes which are expressed in terms of factors, differences or qualitative changes. Table 1 shows the possible combination of adaptation rules. If rules contradict each other, e.g. functions < and >, their combination results in an undefined rule. In that case, adaptation is not possible and the considered experimental result is discarded. The combination of the parameter adaptations is applied to the found experiment result. Using < and > at a metrical result leads to a corresponding open interval. Factors and differences are just applied.

Table 1. Combination of adaptation rules. Functions d_i are differences, f_i are factors.

Fct.	<	>	$d_2 < 0$	$d_2 > 0$	$f_2 < 1$	$f_2 > 1$
<	<	undef.	<	undef.	<	undef.
>	undef.	>	undef.	>	undef.	>
$d_1 < 0$	<	undef.	$d_1 + d_2$	undef.	<	undef.
$d_1 > 0$	undef.	>	undef.	$d_1 + d_2$	undef.	>
$f_1 < 1$	<	undef.	<	undef.	$f_1 * f_2$	undef.
$f_1 > 1$	undef.	>	undef.	>	undef.	$f_1 * f_2$

3.5 Presentation of results

As it can be seen in Fig. 3, the system presents computed results together with a case–based explanation of them. All cases involved in the reasoning process und subprocesses can be reached by a hierarchical explanation component. This enables the domain expert of validating the results und gives him an idea of what publications might be interesting for predicting the time course of a result parameter under a certain healing situation. By experimenting with different healing parameters, the expert gets an idea of which situation might provide successful healing results. Based on that, studies can be planned to validate the quality of the healing method.

3.6 Evaluation

Below we present a few results of OASES. Therefore, one selected publication, typically consisting of more than 12 cases, was removed from the case base and used for testing. By this means about 90 inquiries on the most frequently used experimental parameters were executed and compared with the de facto results of the publication [4]. It is typical for OASES to present more than one result.

In order to evaluate if OASES was able to reproduce the dynamic of a healing process, we removed a publication (Claes et al., 1995 [3]) whose results document the 'interfragmentary movement' over time. The system identifies a matching publication (Claes et al., 1987 [2]) with a similar observation pattern. Figure 4 compares the predicted and real behaviour of the interfragmentary movement over 7 weeks. For approximation, the system employs multiple interpolation of both 'experiment duration' and initial 'interfragmentary movement'.

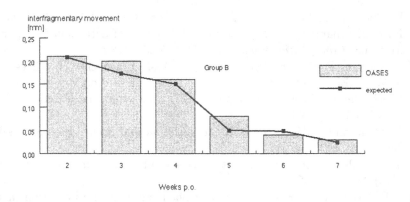

Fig. 4. Actual and approximated course of interfragmentary movement for Claes et al, 1995 [3].

4 Conclusion

OASES predicts the dynamics of a system based on documented experimental studies. It employs consequently the ideas of case based reasoning throughout the whole process of prediction. The heterogeneity of second order data, as shown by experimental studies on bone healing, requires specific, context sensitive methods and knowledge for matching and adaptation. OASES interprets and assesses temporal relations with respect to the given situation and treats time as explicit part of the cases. Due to its explicit representation and case–based processing of time, OASES deviates from other case–based approaches aimed at analysing temporal relations. As only few other case–based approaches [10], OASES benefits during matching and adapting cases from the accuracy of case based methods to deal with idiosyncrasies [8]. This constitutes an essential precondition to forecast the behaviour of systems based on a plethora of rather different and short time series. The promising results of OASES have fostered another medical application. In Anaesthesiology, currently a case base with around 1500 cases from 90 publications is developed to explore postoperative side effects of anaesthesiologic procedures.

References

[1] H.T. Aro and E.Y.S Chao. Bone-healing patterns affected by loading, fracture fragment stability, fracture type, and fracture site compression. *Clinical Orthopaedics and Related Research*, (293):8–17, 1993.

[2] L. Claes, J. Reinmueller, and L. Duerselen. Experimentelle untersuchungen zum einfluss der interfragmentaeren bewegungen auf die knochenheilung. *Hefte zur Unfallheilkunde*, (189):53–58, 1987.

[3] L. Claes, H.-J. Wilke, P. Augat, S. Ruebenacker, and K.J. Margevicius. Effect of dynamization on gap healing of diaphyseal fractures under external fixations. *Clinical Biomechanics*, 10(5):227–234, 1995.

[4] D. Damm, F.W. von Henke, A. Seitz, A.M. Uhrmacher, L. Claes, and S. Wolf. Ein fallbasiertes system f"ur die interpretation von literatur zur knochenheilung. Technical Report 98-01, Ulmer Informatik-Berichte, Universit"at Ulm, 1998.

[5] R. Duda and P. Hart. *Pattern Classification and Scene Analysis*. Wiley, New York, 1973.

[6] T.A. Einhorn. Enhancement of fracture-healing. *J Bone Joint Surg Am*, 77(6):940–56, 1995.

[7] A.E. Goodship J. Kenwright. Controlled mechanical stimulation in the treatment of tibial fractures. *Clin Orthop*, (241):36–47, 1989.

[8] J. Kolodner. *Case-Based Reasoning*. Morgan Kaufman Publishers, San Mateo, CA, 1993.

[9] Phyllis Koton. Integrating case-based and causal reasoning. In *Proceedings of the Tenth Annual Conference of the Cognitive Science Society. Montreal, 17.-19.8.1988*, pages 167–173, Northvale, N.J., 1988. Erlbaum.

[10] D.B. Leake, A. Kinley, and D. Wilson. A case study of case-based cbr. In D.B. Leake and E. Plaza, editors, *Case-Based Reasoning Research and Development, Proceedings of the 2nd International Conference on Case-Based Reasoning*, volume 1266 of *Lecture Notes in Artificial Intelligence*, pages 371–82, Berlin, 1997. Springer.

[11] G. Nakhaeizadeh. Learning prediction of time series - a theoretical and empirical comparison of cbr with some other approaches. In S. Wess, K.-D. Althoff, and M.M. Richter, editors, *Topics in Case-Based Reasoning*, volume 837 of *Lecture Notes in Artificial Intelligence*, pages 65–76, Berlin, 1993. Springer.

[12] A. Nebot, F.E. Cellier, and D.A. Linkens. Controlling an anaesthetic agent by means of fuzzy inductive reasoning. In *Proc. QUARDET'93, IMACS Intl. Workshop on Qualitative Reasoning and Decision Technologies*, Barcelona, Spain, June 1993.

[13] M.E. O'Sullivan, J.T. Bronk, E.Y. Chao, and P.J. Kelly. Experimental study of the effect of weight bearing on fracture healing in the canine tibia. *Clin Orthop*, (302):273–283, 1994.

[14] R. Schmidt, B. Heindl, B. Pollwein, and L. Gierl. Abstractions of data and time for multiparametric time course prognoses. In I. Smith and B. Faltings, editors, *Advances in Case-Based Reasoning*, volume 1168 of *Lecture Notes in Artificial Intelligence*, pages 377–391, Berlin, 1996. Springer.

[15] D. Shepard. A two dimensional interpolation function for irregularly-spaced data. In *Proc. ACM National Conference*, pages 517–524, 1968.

[16] A.M. Uhrmacher, R.J. Frye, and F.E. Cellier. Applying fuzzy based inductive reasoning to analyze qualitatively the dynamic behavior of an ecological system. *The International Journal on Artificial Intelligence in Natural Resource Management*, 11(2):1–10, 1997.

[17] D. Wettschereck, D.W. Aha, and T. Mohri. A review and comparative evaluation of feature weighting methods for lazy learning algorithms. *Artificial Intelligence Review*, 11:273–314, 1997.

Formal Representation of Temporal Items of the Diagnostic and Statistic Manual of Mental Disorders

A Description Logic Approach Based on the CEN Time Standards for Health Care Specific Problems

Cord Spreckelsen[1], Klaus Spitzer[1]

Institut für Med. Informatik der RWTH Aachen

Abstract. As a paradigm for abstract, nested time-references occurring in medical domain knowledge we analyze temporal diagnostic items of the Diagnostic and Statistic Manual of Mental Disorders (DSM–IV). Based on an elicitation of categories of DSM-IV time-references a formal approach to the representation of nested temporal references is proposed. Generic time-related concepts are introduced, which have to be specialized by concepts representing temporal patterns of the diagnostic items. Satisfiability of the knowledge base ensures the conformance to the Time Standards for health care specific problems (a CEN-prestandard).). Terminological inferences support the nosologic analysis of the DSM-IV classification.

1 Introduction

1.1 The Diagnostic and Statistic Manual of Mental Disorders DSM–IV

The Diagnostic and Statistic Manual of Mental Disorders is a comprehensive classification of psychiatric diagnoses developed by the American Psychiatric Association (APA). Apart from the ICD it is the world standard for the psychiatric domain. A revised fourth edition has been published in 1994 (the German translation appeared two years later).

The DSM–IV presents explicit diagnostic criteria for mental disorders in order to operationalize the diagnostic effort in psychiatry and to increase its reliability. Any section of the DSM–IV referring to a mental disorder comprises a detailed and strictly structured description of special aspects such as 'Diagnostic Features, 'Subtypes and/or Specifiers', 'Prevalence', 'Course', 'Familial Pattern' etc. together with a concise, itemized comprehension of the diagnostic criteria. An important source of complexity in the DSM–IV is the existence of temporal diagnostic criteria, which leads to nested temporal references.

Application Problems of the DSM-IV. Application problems of the DSM-IV are caused by the extent and the complexity of the classification, which is extremely difficult to learn and to be handled in the clinical praxis. Moreover in the context of European psychiatry some of the diagnostic criteria are not well-established and the doctors complain about the restrictiveness of DSM-IV categories, which does not cover the subtleties of their clinical descriptions.

1.2 The DSM-IV Assistant

The DSM-IV Assistant[1] is a project, which aims at a knowledge based assistance supporting the application of the DSM-IV. The core of the system is the formally represented taxonomic structure of the DSM–IV classification. The interdependencies of the diagnostic items have been made explicit in order to represent as much as possible of the inherent nosologic knowledge. This paper addresses the problem of the formal representation of the above mentioned nested temporal references, which play an important part in the DSM-IV classification. The approach is based on an elicitation of the different categories of DSM-IV time references. In order to preserve a high degree of explicitness and reusability the formal approach had to meet the following requirements: it should have a clear semantics, respect the European standardization effort and support taxonomic inferences.

2 Basics

2.1 Time Standard for health care specific problems

In 1995 the European Committee for Standardization (CEN) published a draft of an European prestandard for the representation of medical information with explicit references to time. The CEN–Time Standards specify a set of representational primitives and semantic relations aiming at an unambiguous representation of explicit time-related expressions in medical informatics.

As stated in the draft, it not the purpose of the Time Standards (TS) to define a temporal logic or to fix up a temporal inference mechanism. The major aim is to ensure the *explicitness* of the temporal aspects of medical information and to standardize their documentation. Moreover it is stated that the TS do not introduce a specific ontology of time. Indeed this has to be understand cum grano salis, because the TS enforce the distinction of event, episode and temporal relations – thus imposing at least a generic ontology to the representation of medical knowledge.

2.2 Description logics

Concept languages or description logics (DL) have been developed in order to provide a formal reconstruction of frame-based knowledge representation systems. The are widely accepted as an adequate means to represent conceptual

---

[1] funded by the RWTH Aachen within the 'Interdiziplinäres Zentrum ZNS'

and taxonomic knowledge in a way that is semantically clear. Description logics has been used as an unifying framework for several (class based) database and knowledge representation formalisms. We choose here a description logic approach in order to make taxonomic knowledge explicit.

Starting with atomic concepts (logically interpreted as unary predicates) and roles (binary predicates), the syntax of DL allows to define more complex concepts (and eventually even complex roles). The set of concept (and role) definitions forms the terminological component (TBox) of the knowledge base. Additionally in many knowledge representation systems the conceptual scheme of the TBox can be instantiated by sets and relations of individual names, where the names represent individual entities of the domain (ABox).

In the following we will refer to the syntax of the well-known concept language $\mathcal{ALC}$ [3]. In $\mathcal{ALC}$ the following concept forming operations are defined: Given an atomic concept A a role R and two arbitrary concepts C, D a concept can be build using concept conjunction $(C \sqcap D)$, concept disjunction $(C \sqcup D)$, atomic negation $\neg A$, and two kinds of role restrictions: $(\forall R.C)$ and $(\exists R.C)$. A formal semantics is introduced by defining an interpretation function $\mathcal{I}$, which maps every atomic concept A to a subset $(A)^{\mathcal{I}}$ of $\Delta^{\mathcal{I}}$, the domain of $\mathcal{I}$, and every role R to a subset $(R)^{\mathcal{I}}$ of $\Delta^{\mathcal{I}} \times \Delta^{\mathcal{I}}$. The interpretation function is extended compositionally: $(C \sqcap D)^{\mathcal{I}} = (C)^{\mathcal{I}} \cap (D)^{\mathcal{I}}, (C \sqcup D)^{\mathcal{I}} = (C)^{\mathcal{I}} \cup (D)^{\mathcal{I}}$ and $(\neg A)^{\mathcal{I}} = \Delta^{\mathcal{I}} \backslash (A)^{\mathcal{I}}$. The extensions of concept restrictions are given by: $(\forall R.C)^{\mathcal{I}} = \{x \in \Delta^{\mathcal{I}} | \forall y : (\langle x, y \rangle \in (R)^{\mathcal{I}} \rightarrow y \in (C)^{\mathcal{I}})\}$ and $(\exists R.C)^{\mathcal{I}} = \{x \in \Delta^{\mathcal{I}} | \exists y : (\langle x, y \rangle \in (R)^{\mathcal{I}} \wedge y \in (C)^{\mathcal{I}})\}$. Obviously all of the constructions have counterparts in first order predicate logics.

Terminological assertions of the form $A \sqsubseteq D$, $A \doteq D$ or $C][D$ read as $\forall x : (A(x) \Rightarrow D(x)), \forall x : (A(x)) \Leftrightarrow D(x))$ and $\forall x : (C(x) \Leftrightarrow \neg D(x))$, respectively. They are used to define concepts, i.e. to fix the interpretation of an atomic concept by the interpretation of a complex concept description.

The syntax of $\mathcal{ALC}$ has been enhanced in several ways e.g by cardinality restrictions on roles [4] or role forming operators [13].

3 Formal representation of temporal DSM–IV items

3.1 Categories of temporal aspects in the DSM–IV items

An analysis of all diagnostic items contained in the DSM–IV leads to the following categorization of time references. The DSM–IV contains temporal descriptions referring to time points and time intervals and which express a duration, frequency, or rate; there are relative time references leading to nested temporal expressions.

- The representationally simplest category are items which refer to the absolute age of a person. These items refer to the time point, when a patient reaches the age mentioned
  Example: 'Clinically significant loss of ... skills *before age 10 years*' (299.10, Childhood Disintegrative Disorder, Item B).

- Items referring to a time interval may refer to absolute dates. In the DSM-IV all time intervals are defined relative to other situations:
  Example '... symptoms ... developed within a month of Substance Intoxication or Withdrawal' (Substance-Induced Mood Disorder, Item B (1))
- Items expressing an duration may quantify a duration directly or relate the duration in question to the duration of a time interval, specified in the expression. The latter leads to nested temporal references. An example for the former is:
  Example 'Duration of the disturbance is more than 1 month' (309.81 Posttraumatic Stress Disorder, Item E).
- Items expressing a duration with reference to a situation:
  Example '... disturbance does not occur exclusively during the course of a chronic Psychotic Disorder'. (293.83, Mood Disorder Due to ... , Item D)
- Some items express a frequency, i.e.: they denote the change of a property over a time interval
  Example: '... occurring at least once a month ..' (311. Depressive Disorder NOS, Item 3).
- Temporal references of the above categories are nested in the DSM-IV items:
  Example: '...During the above 2-year period (...), the person has not been without the symptoms in Criterion A for more than 2 months at a time.' (301.13, Item B)
- There are no deictic temporal references (references, which can only given an exact meaning in a given context of utterance)

The categories match with the temporal expressions defined in the CEN Time Standards.

3.2 Problems with genericity

As a common experience of different approaches to the representation of medical terminology or taxonomies (e.g. [11]), the extensive use of specialization hierarchies in medicine and the depth of those hierarchies, makes it difficult or even impossible to draw a well-defined line between generic concepts (to be represented in the TBox of the terminological knowledge representation system) and entities (to be represented in the ABox) during the acquisition process: Depending on the actual intention a concept like 'Mood Disorder' may be considered as a generic scheme (prescribing the structure of special entries representing special mood disorders) or as an instance of the more abstract concept 'Mental Disorder', respectively. This problem has been addressed as an interaction between the knowledge representation and the application ([5]); in medicine the problem arises even within a single application (see [11]).

As a consequence important examples of a formal representation of medical terminology - namely SNOMED and GALEN - avoid the separation of a concept and instance layer and concentrate on the TBox. Knowledge representation in the DSM-IV project followed that way, too. In the following we introduce generic time-related concepts, which have to be *specialized* by concepts representing temporal patterns of the DSM–IV items. Satisfiability of the knowledge base implies the conformance to the Time Standards.

3.3 Generic time-related concepts conforming to the Time Standards

The Time Standards come with a BNF-Syntax for so-called standard predications: - nested expressions for time related information (see appendix). The problem with this syntactic scheme is, that it does *not* reflect all of the restrictions (e.g. with respect to the allowed combinations of situations, temporal links and temporal expressions) given by the TS.

In addition to the BNF-description we propose here a set of generic time-related concepts. If they are integrated in a terminological knowledge-base and specialized respecting satisfiability constraints, they lead to conformance with the Time Standards.

$$
\begin{aligned}
\text{Situation} &\sqsubseteq \exists \text{ characterisedBy: } <\text{concept}> \\
&\sqcap \forall \text{ hasComplexTemporalReference: ComplexTempLink} \quad (1) \\
\text{Concept} &] [\text{ Situation} \quad (2) \\
\text{Event} &\sqsubseteq \text{Situation} \sqcap \forall \text{ hasOccurence: EventOccurence} \\
&\sqcap \forall \text{ hasFrequency: Frequency} \quad (3) \\
\text{Episode} &\sqsubseteq \text{Situation} \sqcap \forall \text{ hasOccurence: EpisodeOccurence} \\
&\sqcap \forall \text{ hasFrequency: Frequency} \\
&\sqcap \forall \text{ hasDuration: Duration} \\
&\sqcap \forall \text{ hasRate: Rate} \\
\text{Episode} &] [\text{ Event} \quad (4)
\end{aligned}
$$

The definition of $<$concept$>$ (1) has been left open by purpose. By specializations of $<$concept$>$ the non-temporal facts, which constitute a special situation, could be represented. Such situation pattern are represented by DL concepts, too. Concentrating on the temporal aspects we leave this out here.

$$
\begin{aligned}
\text{EventOccurence} &\sqcap \forall \text{ at: TimePoint} \sqcup \text{TimeSeries} \\
&\sqcap \forall \text{ before: TimeInterval} \sqcup \text{TimePoint} \sqcup \text{TimeSeries} \\
&\sqcap \forall \text{ after: TimeInterval} \sqcup \text{TimePoint} \sqcup \text{TimeSeries} \\
&\sqcap \forall \text{ during: TimeInterval} \\
&\sqcap \forall \text{ nonQualifiedOccurence: TimePoint} \quad (5) \\
\text{EpisodeOccurence} &\sqcap \forall \text{ at: TimeInterval} \sqcup \text{TimeSeries} \\
&\sqcap \forall \text{ before: TimeInterval} \sqcup \text{TimePoint} \sqcup \text{TimeSeries} \\
&\sqcap \forall \text{ after: TimeInterval} \sqcup \text{TimePoint} \sqcup \text{TimeSeries} \\
&\sqcap \forall \text{ during: TimeInterval} \sqcup \text{TimeSeries} \\
&\sqcap \forall \text{ includes: TimeInterval} \sqcup \text{TimeSeries}
\end{aligned}
$$

$$\sqcap \forall \, \text{until: } \, \text{TimeInterval} \sqcup \text{TimePoint} \sqcup \text{TimeSeries}$$
$$\sqcap \forall \, \text{follows: } \, \text{TimeInterval} \sqcup \text{TimePoint} \sqcup \text{TimeSeries}$$
$$\sqcap \forall \, \text{since: } \, \text{TimeInterval} \sqcup \text{TimeSeries}$$
$$\sqcap \forall \, \text{up-to: } \, \text{TimeInterval} \sqcup \text{TimeSeries}$$
$$\sqcap \forall \, \text{co-continues: } \, \text{TimeInterval} \sqcup \text{TimeSeries}$$
$$\sqcap \forall \, \text{co-precedes: } \, \text{TimeInterval} \sqcup \text{TimeSeries}$$
$$\sqcap \forall \, \text{co-starts: } \, \text{TimeInterval} \sqcup \text{TimeSeries}$$
$$\sqcap \forall \, \text{co-ends: } \, \text{TimeInterval} \sqcup \text{TimeSeries}$$
$$\sqcap \forall \, \text{nonQualifiedOccurence:}$$
$$\text{TimeInterval} \sqcup \text{TimeSeries}$$

The concepts EventOccurence and EpisodeOccurence had to be introduced in order to reflect the combinatorial restrictions (see [6], p.12 - 13) of the Time Standards mentioned above.

$$\text{TemporalReference} \sqsubseteq \forall \, \text{refersTo: } \, \text{Situation} \sqcup \text{<concept>})$$
$$\text{TimePoint} \sqsubseteq \text{TemporalReference} \sqcap \forall \, \text{refersToSituation:}$$
$$(\text{Event} \sqcup \text{<concept>})$$
$$\text{TimeInterval} \sqsubseteq \text{TemporalReference}$$
$$\text{TimeSerie} \sqsubseteq \text{TemporalReference}$$
$$\text{Duration} \sqsubseteq \text{TemporalReference}$$
$$\text{Frequency} \sqsubseteq \text{TemporalReference}$$
$$\text{Rate} \sqsubseteq \text{TemporalReference}$$
$$\text{Frequency} \,][\, \text{Rate} \,][\, \text{TimePoint}][\, \text{TimeSerie} \,][\, \text{Duration} \,][\, \text{TimeInterval}$$
$$\text{ComplexTempLink} \sqsubseteq \exists \, \text{Label: <primitive>} \sqcap \exists \, \text{symbol: <primitive>}$$
$$\sqcap \forall \, \text{refersDateDescription: DateDescription}$$

4 Applying the generic time-related concepts

4.1 Representing temporal patterns

The above framework is applied to the representation of temporal patterns occurring in the DSM–IV items. Concepts describing such time patterns have to be explicitly defined as specializations of the generic time related concept (this enables the satisfiability checker to detect a lack of conformance to the TS). The following example gives a synopsis of a time reference within a DSM–IV item, the corresponding standard predication conform to the TS and the formal representation which specializes the generic concepts:

Example. 'Clinically significant loss of ... skills before age 10 years' (299.10, Childhood Disintegrative Disorder, Item B).

Coded as a Time Standard predication this would read:

```
EVENT('clinically significant loss of skills')
(hasOccurence BEFORE TP('Age of Patient is 10 years')))
```

The conceptual description is:

```
Event ⊓ ∀ characterizedBy: <'clinicallySignificantLossOfSkills'>
    ⊓ ∀ hasOccurence: [EventOccurence ⊓∀before:
    (TimePoint ⊓ ∀definedBy:<'AgeOfPatientIs10Years'>)]
```

4.2 Inference

As mentioned above the major aim of the Time Standards is to make time-related aspects explicit. The description logic approach is meant to clarify semantic aspects of the TS Standard Predication. Even here the focus is on an explicit representation of temporal relations. Temporal reasoning, e.g. temporal abstraction, is not the major concern of our approach. Our medical partners are interested in nosology, i.e. in the description and definition of disorders or diseases, their naming and classification. What can be done is a classification of temporal patterns, which takes into consideration the classification of non-temporal facts defining a situation.

To give a very simple (but nevertheless realistic) example:
The DSM–IV defines the 'Substance induced Mood Disorder', which has a defining temporal pattern: '... syndrome ... developed within a month of Substance Intoxication or Withdrawal'. The subsumption algorithm allows to infer that the temporal pattern 'Syndrome developed within a month of Alcohol Intoxication or Withdrawal' is a specialization of the first, given the taxonomic knowledge that alcohol is a substance. As a consequence the subsumption relation between 'Substance-induced Mood Disorder' and 'Alcohol-induced Mood Disorder' (both being part of the DSM-IV classification) is confirmed. However, if we allow general concept inclusions (as it has been done before e.g. in the GRAIL language of GALEN), it is possible to represent abstract temporal axioms leading to temporal inferences via subsumption. General concept inclusion are terminological assertions of the form $C \sqsubseteq D$, where both C and D are non-atomic. A temporal axiom stating that a time pattern referring to an event occurrence after a time interval, which contains a certain type of a time point (it has to be noted that no concrete time point or time stamp can be referenced in the TBox), implies that the time pattern refers to an event occurrence, that takes place after this type of a time point, can be represented as:

```
EventOccurence⊓ (∀ after:(TimeInterval⊓
(∀ refersTo:(Episode⊓ ∀ hasOccurence:
( EpisodeOccurence⊓∀ after: (TimePoint⊓refersTo: <fact1>)))))
⊑ EventOccurence⊓∀ after: (TimePoint⊓refersTo: <fact1>)
```

The abstract classification of time patterns becomes useful in the case of the more complex, nested time references of Schizophrenia and several Mood Disorders and supports the nosological investigation of the diagnostic items of the DSM–IV. It is the fact that time-independent facts and time patterns are both represented as concepts, which allows the use of a uniform inference mechanism combining temporal and time-independent aspects. We consider this a strength of the approach.

4.3 Characteristics of the approach

Obviously the definitions of the generic concepts for time-related aspects contain cycles, because a temporal reference, used to define a situation, may refer to other situations. This reflects the possibility to formulate nested standard predications in the Time Standards. It is feasible to define a formal semantics for non cycle-free terminologies (see the seminal paper of Nebel [10]) and to check subsumption ([3], [7]). Cycles increase the complexity of reasoning (EXPTIME-complete vs. PSPACE-complete in the case of $\mathcal{ALC}$). Nevertheless: cycles do not appear in DSM–IV concept definitions of temporal patterns except for these abstract generic concepts. If satisfiability constraints with respect to the generic concepts are respected by concepts defining more special time patterns - which is supported by the acquisition environment - the cyclic expansion of the latter could be pruned during subsumption checking between the more special time patterns.

The concept language used is $\mathcal{ALC}$ and reasoning is reduced to subsumption checking via testing satisfiability of the terminological assertions, which can be decided by a sound and complete calculus (see e.g. [3]). As mentioned above subsumption checking is at least PSPACE-complete. Therefore the assistance system will present the contents of the DSM-IV on the basis of a concept subsumption lattice, which has been previously inferred.

5 Discussion

Clearly our approach answers to an application problem. The aim has neither been the theoretical investigation of description logics - which has been done extensively by other researchers -, nor to present a new approach to temporal reasoning.

Our leading question was how to find a representation of temporal aspects of nosological knowledge, which 1) is semantically clear and satisfies a certain degree of formal rigor 2) nevertheless meets the requirements of European standardization playing an important role in medical informatics 3) supports taxonomic inferences. Furthermore it has been our effort to acquire a comprehensive knowledge base, which covers a corpus of medical knowledge of high relevance in praxi. Nevertheless the approach should be compared with existing conceptualizations of time-related knowledge:

Situation Calculus represents time in a first order logic (eventually a sorted logic) by additional temporal arguments of predicates. Example: 'isClinicallySignificant(LossOfSkills, PatientA, 11 March)' may be interpreted as: 'PatientA suffers from a significant loss of skills at 11th of March'. An important shortcoming is, that is not possible to express generalities of temporal relations.

Modal temporal logics try to partly shift the representation of temporal aspects to the formal semantics of first order formulas. The common Kribke-style possible world semantics of modal logics is modified. In a modal temporal logic, different times correspond to different possible worlds. Modal Operators are introduced, which qualify the truth of a given formula with respect to times (possible worlds) Example: (P isClinicallySignificant(LossOfSkill, PatientA) signifies, that there is a past world, in which the formula 'isClinicallySignificant(...)' is true.

Reification as an approach to the representation fo temporal aspects introduces so-called temporal occurrence predicates (HOLDS, OCCURS) and the sort of temporal element (e.g. points in time, intervals). The central aspect is, that propositions of a first order language such as *isClinicallySignificant(LossOfSkill, PatientA)* become *names* of the second sort of elements. *OCCURS(isClinicallySignificant(LossOfSkill, PatientA), 11 March)* may be interpreted as follows: the fact (treated as a single entity), that Patient A suffers form a loss of skills occurs at 11th of March.

Some of the most influential approaches to temporal logics in AI, namely the works of Allen [1], McDermott [9], Kowalski and Sergot [8], can be subsumed under the category of reified temporal logics. Reification may be understand as a trick to achieve higher-order expressiveness while staying at a first-order representation. The cost to pay is a somehow unclear semantics, with respect to the reified proposition. Shoam [14] proposed a solution to the interpretation problem, but his approach was criticized for its lack of proof theory and for not being fully reified.

Token reification provides a conceptualization of temporal knowledge, which avoids these semantic difficulties. (Vila and Reichgelt [16]) use a sorted first-order logic with the sorts of individuals, times, state and event tokens. An expression as *isClinicallySignificant(LossOfSkill, PatientA, 11 march)* is not taken as a predicate expression, but as a function expression which returns an event token e. The fact that Patient A suffers form a loss of skills occurs at 11th of March, can now be represented as *OCCURS(isClinicallySignificant(LossOfSkill, PatA, 11 march))*. In contrast to simple reification this approach allows to quantify over the arguments of the functions as far as over event or state tokens leading to the possibility of representing general temporal relation and temporal axioms.

Conclusion. In contrast to these approaches the proposed representation of temporal patterns does not refer to concrete dates or time stamps. Reasoning based on the comparison of time stamps is not within the scope of our approach, which treats time patterns as concept descriptions, in order to make temporal relations explicit. The approach present representational means, which automatically lead to the conformance with the CEN Time Standards. It is straight forward to generate TS standard predications from terminological assertion. Reasoning is reduced to subsumption checking in order to infer taxonomic relations between time patterns. Nevertheless it is possible to represent temporal axioms and to express temporal generalities, as it is possible in the token reification approach.

6 Appendix: BNF description of the CEN-TS Standard Predications

⟨standard predication⟩ ::= (⟨propositional clause⟩⟨temporal references⟩)
⟨propositional clause⟩ ::= ⟨clause label⟩(⟨string⟩)
⟨clause label⟩ ::= SIT| EVENT | EPISODE
⟨temporal references⟩ ::= {⟨temporal reference⟩}*
⟨temporal reference⟩ ::= ⟨temp link⟩[temp-comparator]⟨temp-expression⟩
⟨temporal link⟩ ::= ⟨basic temporal link⟩ | ⟨complex temporal link⟩
⟨basic temporal link⟩ ::= has_duration | has_occurence | has_frequency | has_rate
⟨complex temporal link⟩ ::= ⟨ctl-lable⟩ ⟨symbol⟩
⟨ctl-lable⟩ ::= HO_ | HD_ | HR_ | HF_
⟨temp-comparator⟩ ::= AFTER | AT | BEFORE | DURING | UNTIL | UP-TO | CO-STARTS | CO-ENDS | CO-PRECEDES | CO-CONTINUES | FOLLOWS | SINCE | INCLUDES
⟨temp-expression⟩ ::= ⟨time point expression⟩ | (time intervall expression⟩ | ⟨duration expression⟩ | (frequency expression⟩ | ⟨rate expression⟩ | ⟨time series expression⟩
⟨time point expression⟩ ::= TP(⟨time-ref-descriptor⟩)
⟨time interval expression⟩ ::= TI(⟨time-ref-descriptor⟩)
⟨time series expression⟩ ::= TS(⟨time-ref-descriptor⟩)
⟨duration expression⟩ ::= DR(⟨time-ref-descriptor⟩)
⟨frequency expression⟩ ::= FQ(⟨time-ref-descriptor⟩)
⟨rate expression⟩ ::= RT(⟨time-ref-descriptor⟩)
⟨time-ref-descriptor⟩ ::= ⟨string⟩ | ⟨standard predication⟩

References

1. Allen, J.F.: Towards a general theory of action and time. Artif. Intell. **23** (1984) 123-154.
2. American Psychiatric Association: Diagnostic and Statistic Manual of Mental Disorders, Fourth Edition. American Psychiatric Association, Washington D.C., (1994).
3. Baader, F., Bürckert, H.-J., Hollunder, B., Nutt, W., Siekmann, J.H.: Concept logics. In: Lloyd, J.W. (ed.): Computational Logics, Symposium Proceedings. Springer, Berlin (1990) 177-201.

4. Baader, F., Buchheit, M., Hollunder, B.: Cardinality restrictions on concepts. Artif. Intell. **88** (1996) 195-213.

5. Brachmann, R.J., McGuinness, D.L., Patel-Schneider, P.F., Resnick, L.A., Borgida, A.: Living with Classic: when and how to use a KL-ONE-like language. In Sowa, J.F. (ed.): Principles of Semantic Networks: Exploration in the Representation of Knowledge. Morgan Kaufmann, San Mateo CA (1991) 401-456.

6. Ceusters, W. et. al.: Time Standards for Health Care Specific Problems. European Commitee for Standardization, Technical Comitee 251, Project Team PT2-017, September 1995.

7. De Giacomo, G., Lenzerini, M.: A Uniform Framework for Concept Definitions in Description Logics. Journal of Artificial Intelligence Research **6** (1997) 87-110.

8. Kowalski, R., Sergot, M.: A logic-based calculus of events. New Generation Comput. **4** (1987) 67-96.

9. McDermott, D.: A temporal logic for reasoning about processes and plans. Cognitive Sci. **6** (1982) 101-155.

10. Nebel, B.: Terminological cycles: Semantics and computational properties. In Sowa, J.F. (ed.): Principles of Semantic Networks: Exploration in the Representation of Knowledge. Morgan Kaufmann, San Mateo CA (1991) 331-361.

11. Rector, A.L., Bechhofer, S., Goble, C.A., Horrocks, I., Nowlan, W.A., Solomon, W.D.: The GRAIL concept modeling language for medical terminology. Artificial Intelligence in Medicine **9** (1997) 139-171.

12. Saß, H., Wittchen, H.-U., Zaudig, M.: Diagnostisches und Statistisches Manual Psychischer Störungen DSM-IV.Hogrefe, Göttingen (1996).

13. Sattler, U.: A Concept Language Extended with Different Kinds of Transitive Roles. In: Proc of KI-96. Springer. Berlin , Heidelberg New York (1996) 333-345.

14. Shoam, Y.: Temporal Logics in AI: Semantical and Ontological Considerations. Artif. Intell. **33** (1987) 89-104.

15. Vila, L.: A Survey on Temporal Reasoning in Artificial Intelligence. AICOM **7**(1) (1994) 4-28.

16. Vila, L., Reichgelt, H.: The token reification approach to temporal reasoning. Artif. Intell.**83** (1996) 59-74.

Part-Whole Reasoning in Medical Knowledge Bases Using Description Logics

Stefan Schulz[a,b], Martin Romacker[a,b] & Udo Hahn[a]

[a]Linguistische Informatik / Computerlinguistik
Universität Freiburg, Werthmannplatz 1, D-79085 Freiburg
[b]Abteilung Medizinische Informatik
Universitätsklinikum Freiburg, Stefan-Meier-Str. 26, D-79104 Freiburg
http://www.coling.uni-freiburg.de/

Abstract. The development of powerful, ubiquitous and comprehensive medical ontologies that support formal reasoning on a large scale is one of the key requirements for clinical computing. Taxonomic medical knowledge, a major portion of these ontologies, is fundamentally characterized by is-a and part-whole relationships between concepts. While reasoning in generalization hierarchies is a well-understood process, no fully conclusive mechanism yet exists for part-whole reasoning. We here propose a new representation construct for part-whole relations based on the formal framework of description logics, i.e. the well-known concept language $\mathcal{ALC}$, and show how part-whole reasoning can naturally be emulated via classification-based reasoning without extending the expressiveness of the underlying terminological system.

1 Introduction

In medical informatics research, knowledge representation issues have been emphasized in recent years. It is obvious that efficient classification, processing of structured data and free texts, as well as a broad variety of sophisticated information retrieval services (e.g., fact retrieval, text passage retrieval) and knowledge-based decision support require a common conceptual framework to facilitate semantic interoperability [6, 7].

Concept systems routinely used in medicine and health care are essentially classification systems which have a fixed set of alphanumeric codes for statistical analysis and accounting (e.g., ICD [23]), or thesauri for bibliographies, indexing and retrieval (e.g., MeSH [14]). While ICD has become a world wide standard, many coding systems used in clinical routine are restricted in their scope to national health systems or clinical specialities. Semantic interoperability between these systems is generally not achieved.

Also, ICD and MeSH, as well as more sophisticated composite conceptual systems, such as the SNOMED nomenclature [5], lack a clear semantics as hierarchical links remain untyped. Especially noteworthy is the frequent mixture of generalization (IS-A) and partitive (PART-OF) relations that often occur at the

Syntax	Semantics
C	$\{d \in \Delta^{\mathcal{I}} \mid \mathcal{I}(C) = d\}$
$C \sqcap D$	$C^{\mathcal{I}} \cap D^{\mathcal{I}}$
$C \sqcup D$	$C^{\mathcal{I}} \cup D^{\mathcal{I}}$
$\neg C$	$\Delta^{\mathcal{I}} \setminus C^{\mathcal{I}}$
R	$\{(d,e) \in \Delta^{\mathcal{I}} \times \Delta^{\mathcal{I}} \mid \mathcal{I}(R) = (d,e)\}$
$\forall R.C$	$\{d \in \Delta^{\mathcal{I}} \mid R^{\mathcal{I}}(d) \subseteq C^{\mathcal{I}}\}$
$\exists R.C$	$\{d \in \Delta^{\mathcal{I}} \mid R^{\mathcal{I}}(d) \cap C^{\mathcal{I}} \neq \emptyset\}$

Table 1. Syntax and Semantics for the Language $\mathcal{ALC}$

same hierarchical level. For instance, "blood" subsumes "blood plasma" (partitive) as well as "fetal blood" (generalization) [5]. Conceptually invalid combinations (e.g., "fracture of the blood") are not rejected, and often the same concept can be arbitrarily classified by various code combinations not linked with each other.

An attempt to unify 53 conceptual systems (with a total of 476,313 concepts) is constituted by the UMLS (Unified Medical Language System) project [15, 13]. The designers of UMLS are fully aware of the problems encountered in the existing terminologies, and, although they make considerable efforts to add semantics to concepts and links, UMLS is still far from being a logically sound ontology of medicine. The inconsistencies inherited from the various sources, also concerning part-whole relationships, are crucial and create continuous problems for UMLS.

The Common Reference Model for medical terminology, developed within the GALEN and GALEN-IN-USE projects [16,17] marks, for the time being, the only major attempt to construct a large-scale medical ontology in a strict, i.e., formally founded way. In this context, GRAIL, a KL-ONE-like knowledge representation language, has been developed and, by design, specifically adapted to the requirements of the medical domain [18]. Interestingly enough, GRAIL, unlike most description logics, has been provided with a built-in mechanism which is in particular suitable for part-whole reasoning, according to the outstanding importance of this reasoning pattern in the medical domain.

In our research, the necessity to account for medical knowledge in a principled way arose from the need to make deductive reasoning capabilities available to MEDSYNDIKATE, a natural language text understanding system that processes pathology reports [9,8]. Since MEDSYNDIKATE had been ported from an information technology (IT) report understanding application, the architecture was to be kept as stable as possible. MEDSYNDIKATE makes use of a standard KL-ONE-style terminological representation language (LOOM) [12]. Although the expressiveness of LOOM extends that of the concept language $\mathcal{ALC}$ [20], we will only refer to the latter since its expressiveness is sufficient for our knowledge engineering approach. Note that LOOM does not support the definition of transitive roles [25]. Syntax and semantics of $\mathcal{ALC}$ are given in Table 1.

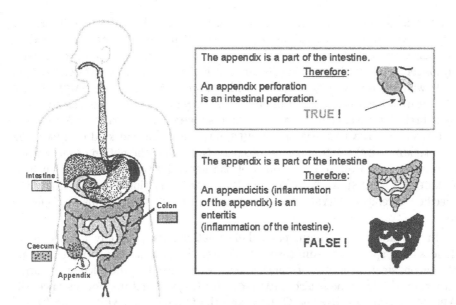

Fig. 1. Digestive Tract and its Parts. Left: Position of the Appendix within a Part-Whole Hierarchy. Right: Disease Concepts related to *Appendix* and to *Intestine*, with and without Part-Whole Specialization along the Part-Whole Hierarchy

In particular, the concept language $\mathcal{ALC}$ provides reasoning about generalization hierarchies but it does not provide special support for part-whole reasoning. Due to the importance of part-whole reasoning in the medical domain, we faced the challenge of accounting for this relevant portion of medical knowledge in a systematic way. One possible solution might have been to introduce particular transitivity operators in order to take account of part-whole reasoning. Suche mechanisms have been proposed by Baader [2] and Sattler [19]. We refrain from such a solution, since we want to preserve the description logics as simple as possible in order to employ off-the-shelves knowledge representation systems (such as LOOM). Second, and more important, it can be shown that transitivity in part-whole reasoning is invalid, in general. Accordingly, we have stepped back and use the terminological classifier for part-whole reasoning in the same way as for taxonomic reasoning along IS-A hierarchies. The solution we arrived at is general in the sense that given a simple encoding schema for meronymic knowledge, versatile part-whole reasoning is made possible, with transitivity switched on and off depending on knowledge engineering needs.

2   The Part-Whole Reasoning Problem

Part-whole (also called meronymic) reasoning has two aspects: *transitivity* and *specialization*.

Transitivity. The transitivity of part-whole reasoning has largely been discussed in the literature, cf. the overview in [1]. Winston et al. [24] argue that part-whole relations can be considered transitive as long as "a single sense of part" is kept. This means that the general PART-OF relation[1] is not transitive, whereas each distinct subrelation of PART-OF is transitive. As soon as more than one single-sense PART-OF subrelation is involved in a relation chain, transitivity no longer holds, in general. For instance, a FINGER is a PHYSICAL-PART-OF an ARM which is a PHYSICAL-PART-OF a MUSICIAN; a MUSICIAN is a MEMBER-OF an ORCHESTRA. Because FINGER and MUSICIAN are related by the same PART-OF subrelation we conclude that a FINGER is a PHYSICAL-PART-OF a MUSICIAN, whereas it is not a PART-OF an ORCHESTRA, since a second kind of a PART-OF (viz. MEMBER-OF) relation comes into play. Note, that the notion of *meronymic* relations refer to all specializations of the general PART-OF relation, such as MEMBER-OF, PHYSICAL-PART-OF etc. By *partitive* relations, however, only the specific subrelation PHYSICAL-PART-OF and all of its subrelations are referred to.

In the anatomy domain, part-whole relations are generally applied to 3-dimensional spaces or 2-dimensional surfaces. If an anatomical object is part of the physical structure of another one, which itself is included in a larger structure, the first one is also a PART-OF this larger structure. For instance, the APPENDIX is a PART-OF the COLON, and the COLON is a PART-OF the INTESTINE. Hence, the APPENDIX is also a PART-OF the INTESTINE (cf. Fig. 1, left side).[2] So, we assume that transitivity generally holds for the PART-OF relation, applied to anatomical objects. We are nevertheless aware of the fact that for certain subrelations of the anatomical PART-OF relation the transitivity assumption is questionable or may even be rejected.

Part-whole specialization. Besides transitivity, so-called *specialization* is the other important issue related to part-whole hierarchies. It is also known as "coordination of multiple taxonomies based on relations other than subsumption" [11]. Incorporating the definition of relations which are inheritable along other domain-specific relations at the level of conceptual modeling constitutes a major desideratum for properly designed medical knowledge bases. Specialization means that from a relation $\mathbf{R}$ specialized by a relation $\mathbf{S}$ it can be deduced that for any objects x, y and z $x\mathbf{R}y \wedge y\mathbf{S}z \Rightarrow x\mathbf{R}z$ holds. This kind of inference must not necessarily include a partitive relation (cf. [4]), but in our domain it occurs generally as a form of inheritance of roles along part-whole taxonomies [1]. For better understanding we will use the term *part-whole specialization* henceforth.

---

[1] We use SMALLCAPS to denote concept and relation identifiers.

[2] As the following example refers to details of the human anatomy, we will introduce some basic concepts for ease of understanding: The *digestive tract* is a part of the human body and constitutes a sequence of tubular organs, one of which is the *intestine*. The *intestine* is divided into the *small intestine* and the *colon*. The *colon* is divided into the *caecum*, the *ascending colon* and some other segments. The *caecum* (localized in the right lower part of the abdomen), has a worm-shaped, dead-ending tubular part called *appendix*. An acute inflammation of this part is generally known as *appendicitis*. The radial division of the digestive tract exhibits an ordered sequence of discrete layers. The innermost layer is called the *digestive mucosa*.

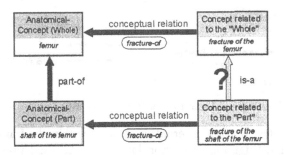

Fig. 2. Inheritance along PART-OF Relations, also called Part-Whole Specialization

Part-whole specialization is furthermore used to compute subsumption relations (IS-A) [16]. As illustrated by Fig. 2, a concept related to a "part" is subsumed by another concept related by the same conceptual relationship to the corresponding "whole". In a medical concept system, e.g., we want to infer that a concept such as FRACTURE-OF-THE-SHAFT-OF-THE-FEMUR is subsumed by a concept FRACTURE-OF-THE-FEMUR given that SHAFT-OF-THE-FEMUR is a PART-OF the FEMUR [11].

Since standard description logics as those implemented within the KL-ONE language family, do not support inheritance other than along taxonomic generalization hierarchies, it is no wonder that due to the importance of part-whole reasoning in medicine, special concept representation languages such as GRAIL [18] have been developed. Here, part-whole specialization is modeled as a property of certain conceptual relations, in the form **R** *specializedBy* **S**, where **S** ⊑ PART-OF. This means that the relation **R** is *always* inherited along hierarchies based on **S**, i.e. the inheritance mechanism is invariably associated with the relation **S**.

However, as a result of our experience with the construction of a pathology knowledge base and based on shared medical expertise we state that

1. Part-whole specialization does *not generally* hold: A PERFORATION-OF the APPENDIX can be classified as an INTESTINAL-PERFORATION, whereas APPENDICITIS (INFLAMMATION-OF the APPENDIX) is certainly not an ENTERITIS (INFLAMMATION-OF the INTESTINE), cf. Fig. 1, right side.
2. The *same* relation (here: INFLAMMATION-OF) may support part-whole specialization in one case, though not in the other: In contradistinction to the fact that APPENDICITIS is not an ENTERITIS, the same relation INFLAMMATION-OF, applied to another organ, e.g. the KIDNEY, exhibits a different behavior: PYELONEPHRITIS, an INFLAMMATION-OF the PYELON (a part of the kidney) can be subsumed consistently by NEPHRITIS (INFLAMMATION-OF the KIDNEY).

We claim that in a medical ontology all phenomena typical of part-whole hierarchies should be represented adequately. As we have shown, neither established large-scale terminologies, nor dedicated medical knowledge representation languages such as GRAIL (cf. the KIDNEY example) achieve this goal.

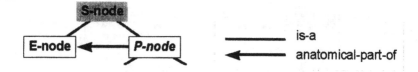

Fig. 3. Basic Construct of Part-Whole Hierarchies

Therefore, we developed an alternative solution within the framework of the terminological knowledge representation language $\mathcal{ALC}$, and present a formal model that accounts for the phenomena described. It incorporates both previous work on description logics [21] and large-scale medical coding systems [22].

3 Terminological Part-Whole Reasoning - An Alternative

Part-Whole Hierarchies and SEP Triplets. In contradistinction to language extensions providing dedicated operators for the definition of transitive roles [2, 19], we present a knowledge engineering methodology for reasoning along transitive part-whole relations that can be achieved using plain $\mathcal{ALC}$. We use the generalization hierarchy to emulate useful inferences that are typical of transitive relations and show, moreover, how the same formalism allows conditioned part-whole specialization.

In our domain model, the relation ANATOMICAL-PART-OF describes the partitive relation between physical parts of an organism and is embedded in a specific triplet structure by which anatomical concepts are modeled (cf. Fig. 3).

A triplet consists, first of all, of a composite "structure" concept, the so-called **S-node** (e.g. INTESTINE-STRUCTURE). The S-node subsumes pairs of concept siblings, namely the **E-nodes** and the **P-nodes**, that are conceptually related by the relation ANATOMICAL-PART-OF. The E-node denotes the *whole* anatomical entity to be modeled (e.g. INTESTINE), whereas the P-node stands for any *part* of the corresponding E-node. As an example, Fig. 4 illustrates the model of a segment of the gastro-intestinal anatomy subdomain. Note that the formalism supports the definition of concepts as conjunctions of more than one P-node concept, as illustrated by the concept CAECUM-EPITHELIUM.

Let C and D be E-nodes (e.g., the organs CAECUM and APPENDIX), and *AStruct* be the top-level concept of a domain subgraph (e.g., ORGANISM-STRUCTURE). *CStruct* and *DStruct* are the S-nodes that subsume C and D, respectively, just as *CPart* and *DPart* are the P-nodes related to C and D, respectively, via the role ANATOMICAL-PART-OF. All these concepts are embedded in a generalization hierarchy:

$$D \sqsubseteq DStruct \sqsubseteq CPart \sqsubseteq CStruct \sqsubseteq .. \sqsubseteq APart \sqsubseteq AStruct \qquad (1)$$

$$C \sqsubseteq CStruct \sqsubseteq .. \sqsubseteq APart \sqsubseteq AStruct \qquad (2)$$

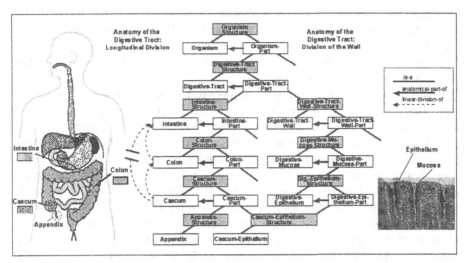

Fig. 4. Segment of the Part-Whole Taxonomy of the Gastrointestinal Tract, using Triplets. Left: Longitudinal Division, Right: Radial Division

The P-node is defined as follows:

$$CPart \doteq CStruct \sqcap \exists\text{ANATOMICAL-PART-OF}.C \qquad (3)$$

Since D is subsumed by $CPart$ (1) we infer that D is an ANATOMICAL-PART-OF the organ C :

$$D \sqsubseteq \exists\text{ANATOMICAL-PART-OF}.C \qquad (4)$$

It is obvious that this pattern of *part-of inheritance* holds at any level of the part-whole hierarchy. In our example (cf. Fig. 4), formula (1) may be illustrated by identifying the concept D with APPENDIX that is a subconcept of APPENDIX-STRUCTURE, CAECUM-PART, CAECUM-STRUCTURE etc. up to ORGANISM-PART and ORGANISM-STRUCTURE in ascending order. In the same way, C is identified with CAECUM which is a subconcept of CAECUM-STRUCTURE, etc. (2). Between CAECUM-PART and CAECUM, there exists an ANATOMICAL-PART-OF relation (3). Consequently, it can be concluded that a relation of the type ANATOMICAL-PART-OF holds between APPENDIX and CAECUM (4), but also between AP-PENDIX and COLON, APPENDIX and INTESTINE, COLON and INTESTINE, etc.

Analyzing the ontological structure of the medical domain reveals an interesting observation. A number of specializations of the ANATOMICAL-PART-OF are not transitive although transitivity seems to hold for the general ANATOMICAL-PART-OF relation. Thus, defining transitivity as a role property would lead to an inappropriate inheritance of this property to all subrelations. The *part-of inheritance* mechanism is able to cope with this phenomenon. This additional feature is shown by the dotted arrows in Fig. 4. *Part-of inheritance* can be selectively obviated in case of certain subrelations of ANATOMICAL-PART-OF, such as LINEAR-DIVISION-OF: COLON can be described as a LINEAR-DIVISION-OF INTES-TINE, CAECUM as a LINEAR-DIVISION-OF COLON, but CAECUM can definitely not be described as a LINEAR-DIVISION-OF INTESTINE (cf. Fig. 1, left side).

Thus, we provide an easily applicable ontology engineering methodology which incorporates part-whole reasoning by introducing a single "proto node" (*viz.* S-node) as a means to introduce reasoning about partonomies simply into Is-A taxonomies, producing similar results as those obtained by an extension of the language with transitive roles.

Coordination of taxonomies (part-whole specialization). Part-whole specialization is a more generalized part-of inheritance that includes relations other than PART-OF, using the same triplet structures made of E-node, P-node and S-node. Whenever a disease concept is related to an anatomical concept, the knowledge engineer must explicitly determine whether it includes part-whole specialization or not (see the FEMUR example from Fig. 2). Part-whole specialization is inferred when a disease concept is linked to an S-node. In order to prevent part-whole specialization it has to be connected to an E-node.

An example is shown in Fig. 5 (top, right side). The concept INTESTINAL-PERFORATION - meant as the perforation of any part of the INTESTINE - is linked via the PERFORATION-OF relation to INTESTINE-STRUCTURE - an S-Node. This way, PERFORATION-OF-APPENDIX, PERFORATION-OF-CAECUM and PERFORATION-OF-COLON are all classified as INTESTINAL-PERFORATION.

Applied to the same anatomical concepts (Fig. 5: top, left side) the concept ENTERITIS (an INFLAMMATION-OF the whole INTESTINE) is linked via the INFLAMMATION-OF relation to an E-node. Thus, an APPENDICITIS as an INFLAMMATION-OF the APPENDIX is *not* classified as being subsumed by ENTERITIS. This corresponds to the usage of these terms and, consequently, the meaning of the concepts in clinical practice.

We consider the same taxonomy as described in the terminological statements (1) to (4). Let R and S be relations that link the PATHOLOGICAL-PHENOMENON concept to the anatomical hierarchy, and W, X, Y, Z concepts that stand for a PATHOLOGICAL-PHENOMENON. From

$$W \doteq \exists S.CStruct \tag{5}$$
$$X \doteq \exists S.DStruct \tag{6}$$
$$DStruct \sqsubseteq CStruct \tag{7}$$

we conclude that

$$X \sqsubseteq W \tag{8}$$

This "S-node pattern" allows part-whole specialization, whereas the following "E-node pattern" does not:

$$Y \doteq \exists R.C \tag{9}$$
$$Z \doteq \exists R.D \tag{10}$$

The conclusion

$$Z \sqsubseteq Y \tag{11}$$

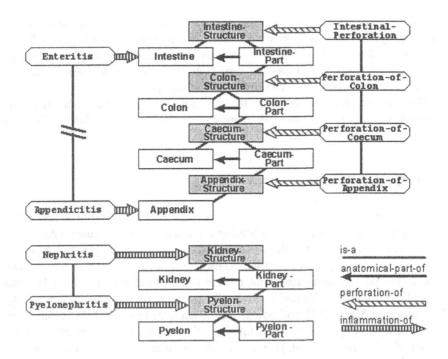

Fig. 5. Conditioned Part-Whole Specialization in a Part-Whole Hierarchy. Top, Left Side: "E-node Pattern" – Disabled Part-Whole Specialization (applied to the role inflammation-of, in the digestive tract subdomain) Top, Right Side: "S-node Pattern" – Enabled Part-Whole Specialization (applied to the role perforation-of, in the same subdomain), Bottom: "S-node Pattern" – Enabled Part-Whole Specialization (the same role inflammation-of, applied to the kidney subdomain)

cannot be drawn, since the extension of D is not a subset of the extension of C.

In our example, (5) and (6) can be interpreted as follows:
The INTESTINAL-PERFORATION is a PERFORATION-OF an INTESTINE-STRUCTURE and the PERFORATION-OF-APPENDIX is a PERFORATION-OF an APPENDIX-STRUCTURE. Since APPENDIX-STRUCTURE is subsumed by INTESTINE-STRUCTURE (7) it follows that a PERFORATION-OF-APPENDIX is an INTESTINAL-PERFORATION (8) (S-node pattern).

The concept ENTERITIS, however, is not linked to the S-Node INTESTINE-STRUCTURE by the role INFLAMMATION-OF, but to the E-node INTESTINE instead (9), just as APPENDICITIS is linked to the E-node APPENDIX (10). As INTESTINE does not subsume APPENDIX, no subsumption relation between APPENDICITIS ($= Z$) and ENTERITIS ($= Y$) can be inferred. (11) (E-node pattern).

It is therefore only the difference in the modeling patterns (linkage to S-node vs. E-node) that liberates or obviates part-whole specialization, since there is no difference in the type of the relations R and S. Thus, the use of the same relation in both patterns is possible as required by the structure of domain knowledge.

This is the case with the relation INFLAMMATION-OF, comparing its use in two subgraphs, illustrated by Fig. 5. Here, the S-node pattern (formula 5 – 8) is applied to the KIDNEY subgraph, in order to define the concepts NEPHRITIS and PYELONEPHRITIS, whereas the definition of ENTERITIS and APPENDICITIS obeys the E-node pattern in the INTESTINE subgraph.

This example shows clearly how the same relation (here: INFLAMMATION-OF) supports part-whole specialization in one case (here: KIDNEY), while in the other it does not (here: INTESTINE).

4 Related Work

For the medical domain, Haimowitz, Patil and Szolovits [10] first raised the claim for the necessity of a representation formalism for *part-whole* relations and corresponding reasoning capabilities as an extension to terminological logics, motivated by the ontological structure of medical domain knowledge. Baader [2] and Sattler [19] discuss such extensions, i.e. the transitive closure of role definitions as needed for part-whole, and their implications on computational complexity. Schmolze and Marks [21] worked out a solution similar to ours using subsumption in order to obtain inferences similar to that of transitive roles or transitive closure of roles. Artale et al. [1] criticize the "proliferation of concepts" in their approach. We argue, however, that many of these additional concepts are by no means "artificial". On the contrary, we even claim that they are necessary, as the distinct mechanisms for conditioned specialization modeling show (cf. Fig. 5). Our model, however, implies to trade off the number of "proto nodes" (the S-nodes for the structures) and the additional complexity due to the internal structure of the triplets against other forms of complexity, e.g., the supply of special-purpose, ie., *part-whole*-specific reasoning procedures. The latter is the case in the GRAIL formalism underlying the GALEN [18] project. This framework constitutes the most far-reaching approach to serve the needs of *part-whole* reasoning, and to incorporate the specialization feature into a medical ontology.

5 Conclusion

We sketched a general representation construct for *part-whole* modeling in the medical domain that is fully embedded in the framework of a parsimonous variant of description logics, using only the constructs of $\mathcal{ALC}$. This allows us to use the built-in terminological classifier for emulating reasoning across *part-whole* hierarchies. Emphasis was laid on the simulation of transitivity and the construction of part-whole specialization. In contrast to approaches that extend description logics by transitive roles, we do not consider transitivity an inheritable property of the ANATOMICAL-PART-OF relation. This way, a serious limitation of the GALEN method is overcome, *viz.* that part-whole specialization is invariably linked to a conceptual relation [3]. This is due to the fact that we realize conditioning (i.e., enabling and disabling) of specialization by modifying the range of the respective conceptual role: if the type of its range is an S-node, specialization is enabled, if it is an E-node, specialization is "switched off". Again, the specialization property is not contained in the conceptual relation itself, but in the structure of the ontology.

In a strict sense, our model does not implement transitivity, but it emulates inferences typical of transitive part-whole reasoning through the taxonomy itself. This approach proved to be completely sufficient for our purposes and seems to generalize to other domains. Consider a simple commonsense scenario like the following. The car-body is clearly a part of the car. From the car-body's color we may infer the color of the car. So are the seats part of a car. The color of the car, however, would not be inferred from that of the seats.

Acknowledgements. We would like to thank our colleagues in the CLIF group and of the Department of Medical Informatics for fruitful discussions. Martin Romacker and Stefan Schulz are supported by a grant from DFG (Ha 2097/5-1).

References

1. A. Artale, E. Franconi, N. Guarino, and L. Pazzi. Part-whole relations in object-centered systems: an overview. *Data and Knowledge Engineering*, 20(3):347–383, 1996.
2. F. Baader. Augmenting concept languages by transitive closure of roles: An alternative to terminological cycles. In J. Mylopoulos and R. Reiter, editors, *IJCAI'91 - Proc. 12th Intl. Joint Conf. on Artificial Intelligence*, pages 446–451. San Mateo/CA: Morgan Kaufmann, 1991.
3. J. Bernauer. Analysis of part-whole relation and subsumption in the medical domain. *Data and Knowledge Engineering*, 20(3):405–415, 1996.
4. P. R. Cohen and C. L. Loiselle. Beyond ISA: structures for plausible inference in semantic networks. In J. Sowa, editor, *AAAI'88 - Proceedings of the 7th National Conference on Artificial Intelligence*, pages 415–420. San Mateo, CA: Morgan Kaufmann, 1988.
5. R. Cote. *SNOMED International.* Northfield, IL: College of American Pathologists, 1993.
6. D. A. Evans, J. J. Cimino, W. R. Hersh, S. M. Huff, and D. S. Bell. Toward a medical-concept representation language. *Journal of the American Medical Informatics Association*, 1(3):207–217, 1994.
7. C. Friedman, S. M. Huff, W. R. Hersh, E. Pattison-Gordon, and J. J. Cimino. The Canon group's effort. Working towards a merged model. *Journal of the American Medical Informatics Association*, 2(1):4–18, 1995.
8. U. Hahn and M. Romacker. Text structures in medical text processing: empirical evidence and a text understanding prototype. In R. Masys, editor, *Proc. of the 1997 AMIA Annual Fall Symposium*, pages 819–823. Philadelphia, PA: Henley & Belfus, 1997.
9. U. Hahn, K. Schnattinger, and M. Romacker. Automatic knowledge acquisition from medical texts. In *Proc. of the 1996 AMIA Annual Fall Symposium*, pages 383–387. Philadelphia, PA: Henley & Belfus, 1996.
10. I. J. Haimowitz, R. S. Patil, and P. Szolovits. Representing medical knowledge in a terminological language is difficult. In R.A. Greenes, editor, *SCAMC'88 - Proc. 12th Annual Symposium on Computer Applications in Medical Care*, pages 101–105. New York: IEEE Computer Soc. Pr., 1988.

11. I. Horrocks, A. Rector, and C. Goble. A description logic based schema for the classification of medical data. In F. Baader, M. Buchheit, M.A. Jeusfeld, and W. Nutt, editors, *KRDB'96 - Knowledge Representation Meets Databases. Proc. of the 3rd Workshop*, pages 24–28, 1996.

12. R. MacGregor. A description classifier for the predicate calculus. In *AAAI'94 - Proc. 12th National Conf. on Artificial Intelligence.*, pages 213–220. Menlo Park: AAAI Press/MIT Press, 1994.

13. A. T. McCray and A. Razi. The UMLS knowledge source server. In *MEDINFO'95 - Proc. of the 8th World Congress on Medical Informatics*, pages 144–147. Amsterdam: North-Holland, 1995.

14. NLM. *Medical Subject Headings*. Bethesda, MD: National Library of Medicine, 1997.

15. NLM. *Unified Medical Language System*. Bethesda, MD: National Library of Medicine, 1998.

16. A. Rector and I. R. Horrocks. Experience building a large, re-usable medical ontology using a description logic with transitivity and concept inclusions. In *AAAI Spring Symposium on Ontological Engineering*, 1997.

17. A. Rector, W. Solomon, W. Nowlan, and T. Rush. A terminology server for medical language and medical information systems. *Methods of Information in Medicine*, 34(2):147–157, 1995.

18. A. L. Rector, S. Bechhofer, C. A. Goble, I. Horrocks, W. A. Nowlan, and W. D. Solomon. The GRAIL concept modelling language for medical terminology. *Artificial Intelligence in Medicine*, 9:139–171, 1997.

19. U. Sattler. A concept language extended with different kinds of transitive roles. In G. Görz and S. Hölldobler, editors, *KI'98 - Proc. 20th Annual German Conference on Artificial Intelligence*, pages 333–345. Berlin: Springer, 1996.

20. M. Schmidt-Schauss and G. Smolka. Attributive concept descriptions with complements. *Artificial Intelligence*, 48(1):1–26, 1991.

21. J. G. Schmolze and W. S. Marks. The NIKL experience. *Computational Intelligence*, 6:48–69, 1991.

22. E. B. Schulz, C. Price, and P. J. B. Brown. Symbolic anatomic knowledge representation in the Read Codes Version 3: structure and application. *Journal of the American Medical Informatics Association*, 4(1):38–48, 1997.

23. WHO. *International Statistical Classification of Diseases and Health Related Problems. Tenth Revision*. Geneva: The World Health Organization, 1992.

24. M. Winston, R. Chaffin, and D. Herrmann. A taxonomy of part-whole relationships. *Cognitive Science*, 11:417–444, 1987.

25. W. Woods and J. Schmolze. The KL-ONE family. *Computers & Mathematics with Applications*, 23(2-5):133–177, 1992.

Part II

Selected German AI Research Projects

E. Sandner and Prof. Dr. S. Hölldobler, both from the AI Institute at the Technical University of Dresden, have undertaken the difficult task of soliciting AI project descriptions from the German AI community. A considerable (and representative) number of AI research groups responded. Our thanks go to E. Sandner and S. Hölldobler for the compilation of the material and to all of those who have contributed.

The project descriptions in section 1 are sorted by the name of the contact person. An alphabetical list of the contact persons can be found in section 2.

O. Herzog
A. Günter

1 Selected German AI Research Projects

Knowledge based image analysis
(http://www-sfb.informatik.uni-erlangen.de/Internal/D1/)
(SFB 182)

Partner: none	Supported by: DFG
Active: 01/1996 – 01/1999	Contact: U. Ahlrichs

Objective:

The goal of our work is the visual exploration of an office scene with an active camera in real-time. Therefore an explicit representation of knowledge about objects and the actions which are necessary to solve a certain task is used. Actions are changes of the camera settings as well as the selection of suitable processing steps from a variety of available options during analysis. The knowledge about objects and actions is represented using *one* semantic network based on the ERNEST-Philosophy. In order to exploit the knowledge, a problem independent A* graph search algorithm is applied. The task of this control algorithm is the selection of the optimal action at each processing step. In addition, for complex tasks like navigation a closed loop of perception and action has to be realized. We also provide an iterative control algorithm, which operates in parallel.

In the low–level part of the system presently red objects are hypothesized and then fovealized by moving the camera and varying the camera's focal length. The zoom adjustment is chosen in such a way, that the objects appear in a previously defined size. The necessary 3D–information is computed by tracking point features in color images during a translational movement of the camera. Color regions which are computed on these detail views of the scene are passed to the primitive concepts of the semantic network.

Results:

Experiments have been performed for the part of the knowledge base which represents the knowledge about the scene using an A*–based control. In 17 experiments the data driven hypotheses located 71 of 90 of three different objects correctly. correctly. The rate of assignments of a region to the correct object was 68%.

Selected publications:

References

1. U. AHLRICHS. Semantic Networks in Active Vision Systems – Aspects of Knowledge Representation and Purposive Control. In H. Christensen, D. Hogg, B. Neumann (eds.): Knowledge Based Computer Vision, Dagstuhl–Seminar–Report, Dagstuhl, 1998.
2. B. HEIGL, D. PAULUS. Punktverfolgung in Farbbildsequenzen. In D. Paulus, T. Wagner (eds.): Dritter Workshop Farbbildverarbeitung, IRB-Verlag, Stuttgart, 1997, 87–92 & 105.
3. H. NIEMANN, V. FISCHER, D. PAULUS, J. FISCHER. Knowledge based image understanding by iterative optimization. In G. Görz, S. Hölldobler (eds.): KI–96: Advances in Artificial Intelligence, 287 – 301. Springer, LNAI 1137, 1996.

MSDoS (Modeling Spontaneous Dialogues of Speech)
(Human Capital Mobility Post-Doctoral Fellowships)

Partner: LME, Erlangen University	**Supported by:** EC
Active: 04/1996 – 10/1997	**Contact:** Dr. M. Aretoulaki

Objective:

The goal of this project was to incorporate *meta-knowledge* in the EVAR Train Information system [2], so that the system knows when it does not know something and why. The focus was placed on location names which are uttered by the user, but are not contained in the lexicon of the system (Out-of-Vocabulary words or OOVs) [3]. Before the incorporation of OOV information, when such a word was uttered in relation to one of the task parameters, e.g. the goal location, EVAR would process an acoustically similar city name, even after the user had tried to correct it by repeating and spelling the problematic word. As a result, the user would either acquire the wrong information or would be referred to a human operator. Extending EVAR with OOV information should give the user more control over the flow of the dialogue leading to greater user satisfaction.

Results:

In the extended version of the system, the detection of an OOV leads to EVAR first asking the user to repeat the problematic word. A repeated OOV triggers the default spelling mode. The identification of an OOV at this point produces a warning to the user that there exists no relevant information in the database and a prompt for a new query or the interruption of the dialogue [1]. OOV detection and classification has been proved to increase Word Accuracy by 5% to reach 78.3% and Concept Accuracy by 7% to 75.1% [1]. The new version of EVAR was tested during the ELSNET Spoken Dialogue System Olympics during Eurospeech'97 attaining a middle score, although an absolute comparison to the other systems is impossible, given that EVAR was the only one that could process OOV words. The majority of the subjects who used the system thought that its reactions were appropriate and that the selected task was completed more or less successfully, listing among EVAR's strong points the intelligibility of its behaviour, the provision of feedback and the flexibility in the dialogue structure. This version of the system has been connected on the public phone network (+49 9131 16287) for the collection of dialogues under realistic conditions.

Selected publications:
References

1. M. BOROS, M. ARETOULAKI, F. GALLWITZ, E. NÖTH, H. NIEMANN. Semantic processing of out-of-vocabulary words in a spoken dialogue system. In Proc. of EUROSPEECH '97, volume 4, 1887–1890, Rhodes, Greece.
2. W. ECKERT, T. KUHN, H. NIEMANN, S. RIECK, A. SCHEUER, E. G. SCHUKAT-TALAMAZZINI. A spoken dialogue system for german intercity train timetable inquiries. In Proc. of EUROSPEECH'93, 1871–1874, Berlin.
3. F. GALLWITZ, E. NÖTH, H. NIEMANN. A category-based approach for recognition of out-of-vocabulary words. In Proc. of ICSLP-96, 228–231, Philadelphia.

Generic Spoken Dialogue Management

http://www.forwiss.uni-erlangen.de/fg-wv/

(Language Engineering)

Partner: none	Supported by: FORWISS
Active: 1998 – 1999	Contact: Dr. M. Aretoulaki

Objective:

The goal of this research is to take advantage of the flexible and generic architecture of the EVAR Train Information system [2] and extend it to different domains, applications and languages.

Results:

EVAR was indeed ported to the domain of Metro queries for Nuremberg in less than a month, indicating that the existing environment is sufficiently generic and extensible to cover modified data and to allow the integration of various new modules [2]. The same Dialogue Manager was used with a slightly modified domain representation. The system was also connected to the WWW so that it can dynamically consult more than a single database. This version of EVAR was installed on the public telephone network for about 2 months during which time 104 dialogues (phonecalls) were collected which showed that the desired behaviour was exhibited. Moreover, in the context of the EC SQEL project [3], a multilingual (German, Slovak, Slovenian and Czech) and multi-functional (train and flight information queries) version of EVAR was implemented [1]. Apart from the language identification issues, the Dialogue Manager of EVAR was adapted to flexibly switch between domains and language-specific modules. 175 dialogues have been collected with a version which works for the train domain (German and Slovak) and the flight domain (Slovenian). The system starts up in a default language and domain and the user is free to use whichever language they want. Once the language has been identified by the word recogniser, it is associated with the corresponding domain and database. Both domains are accommodated for concurrently in the generic ontology employed by the system. Both versions of EVAR described here will be installed on the public phone network in order to collect more data for their precise evaluation.

Selected publications:

References

1. S. HARBECK, E. NÖTH, H. NIEMANN. Multilingual Speech Recognition. In Proc. of the 2nd SQEL Workshop on Multi-Lingual Information Retrieval Dialogs, 1997. Pilsen, Czech Republic, 9–15.
2. R. KOMPE, W. ECKERT, ET AL. Towards domain-independent understanding of spontaneous speech. In EUFIT'95, 2315–2319, Aachen, Germany, August.
3. Proc. of the 2nd SQEL Workshop on Multi-Lingual Information Retrieval Dialogs, 1997. Pilsen, Czech Republic.

Methods for combining special problem solvers in deduction
(Schwerpunkt Deduktion)

Partner: 1. Theoretische Informatik,	Supported by: DFG
RWTH Aachen	
2. CIS, Universität München	
Active: 09/1994 – 10/1998	Contact: Prof. Dr. F. Baader

Objective:

In contrast to general purpose deductive procedures, special inferences methods are usually rather efficient, but they only apply to the restricted class they have been designed for. The integration of special methods into general purpose deductive systems tries to combine the efficiency of the former with the universality of the latter. When integrating more than one special procedure, one is faced with the problem of how to combine different special inference methods with each other. The long-term objective of this project was to gain a better understanding of the fundamental logical, algebraic, and algorithmic problems that occur in this situation.

More concretely, our aim was, on the one hand, to implement, optimize and evaluate the known methods for combining decision procedures for unification modulo equational theories over disjoint signatures. On the other hand, we wanted to generalize these combination methods such that they can handle more general constraints and solution structures.

Results:

In a series of publications, the combination method was first extended from unifica-

PSYLOCK – Identifikation eines Tastaturbenutzers anhand des Tippverhaltens
http://wwwbrauer.informatik.tu-muenchen.de/~bartmann/project.html

Partner: none	Supported by: IBI[1]
Active: 04/1996 – 04/1999	Contact: D. Bartmann

Objective:
Ziel des Projekts ist die Entwicklung eines neuartigen Authentifikationssystems, das auf dem biometrischen Merkmal Tippverhalten basiert. Durch Analyse von Schreibrhythmus, Anschlagfolge und anderen Aspekten des Tippverhaltens wird es damit möglich, auf Grund eines beliebigen kurzen Eingabestrings, eine Person sicher zu identifizieren.
Die Einsatzmöglichkeiten für ein derartiges System sind vielfältig: Angefangen vom Zugangsschutz zum Rechner bzw. Netzwerk (Biometrie als Paßwortersatz) über sicheres Homebanking und Handel im Internet bis hin zur Absicherung der Chipkarte.

Results:
Das derzeitige System besteht aus drei Komponenten. Die erste untersucht die, in einer anfänglichen Enrolmentphase erhobenen Lerndaten eines Probanden, und extrahiert daraus einen Merkmalsvektor, der das Tippverhalten der entsprechenden Person beschreibt. Die zweite berechnet aus einem derartigen Vektor und aufgenommenen Meßdaten (typischer Weise durch Tippen von 100 Zeichen Text entstanden) eine Reihe von Maßzahlen, die angeben, in wie weit das durch den Vektor beschriebene und das bei der Generierung der Meßdaten an den Tag gelegte Tippverhalten übereinstimmen. Die dritte Komponente führt schließlich die gewünschte Klassifikation durch: Sie entscheidet anhand der berechneten Maßzahlen, ob die beiden involvierten Personen (Urheber des Vektors und Urheber der Meßdaten) identisch sind oder nicht.
Der Schwerpunkt der derzeitigen Forschung liegt auf dem letzten Teil. Es wird die Eignung verschiedener neuronaler Architekturen zur Bewältigung dieser speziellen Klassifikationsaufgabe untersucht.

Selected publications:
References

1. D. BARTMANN. PSYLOCK - Identifikation eines Tastaturbenutzers durch Analyse des Tippverhaltens. Informatik '97: Informatik als Innovationsmotor, Aachen, September 1997, M. Jarke et al. (eds.), 327-334. Springer 1997.

---

[1] Institut für Bankinformatik an der Universität Regensburg

Analysis and verification of annotated logic programs

http://www.informatik.fernuni-hagen.de/pi8/aval/

(DFG Schwerpunktprogramm Deduktion)

Partner: none	**Supported by:** DFG
Active: 02/1997 - 02/1999	**Contact:** Prof. Dr. C. Beierle

Objective:

The concept of enriching programs with annotations for analysis and verification is applied to logic programs. Thus complex conditions like consistency constraints or correctness issues can be checked and many programming errors can be detected before execution time of a program. Different classes of annotations can be distinguished, e.g. type annotations, domain-specific annotations like arithmetic constraints, or annotations containing formulas in predicate logic. In order to promote the approach and to be able to exploit the runtime efficiency of commercial systems, the annotations are applied to standard Prolog.

Results:

The system Typical provides static type-checking for full standard Prolog. Additional features provided by specific Prolog systems like Sicstus Prolog can be taken care of via type libraries. The software checks Prolog programs with (semantically neutral) type declarations added. The type system includes subtyping and parametric polymorphism. The key novelties of the approach are new, more precise type declarations based on type constraints, and a better suited notion of well-typing in the presence of type parameters ('type consistency').

The recent development of Typical includes a better support for meta programming by means of meta types. Another line of research aims towards capturing procedural aspects of a Prolog program in a declarative way. We provide Prolog predicate annotations expressing dataflow properties, backtracking behaviour, etc. The annotations are executable comments, which are currently automatically checked at runtime.

Selected publications:

References

1. G. MEYER, C. BEIERLE. Dimensions of Types in Logic Programming. In W. Bibel, P.H. Schmitt (eds): Automated Deduction. A basis for applications. Kluwer Academic Press, 1998 (to appear).

Computational Dialectics
(DFG Forschergruppe Kommunikatives Verstehen)

Partner: Project within the DFG-Forschergruppe Kommunikatives Verstehen Active: 04/1998 – 04/2001	Supported by: DFG Contact: Prof. Dr. G. Brewka

Objective:

The goal of the project is to combine results from AI, in particular nonmonotonic reasoning, and philosophical argumentation theory in order to formalize decision making processes based on dialogues. The focus will be on models of argumentation contexts which regulate the role of the dialogue partners, their rights and obligations, burdens of proof etc. The major goal is to come up with a realistic model of argumentation which captures aspects like fairness, efficiency and resource limitation.

Case-based Diagnosis of Technical Systems

http://www.informatik.hu-berlin.de/Institut/struktur/ki/forschung/research-
fbs.html#DFG

(Case-based Diagnosis for Technical Systems)

Partner: Prof. Dr. Bernd Neumann, University of Hamburg	**Supported by:** DFG
Active: 1992 – 1998	**Contact:** Prof. Dr. H.-D. Burkhard

Objective:

Studies about the usability of AI methods for case data in technical diagnosis.

Results:

Diagnostic cases and their modeling have been analyzed for networks. The system ExperienceBook has been developed with concrete trouble case data. Via the internet, system administrators have access to a collection of problem cases being already solved. It is possible for them to add new cases to the system. The cases consist of several sections in natural language and some attributes. By means of textual CBR techniques, they are internally organized as a case retrieval net. In another prototypical implementation, an object oriented case retrieval net has been developed for case-based diagnosis. In connection with a rule-based system, cases are evaluated for the selection of appropriate symptoms being checked in the process of diagnosis.

Selected publications:
References

1. H.-D. BURKHARD, R. KÜHNEL, P. PIRK. Case based diagnosis in a technical domain. In I. Plander, editor, Artificial Intelligence and Information-Control Systems of Robots, 241–246, Singapore, 1994. World Scientific Publishing.
2. G. KAMP, P. PIRK, H.-D. BURKHARD. Falldaten: Case-based reasoning for the diagnosis of technical devices. In G. Görz, S. Hölldobler, editors, KI-96: Advances in Artificial Intelligence, LNAI 1137, 149–161. Springer 1996.
3. M. KUNZE. Das ExperienceBook – Dokumentation eines fallbasierten Systems zur Unterstützung der Systemadministration. Master's thesis, Humboldt-Universität zu Berlin, 1998.
4. M. KUNZE, A. HÜBNER. CBR on Semi-structured Documents: The ExperienceBook and the FAllQ Project. In L. Gierl, M. Lenz, editors, 6th German Workshop on CBR, 77–85, Rostock, 1998. Universität Rostock. IMIB Series Vol. 7.
5. M. LENZ, H.-D. BURKHARD, P. PIRK, E. AURIOL, M. MANAGO. CBR for Diagnosis and Decision Support. AI Communications, 9(3):138–146, 1996.
6. M. LENZ, A. HÜBNER, M. KUNZE. Textual CBR. In M. Lenz, H.-D. Burkhard, B. Bartsch-Spörl, S. Weß, editors, Case-Based Reasoning Technology — From Foundations to Applications, LNAI 1400. Springer 1998.

FAllQ

http://www.informatik.hu-berlin.de/Institut/struktur/ki/forschung/research-fbs.html#FAllQ

Partner: LHS Verwaltungs GmbH, Dreieich-Sprendlingen; TecInno GmbH Kaiserslautern	Supported by: Partners
Active: 1996 –	Contact: Prof. Dr. H.-D. Burkhard

Objective:
Studies about the usability of AI methods to obtain knowledge from textual documents.

Results:
Knowledge of a company, usually stored in textual documents can be made accessible using Textual Cased Based Reasoning methods. The FAllQ project has been developed with LHS as industrial partner. Knowledge of the company is stored in documents of different formats (e.g. FAQs, manuals, documentations). To make this knowledge available the domain has to be modeled very carefully. Each document is to be considered as a case. These cases are organized in the system as a case retrieval net. It has been shown that case retrieval nets can handle large knowledge bases, and access them very fast (40.000 documents, 45 MB data, retrieval time 2 sec.).

Selected publications:

References

1. M. KUNZE, A. HÜBNER. CBR on Semi-structured Documents: The ExperienceBook and the FAllQ Project. In L. Gierl, M. Lenz, editors, 6th German Workshop on CBR, 77 – 85, Rostock, 1998. Universität Rostock. IMIB Series Vol. 7.

2. M. LENZ, H.-D. BURKHARD. Lazy propagation in Case Retrieval Nets. In W. Wahlster, editor, 12th European Conf. on Artificial Intelligence (ECAI-96), 127 – 131. John Wiley & Sons, 1996.

3. M. LENZ, H.-D. BURKHARD. Applying CBR for Document Retrieval. In Y. Nakatani, editor, Proc. Workshop Practical Use of CBR at IJCAI97, 1997.

4. M. LENZ, H.-D. BURKHARD. CBR for Document Retrieval – The FAllQ Project. In D. B. Leake, E. Plaza, editors, Case-Based Reasoning Research and Development, Proc. ICCBR-97, LNAI 1266, 84–93. Springer 1997.

5. M. LENZ, A. HÜBNER, M. KUNZE. Textual CBR. In M. Lenz, H.-D. Burkhard, B. Bartsch-Spörl, S. Weß, editors, Case-Based Reasoning Technology – From Foundations to Applications, LNAI 1400. Springer 1998.

Autonomic Function and Artificial Neural Networks
(Neurolab 4, NASA-Mission)

Partner: DLR Institute for Aerospace Medicine, Cologne, GER, and Univ. of Texas, Dallas, TX, USA, Hunter Holmes Medical Center Richmond, VA, USA, Vanderbilt University, TN, USA	**Supported by:** NASA/NIH
Active: 1994 – 1998	**Contact:** Prof. Dr. A.B. Cremers

Objective:

Cardiovascular regulation and its alterations in micro-G.

Results:

First, a flexible tool (named CARDIO) for the construction of cardiovascular models was developed. It separates between anatomy and dynamics. Different formulations of the hemodynamics can be combined within a model. Vessel systems may be hierarchically structured. CARDIO is based on the agent system shell MARC, a message-based micro-kernel that allows distributed computing on a network. LBNP-models were developed and simple artificial neural network controllers were trained to reproduce the cardiovascular reactions patterns of astronauts after return to earth.

Selected publications:

References

1. M. CONTZEN, J. FRINGS, K. MÖLLER, C. REINER. MARC – Eine Agentensystemshell zur verteilten Programmierung. In C. Cap (ed.) SIWORK'96, vdf, Zürich.
2. K. MÖLLER, L. BECK, F. BAISCH. Cardiovascular Control with Artificial Neural Networks. J. Gravitational Physiology, 1996.
3. A. ASTEROTH, K. MÖLLER, F. BAISCH, L. BECK, J. DRESCHER. Cardiovascular Regulation: A Modelling approach. J. Grav.Physiol.1997

Automated Identification of Solitary Bees

Partner: Institute of Agricult. Zoology University of Bonn **Active:** 1996 – 2000	**Supported by:** DFG **Contact:** Prof. Dr. A. B. Cremers

Objective:

Solitary bees (Hymenoptera: Apoidea) are endangered by extinction. Furthermore they are highly suited for nature conservancy indication purposes. Nevertheless their appearance in development and ecological planning tasks is quite seldom due to their difficult classification. Our approach to classification of solitary bees is based on two ideas: (1) to use only the veining of the forewings for discrimination, (2) to automate measurement, evaluation, and classification using image analysis and a hierarchical classification approach.

Results:

We have developed a hierarchical approach to classify solitary bees by analyzing digital images of their forewings. Feature extraction derives a vein graph of a forewing. We apply three classification steps: (1) graph isomorphism with a prototype graph of the data base results in a set of genera, (2) the traversal of a taxonomical key encoded as a fuzzified decision tree results in a genus or a small group of genera, (3) statistical analysis of numerical attributes and relations of the extracted image features results in species.

Our approach has proven to work successfully even for the classification of species within genera like *Andrena* where all species look very similar and are very difficult to classify. We currently work on non-linear classification schemes to handle also species with significant intra-class differences due to different sex or generation.

Selected publications:

References

1. S. SCHRÖDER, W. DRESCHER, V. STEINHAGE. Applications of Automated Image Processing and Computer-Based Information Processing for Biometrical Taxonomy of Solitary Bees (Hymenoptera, Apoidea). Apidologie, No. 5, 1994.
2. S. SCHRÖDER, W. DRESCHER, B. KASTENHOLZ, V. STEINHAGE. An Automated Method for the Identification of Bee Species (Hymenoptera: Apoidea). Proc. Intern. Symp. on Conserving Europe's Bees, Int. Bee Research Ass. & Linnean Society London, UK, 1995.
3. V. STEINHAGE, B. KASTENHOLZ, S. SCHRÖDER, W. DRESCHER. A Hierarchical Approach to Classify Solitary Bees Based on Image Analysis. Mustererkennung 1997, 19. DAGM-Symposium, Braunschweig, Informatik aktuell, Springer, 419-426, 1997.

Computer-based simulation and intra-operative validation of cerebrovascular flow and pressure.

Partner: Clinic of Neurosurgy, Univ. of Bonn, and Neuroradiology, Univ. of Bonn
Active: 1998 – 1999

Supported by: BONFOR

Contact: Prof. Dr. A.B. Cremers

Objective:

Prediction of intra-operative changes to the cerebrovascular blood-flow.

Results:

CARDIO, the agent-based simulations system was enhanced with a 3D-front-end to allow the efficient construction of complex (hierarchically organized) vascular structures. Various approximations of hemodynamics were incorporated and are currently under validation.

Selected publications:

References

1. K. MÖLLER, B. MEYER, C. SCHALLER. Towards realistic simulation of cerebrovascular arteriovenous malformations. To appear.

Extraction of Buildings from Digital Images
(Semantic Modelling and Extraction of Spatial Objects)

Partner: Institute of Photogrammetry (Bonn)	**Supported by:** DFG
Active: 1993 – 1999	**Contact:** Prof. Dr. A.B. Cremers

Objective:

We propose a model-based approach to automated 3D extraction of buildings from aerial images. We focused on a reconstruction strategy that is not restricted to a small class of buildings. Therefore, we employ a generic modelling approach which relies on the well defined combination of building part models. Building parts are classified by their roof type. Starting from low-level image features we combine data-driven and model-driven processes within a multi-level aggregation hierarchy, thereby using a tight coupling of 2D image and 3D object modelling and processing, and ending up in complex 3D building estimations of shape and location. Due to the explicit representation of well defined processing states in terms of model-based 2D and 3D descriptions at all levels of modelling and data aggregation our approach reveals a great potential for a reliable building extraction.

Results:

We have developed an iterative approach to building reconstruction which executes three main tasks: (1) 2D → 3D: model-driven reconstruction of 3D object features from 2D image features by bundle adjustment, (2) 3D → 3D: indexing into a library of parameterized models of building parts and aggregation of part models to complete 3D building hypotheses, (3) 3D → 2D: image verification of building hypotheses back projected into the original aerial images. The successful sequence of matching steps results in an iteratively improved gain in knowledge. The three steps are repeated until no further hypotheses can be generated. Our approach has been proven to work successfully on test data sets provided by the Landesvermessungsamt Bonn and the ETH Zürich.

Selected publications:
References

1. A. FISCHER, T. H. KOLBE, F. LANG, A.B. CREMERS, W. FÖRSTNER, L. PLÜMER, V. STEINHAGE. Extracting Buildings from Aerial Images using Hierarchical Aggregation in 2D and 3D, 1998. To appear.
2. A. FISCHER, T. H. KOLBE, F. LANG. Integration of 2D and 3D Reasoning for Building Reconstruction Using a Generic Hierarchical Model. Workshop on Semantic Modeling for the Acquisition of Topographic Information from Images and Maps, SMATI '97, 159-180, 1997.
3. A. FISCHER, V. STEINHAGE. Solid Modeling for Building Extraction from Aerial Images. Proc. 5th Int. Conf. in Central Europe on Computer Graphics and Visualization 97, WSCG'97, Plzen, 114-123, 1997.
4. T. H. KOLBE, L. PLÜMER, A. B. CREMERS. Using Constraints for the Identification of Buildings in Aerial Images. Porc. Practical Applications of Constraint Technology, PACT'96, London, 143-154, 1996.
5. F. LANG, W. FÖRSTNER. Surface Reconstruction of Man-Made Objects using Polymorphic Mid-Level Features and Generic Scene Knowledge. Zeitschrift für Photogrammetrie und Fernerkundung, Vol. 6, 193-201, 1996.

MOBOCOL
(MIR'97- German-russian Space mission)

Partner: DLR, Institute of Aerospace medicine	Supported by: BMBF/DARA GmbH
Active: 1996 – 1998	Contact: Prof. Dr. A.B. Cremers.

Objective:

Model based evaluation of cardiovascular alterations in astronauts.

Results:

An approximation of cardiovascular dynamics with linear differential equations was developed by separating the heart cycle into four phases. Models were fitted to reproduce obtained data from BDC-experiments (individualization of cardiovascular models). Optimization techniques were employed to estimate control parameters that best "explain" alterations in post-flight reaction patterns. This complex optimization task was sped up with the help of artificial neural networks. An initial guess was computed with network-inversion on differentiable backpropagation networks.

Selected publications:
References

1. K. MÖLLER, L. BECK, F. BAISCH, A. DIEDRICH, J. DRESCHER. MOBOCOL: Model based optimization of countermeasures using LBNP. In P. Sahm, M. Keller, B. Schiewe (eds.) Research Program of the German-Russian Space Mission MIR '97 WPF, Köln, 1997.
2. A. ASTEROTH, K. MÖLLER, L. BECK, J. DRESCHER. Model based characterization of micro-G induced alterations of CVS-regulation, J. Grav. Physiol., 1998. To appear.

Multi-Robot Navigation
(Navigation Strategies in Multi-Robot Scenarios)

Partner: Research Establishment for Applied Science Active: 08/1997 – 12/1999	Supported by: Research Establishment for Applied Science Contact: Prof. Dr. A. B. Cremers

---

Objective:

The project Multi Robot Navigation is concerned with navigation strategies allowing several mobile robots to navigate safely in their environment. It furthermore addresses techniques for multi-robot exploration, mapping and localization.

Results:

Within this research project we developed a technique for concurrent map building and localization, which can easily be adopted to a multi-robot scenario in which multiple agents concurrently map an unknown environment.

Selected publications:

References

1. F.E. SCHNEIDER, D. WILDERMUTH. Simulation von Mehrrobotersystemen. Fachgespräch Autonome Mobile Systeme, Stuttgart, Springer Verlag, Oktober 1997.
2. F.E. SCHNEIDER, K.-P. GÄRTNER, D. WILDERMUTH. Einsatz einer verteilten Simulation beim Entwurf von Mensch-Mehrroboter-Systemen. Symposium Neue Technologien in der Simulation, Mannheim, September 1997.
3. F.E. SCHNEIDER, K.-P. GÄRTNER. Mensch-Mehrroboter-Systeme im Bereich autonomer mobiler Systeme. Deutsch-Französischer Workshop Robotik, Ludwigshafen, Juni 1997.
4. S. THRUN, D. FOX, W. BURGARD. Probabilistic mapping of an environment by a mobile robot. In Proc. of the IEEE International Conference on Robotics and Automation, 1998.

RTL
(Robotic Tele-Lab)

Partner: Virtuelle Wissensfabrik NRW	Supported by: MWF-NRW
Active: 07/97:12/99	Contact: Prof. Dr. A. B. Cremers

Objective:

The objective of the RTL project is the development of a multi-media interface allowing multiple researchers to carry out joint experiments with a mobile robot over the Internet.

Results:

So far, we developed a client server architecture for the visualization of joint robot navigation experiments over the Internet. The visualization tool applies predictive simulation techniques to provide smooth animations at the client side. Special abstract sensors are used to quickly adopt the scene according to changes in the environment such as opened or closed doors.

Selected publications:
References

1. A. B. CREMERS, W. BURGARD, D. SCHULZ. Architecture of the robotic tele-lab. In Proc. of the 1997 HFESEC Annual Conference on Advances in Multimedia and Simulation, 1997.
2. A. HOPP, D. SCHULZ, W. BURGARD, A. B. CREMERS, D. FELLNER. Virtual reality visualization of distributed tele-experiments. In Proc. of the 24th Annual Conference of the IEEE Industrial Electronics Society (IECON'98), 1998. To appear.
3. W. BURGARD, A. B. CREMERS, D. FOX, D. HÄHNEL, G. LAKEMEYER, D. SCHULZ, W. STEINER, S. THRUN. The interactive museum tour-guide robot. In Proc. of the Fifteenth National Conference on Artificial Intelligence, 1998. To appear.

VIRGO

http://www.ics.forth.gr/virgo/
(Vision-based robot navigation research network)

Partner: Foundation for Research and Technology – Hellas, Greece*; Aalborg University, Denmark; University of Genova, Italy; Technical University, Graz, Austria; Kungl Tekniska Hogskolan, Sweden; National Institute for Research in Computer Science and Control, France; Universität Bonn, Germany; Forschungszentrum Informationstechnik, GmbH, (GMD), Germany; University of Copenhagen, Denmark; University of Zurich, Switzerland. *Coordinator.	**Supported by:** EU
Active: 08/1996-08/1999	**Contact:** Prof. Dr. A. B. Cremers

Objective:

The stated goal of the whole VIRGO project is to coordinate European research and post-graduate training activities that address the development of intelligent robotic systems able to navigate in (partially) unknown and possibly dynamic environments. Bonn University is an active participant in this project.

Results:

Bonn university is implementing the RECIPE system – the Reconfigurable Extensible Capture and Image Processing Environment. RECIPE (http://www.cs.uni-bonn.de/~arbuckle/recipe/) is being developed to provide a robust, standardised and extensible means of capturing and processing images on robots. Designed to be largely platform independent, it has a modular multi-threaded architecture which is specifically tailored to the needs of autonomous robots. Functionality is loaded and unloaded at run-time and the system employs automatic restart, reconfiguration and persistent storage to improve its overall reliability. Additional contributions within the VIRGO project lie in the area of active localisation. We have shown how active localisation can be integrated within a high-level robot control system.

Selected publications:

References

1. M. BEETZ, W. BURGARD, D. FOX, A.-B. CREMERS. Integrating Active Localization into High-level Robot Control Systems. Robotics and Autonomous Systems, Special Issue for SIRS'97 (to appear).
2. M. BEETZ, T. ARBUCKLE, A. B. CREMERS, M. MANN. Transparent, Flexible and Resource-adaptive Image Processing for Autonomous Service Robots. Proc. European Conference on Artificial Intelligence, Brighton, U.K., 1998. to appear.
3. M. BEETZ, W. BURGARD, A. B. CREMERS, D. FOX. Active Localization for Service Robot Applications. Proc. 5th International Symposium on Intelligent Robotic Systems, (SIRS'97), Stockholm, Sweden, 1997.

Programming by Demonstration using an Active Stereo-Vision System and a Data-Glove

Partner: IPR, University of Karlsruhe **Supported by:** DFG

Active: 02/1996 – 02/2000   **Contact:** Prof. Dr. R. Dillmann

Objective:

The project's goal is to develop an innovative programming system which follows the *Programming by Demonstration* paradigm. It allows a user to create robot programs based on demonstrations of the task given by the user itself. However, unlike state-of-the-art *PbD* systems this project aims at developing methods which enable the generation of flexible, i.e. generalized, programs. These contain variables and branches, are widely applicable, and reusable as modules for other task solutions. In order to achieve this research in the fields of image processing, knowledge representation, interactive machine learning, and human-computer interaction is carried out.

Results:

On the vision side methods for identifying the user's hand and objects in the environment as well as methods for tracking these during the demonstration were developed. Furthermore neural network based classifiers were generated which allow to classify grasps carried out by the user. Classification is based on the flexion of the finger joints which is measured using the data-glove. These tools were integrated into the programming system set up. Based on an environment model, the measured trajectory of a demonstration, and the poses of the user's hand a demonstration is analyzed. Hypotheses about un-/grasping actions, manipulated objects, preferred motion types and last not least the intention the user followed with a demonstration are derived. These hypotheses are checked back with the user using a multi-modal user interface. Finally, using a newly developed method, a program which represents the generalized intended task solution is generated automatically.

Selected publications:
References

1. H. FRIEDRICH. Robot programming meets virtual reality. In Proceedings of the 7th International Conference on Human-Computer Interaction (HCI'97), San Francisco, USA, 24-29 August 1997.
2. H. FRIEDRICH, M. RIEPP, R. DILLMANN. Knowledge based parameterization of operator sequences. In R. Engels, H. Friedrich, M. Wiese, editors, Proceedings of the 11th Meeting GI Special Interest Group Machine Learning, Karlsruhe, Germany, August 6-8 1997.
3. H. FRIEDRICH, J. HOLLE, R. DILLMANN. Interactive generation of flexible robot programs. In Proceedings of the IEEE International Conference on Robotics and Automation, Leuven, Belgium, May 16-21 1998.

Skill-Mart, Skilled Multi-Arm Robots
(BRITE/EuRAM)

Partner: IPR, University of Karlsruhe, University of Parma, University of Malaga, University of Bristol, Propack Data, Scienzia Machinale British Aerospace	**Supported by:** EU
Active: 05/1996 - 05/1999	**Contact:** Prof. R. Dillmann

Objective:

The project addresses the issue of defining a 'skilled' multi-arm robotics system for handling non-rigid material such as textile, food, plastic foam, wire and flexible containers. The research objectives of SKILL-MART are to define what skill is, to investigate if and how programming by demonstration can be used to teach skill, and how non-rigid product behaviour can be interpreted in terms of skilled manipulation. Moreover, the project intends to investigate how state-of-the-art Hard-and Software need to be enhanced to enable the skilled manipulation of flexible material in general, and to research techniques and methods enabling the required enhancements. The project intends to contribute towards the problem of high cost of robotics system development and the lack of knowledge on the practical implementation of 'skilled' and adaptive systems that have been the major limiting factors for the automation of a large variety of tasks.

Results:

Regarding the simulation of non-rigid material advances in modeling different material were made. Moreover, simulation speed was enhanced significantly by optimizing the code of the simulation system. On the vision side methods for identifying, classifying, and localizing different types of non-rigid objects were developed. Regarding the representation and execution of solutions of manipulation tasks that require skilled manipulation a representation formalism was developed. Furthermore, a concept for mapping robot neutral task solutions to specific execution robot systems was developed. Finally, a two arm robot system was set up as platform for experiments. Controllers for skillful manipulation of wires were designed for the robot system.

Selected publications:
References

1. O. ROGALLA, M. EHRENMANN, R. DILLMANN. A Sensor Fusion Approach for PbD. In Proceedings of the 11th IEEE/RSJ International Conference on Intelligent Robots and Systems (IROS '98), Victoria, B.C., Canada 1998.
2. H. FRIEDRICH, O. ROGALLA, R. DILLMANN, N. GUIL, P. TRABADO. Knowledge representation and efficient image processing for high-level skill acquisition. In Human Skill Acquisition for Service Robots, Workshop at the 10th IEEE/RSJ International Conference on Intelligent Robots and Systems IROS'97, Grenoble, France, September 7-11 1997.

DisLoP: Ein Forschungsprojekt zu Disjunktiver Logikprogrammierung

| **Partner:** Universität Koblenz–Landau | **Supported by:** DFG |
| **Active:** 07/1995 – 09/2000 | **Contact:** Dr. J. Dix |

Objective:

Ziel dieses Forschungsvorhabens ist die Untersuchung und Entwicklung eines Programmiersystems für *erweiterte Disjunktive Logikprogramme mit Negation*. Dies soll durch Kombination von Methoden aus dem Bereich der klassischen Deduktion mit nichtmonotonen Ansätzen der Wissensrepräsentation erreicht werden. Insbesondere sollen Prolog-artige Sprachen durch *Disjunktionen* und verschiedenartige *nichtmonotone Negationen* erweitert, effiziente (und praktisch anwendbare) Implementierungen entwickelt und deren Einsatz an mehreren nichttrivialen Anwendungen untersucht werden. Das Ziel des DISLoP-Projekts insgesamt ist die Etablierung der Logikprogrammierung mit Disjunktionen, Negationen und Constraints für Anwendungen z.B. in Informationsmanagement-Systemen (IMS), bei der Analyse von Regelwerken und im Diagnose-Bereich. Info:http://www.uni-koblenz.de/ag-ki/DLP/dlp-d.html

In der erst kürzlich begonnenen zweiten Phase (Januar 1998), werden wir insbesondere auf Anwendungen eingehen: Disjunktive Programme als Anfragesprachen im www, NetBots als logische Programme, Data-Mining und Deduktion.

Results:

Die Ergebnisse der ersten Projektphase sind in [1] detailliert aufgeführt. Mitarbeiter hier: C. Aravindan und I. Niemelä. Insbesondere wurde eine disjunktive Version D-WFS der wohlfundierten Semantik mit guten Eigenschaften entwickelt (konfluenter Kalkül, modular, relevant, goal-orientiert: siehe [3,2]). Außerdem wurde ein sehr effizientes System zur Berechnung von minimalen und stabilen Modellen entwickelt: smodels ([6]). Mitarbeiter in der zweiten Phase: I. Dahn, M. Kühn und B. Thomas

Selected publications:

References

1. C. Aravindan, J. Dix, I. Niemelä. Dislop: A research project on disjunctive logic programming. AI Communications, 10:151–165, 1997.
2. S. Brass, J. Dix. Characterizations of the Disjunctive Stable Semantics by Partial Evaluation. Journal of Logic Programming, 32(3):207–228, 1997.
3. S. Brass, J. Dix. Characterizations of the Disjunctive Well-founded Semantics: Confluent Calculi and Iterated GCWA. Journal of Automated Reasoning, 20(1):143–165, 1998.
4. J. Dix, U. Furbach, I. Niemelä. Nonmonotonic Reasoning: Towards Efficient Calculi and Implementations. In A. Voronkov, A. Robinson (eds.) Handbook of Automated Reasoning. Elsevier-Science-Press, 1998. To appear.
5. J. Dix, F. Stolzenburg. A Framework to incorporate Nonmonotonic Reasoning into Constraint Logic Programming. Journal of Logic Programming, 36(1,2,3):5—37, 1998. Special Issue on Constraint Logic Programming, Guest Editors: K. Marriott, P. Stuckey.
6. I. Niemelä, P. Simons. Efficient Implementation of the Well-founded and Stable Model Semantics. In M. Maher (ed.) Proceedings of the JICSLP, 289–303, Bonn, Germany. The MIT Press.
7. F. Stolzenburg, B. Thomas. Analysing Rule Sets for the Calculation of Banking Fees by a Theorem Prover. In W. Bibel, P. H. Schmitt (eds.), Automated Deduction — A Basis for Applications. Kluwer Academic Publishers, 1998. To appear.

Knowledge Based Scene Exploration and Visual Navigation
(DIROKOL – A lightweight lowcost service robot)

Partner: DLR	Supported by: Bay. Forschungsstiftung
Active: 1998 – 2000	Contact: C. Drexler

Objective:

The objective is to develop a servicerobot which serves as an aid for handicapped people in public health facilities (hospitals, nursing homes) and home care. It should help to facilitate their daily live, especially with fetch and deliver services, simple nursing tasks, and handling gadgets and objects.

Navigation and object recognition is done by visual information acquired by a stereo camera system mounted on top of the robot. It has four degrees of freedom (pan, tilt, left and right vergence) and motorized zoom/focus/aperture lenses enabling human-like head movements. In order to achieve a reliable sensing–control loop active vision algorithms like active contours and resolution hierarchies are applied for fast selective stereo image processing.

For being able to perform the mentioned tasks, the robot has to navigate in man-made environments and interact with different objects. As it is not desirable to store sophisticated environmental maps on the robot, because the adaptation for different surroundings would be difficult, the robot is going to "learn" about the environment himself. This is done by adaptive exploration based on knowledge bases which describe the fundamental structure of the environment. A map is build on the features extracted from the stereo images, according to the stored knowledge, and will be updated upon detected changes.

Results:

There exist a stationary system for real–time pedestrian tracking using active rays and a featureless depth estimation from stereo images based on gabor filter hierarchies. Also an autonomous RC–car has been developed which solves a slalom parcour with visual information from a mounted camera.

Selected publications:
References

1. U. AHLRICHS, U. Semantic Networks in Active Vision Systems – Aspects of Knowledge Representation and Purposive Control. In H. Christensen, D. Hogg, B. Neumann (eds.), Knowledge Based Computer Vision, Dagstuhl–Seminar–Report, Dagstuhl, 1998.

2. J. DENZLER, H. NIEMANN. Real-time pedestrian tracking in natural scenes. In G. Sommer, K. Daniliidis, J. Pauli (eds.), Computer Analysis of Images and Patterns, CAIP'97, 42–49, 1997.

3. J. DENZLER. The Dialogue with the Scene: Probabilistik Knowledge Based Active Vision. In H. Christensen, D. Hogg, B. Neumann (eds.), Knowledge Based Computer Vision, Dagstuhl–Seminar–Report, Dagstuhl, 1998

Interpretative and Constructive Processes in Spatially Organized Knowledge Structures
(Spatial Structures in Aspect Maps)

Partner: none	**Supported by:** DFG
Active: 1996 – 2002 (planned)	**Contact:** Prof. C. Freksa, Ph.D.

Objective:

The objective of this project is the development of an architecture for processing pictorial and symbolic knowledge represented in an integrated way [1]. Complex external knowledge representations like geographic maps contain spatial information in spatio-analogical form as well as non-spatial information represented in symbolic form. Aspect-specific basic representational elements shall be identified and extracted by appropriate operators. The aspects are stored in separate representation structures organized analogically in correspondence to the underlying spatial structure. Thus, relevant information can easily be accessed depending on the task at hand. The common spatial structure of the different maps makes it possible to recombine different aspects selectively to yield knowledge about new aspects of specific states of affairs. The main emphasis of the project lies on investigating knowledge structures from a computer science perspective. The project is carried out in cooperation with cognitive psychologists to enable the use of the architecture for psychological modeling.

Results:

- Investigation of schematic public transportation network maps: identification of construction principles, problems, and approaches to resolutions [2].
- Theoretical investigation of map interpretation and inference processes [3].
- Empirical study on human map reasoning [4].
- Implementation of a shell system in Macintosh Common Lisp.
- Prototypical realization of interpretation and inference processes.

Selected publications:
References

1. T. BARKOWSKY, C. FREKSA, B. BERENDT, S. KELTER. Aspektkarten - Integriert räumlich-symbolische Repräsentationsstrukturen. In C. Umbach, M. Grabski, R. Hörnig (eds.), Perspektive in Sprache und Raum, 147-168. Deutscher Universitäts-Verlag, 1997.
2. T. BARKOWSKY, C. FREKSA. Cognitive requirements on making and interpreting maps. In S. Hirtle, A. Frank (eds.), Spatial information theory: A theoretical basis for GIS, 347-361. Springer, 1997.
3. B. BERENDT, T. BARKOWSKY, C. FREKSA, S. KELTER. Spatial representation with aspect maps. In C. Freksa, C. Habel, K. F. Wender (eds.), Spatial cognition - An interdisciplinary approach to representing and processing spatial knowledge, 313-336. Springer, 1997.
4. B. BERENDT, R. RAUH, T. BARKOWSKY. Spatial thinking with geographic maps: an empirical study. In H. Czap, P. Ohly, S. Pribbenow (eds.), Herausforderungen an die Wissensorganisation: Visualisierung, multimediale Dokumente, Internet-strukturen, 63-74. Würzburg: ERGON-Verlag, 1998

Qualitative Knowledge About Space and Time Spatial Inference

(DFG Priority Program on Spatial Cognition)

Partner: none	Supported by: DFG
Active: 1996 – 2002 (planned)	Contact: Prof. C. Freksa, Ph.D.

Objective:

The scientific goal of the project is the development of approaches to qualitative spatial and temporal reasoning. A basic hypothesis of our approach is that the integration of perception and action with processes of reasoning and cognition creates a foundation for intelligent bahavior. For this reason, our approaches are based on perception-related representations of partial knowledge about spatio-temporal environments. The work in the Spatial Inference project is carried out on a theoretical level (development and analysis of representation and reasoning structures), on a modelling level (computer implementation and testing of synthetic environments), and on an experimental level (robot navigation using various spatial inference strategies). In this way, we can isolate and integrate individual aspects involved in spatial reasoning and we can explore how realistic certain assumptions are in the setting of a real environment.

Results:

Specific topics for integrating qualitative spatial and temporal calculi have been: the integration of orientation calculi [3], axiomatization of qualitative topological theories [1], and qualitative spatial reasoning using cell matrices. The approaches based on the notion of conceptual neighborhoods, which have been developed in the project form the basis for an inference engine capable of reasoning with incomplete, fuzzy, uncertain, and contradictory knowledge [2, 4].

Selected publications:

References

1. C. DORNHEIM. Undecidability of Plane Polygonal Mereotopology. In A.G. Cohn, L.K. Schubert, S.C. Shapiro (eds.): Principles of Knowledge Representation and Reasoning: KR-98. San Francisco, CA: Morgan Kaufmann Publishers, 1998.

2. R. MORATZ, C. FREKSA. Spatial Reasoning with Uncertain Data Using Stochastic Relaxation. In W. Brauer, (Eds.) Fuzzy-Neuro Systems-98, 106-112. Infix-Verlag, 1998.

3. R. RÖHRIG. Representation and Processing of Qualitative Orientation Knowledge. In G. Brewka, C. Habel, B. Nebel (eds.), KI-97: Advances in Artificial Intelligence, 219-230. Springer, 1997.

4. K. ZIMMERMANN, C. FREKSA. Qualitative spatial reasoning using orientation, distance, and path knowledge. Applied Intelligence 6, 49-58, 1996. Springer.

Data-Mining im World-Wide-Web mit KI-Methoden
(Neue Technologien und Umwelt)

Partner: Universität Koblenz–Landau	**Supported by:** das Land Rheinland-Pfalz
Active: 01/1998 – 01/1999	**Contact:** Prof. Dr. U. Furbach

Objective:

Mit diesem Vorhaben wollen wir neue Technologien aus der Künstlichen Intelligenz zum Data-Mining im World-Wide-Web anwenden. Denn oft liefern herkömmliche Suchmaschinen zu einer Suchanfrage an das World-Wide-Web eine unübersehbare Menge von Daten. Da die eigentliche Information häufig nur implizit in einem Dokument oder verteilt auf mehrere Dokumente vorliegt, ist es oft schwierig, überhaupt noch Informationen aus der Datenflut zu gewinnen. In unserem Vorhaben wollen wir daher diesem Problem mit Hilfe von Methoden aus der Künstlichen Intelligenz (insbesondere aus der Logikprogrammierung) und dem sich gerade etablierenden Gebiet des Data-Minings entgegentreten. Aus der Logikprogrammierung können die Techniken zur Kodierung, Verarbeitung und Beantwortung von Anfragen, aus dem Data-Mining Techniken des Maschinellen Lernens und der Induktiven Logikprogrammierung erfolgversprechend eingesetzt werden. Es ist zu erwarten, daßdie dabei neu zu entwickelnden Methoden und Werkzeuge einen wesentlichen Beitrag zur Forschungs-

Deduktive Techniken für
Informations-Management-Systeme

Partner: Universität Koblenz–Landau; Joseph Raab GmbH&Cie KG, Neuwied; R. Wolfrum Consulting, Mülheim-Kärlich; Ing.Büro W. Lehnigk-Emden jun., Ochtendung; Schlaadt Plastics GmbH, St.Goarshausen	**Supported by:** Das Ministerium für Wirtschaft Verkehr, Landwirtschaft und Weinbau des Landes Rheinland-Pfalz
Active: 09/1995 - 03/1998	**Contact:** Prof. Dr. U. Furbach

Objective:

Das Ziel dieses Projektes ist die Anwendung deduktiver Techniken als eine Basis für Informations-Management-Systeme. Die Anwendungen hierzu können in mittelständischen Unternehmen gesehen werden. Hier liegt das Problem in der Bereitstellung eines einheitlichen Zugriffs auf verschiedene Quellen heterogener Daten. Zusätzlich mu"s eine flexible Verarbeitung und adäquate Darstellung bereitgestellt werden. Die Ergebnisse werden prototypisch in das System GLUE integriert [3].

Results:

Es wurde ein prototypisches System [2] [4] für den einheitlichen Zugriff auf verschiedenste Datenbank- und Dateisysteme implementiert und auf reale Datenmengen aus mittelständischen Unternehmen angewendet. Eine Weiterentwicklung des Systems wird derzeit zum Entwurf von intelligenten Internet-Agenten bearbeitet. Neue Verfahren zur Informationsextraktion aus dem World Wide Web und die Integration dieser Daten in Informations-Management-Systeme wurden in diesem Projekt mit Hilfe deduktiver Techniken entwickelt [5]. Die aus diesem Projekt gewonnenen Verfahren bilden die Basis für die weitere Forschung auf den Gebiet der intelligenten Internet-Agenten (*LogicRobots*), die mit deduktiven Methoden und verwandten Gebieten der *Künstlichen Intelligenz* autononme, wissensbasierte Informationsagenten darstellen. Ein *LogicRobot* zur Kleinanzeigensuche wurde mit diesen Verfahren implementiert [1].

Selected publications:

References

1. LogicRobot:. http://www.uni-koblenz.de/~bthomas/such_und_find.html.
2. G. NEUGEBAUER. Glue: Using heterogeneous sources of information in a logic programming system. In *International Workshop: Intelligent Information Integration,,* 1997. during the 21st German Annual Conference on Artificial Intelligence, KI-97. Freiburg, Germany.
3. G. NEUGEBAUER, D. SCHÄFER. Glue - opening the world to theorem provers. In *Logic Programming and Non-Monotonic Reasoning*, volume 1165, 1997.
4. B. THOMAS. GLUE: Heterogeneous Sources of Information in a Logic Programming System. Technical report, Jahrestreffen der GI-Fachgruppe 1.2.1 'Deduktionssysteme', Fachberichte Informatik, Uni Koblenz 23/97, 1997.
5. B. THOMAS. Token-Templates und Logisches Programmieren im World-Wide-Web. Master's thesis, University of Koblenz-Landau, Abteilung Landau, Institut für Informatik, 1998. http://www.uni-koblenz.de/~bthomas/doc/diplom.ps.

EPK-fix

Support for Engineering Electronic Product Catalogues

http://www.forwiss.de/fg-we/EPK-fix.html

Partner: FORWISS, mediatec GmbH	**Supported by:** BMBF
Active: 05/1995 – 10/1997	**Contact:** B. Gaede

Objective:

The goal of the EPK-fix software engineering project has been the development of methods and integrated tools for efficient specification, production, and validation of software, here Electronic Product Catalogues (EPCs). The tools must be easy to use, reduce the amount of EPC development time and permit a low-cost production of catalogues to guarantee the acceptance of the EPK-fix system especially in small and medium size organizations. The methodologies and specific tools support the complete life cycle of EPCs starting from the acquisition of catalogue providers' requirements, continuing with the design and implementation up to functional tests.

Results:

The EPK-fix system components comprise the formal description markup language for EPCs (EPKML) and the four tools: RASSI, SASSI, GASSI, and TASSI. EPKML is a specification language to describe static and dynamic aspects of EPCs. A Requirements ASSIstant supports the recording of information (text, images) based on structured interviews during the requirements analysis stage. It is a tool for structured elicitation of knowledge. A Specification ASSIstant is responsible for the EPC design based on the results of the RASSI tool. It converts them in a catalogue specification in EPKML. Efficient and powerful editors that assist the catalogue developer are part of this component. Generation ASSIstants make use of the EPC description that has been generated by SASSI and transform this EPKML specification into a Java program. This step automates the implementation of EPCs. Testing ASSIstants realize static tests on the catalogue description in EPKML and a dynamic validation via direct communication with the EPC generated by GASSI. Generated test data is derived from statecharts with respect to test strategies and other criteria, e.g. path or node coverage. A horn clause interpreter allows to check specified object properties. AI-relevant topics in the EPK-fix project comprise natural language knowledge-acquisition as well as rule-based completion and validation of formal specifications.

Selected publications:

References

1. A. KNAPP ET AL. EPKfix: Methods and Tools for Engineering Electronic Product Catalogues. In E. Paulus, F. M. Wahl (eds.). European Workshop on Interactive Distributed Multimedia Systems and Telecommunication Services (IDMS), LNCS. Springer 1997.
2. A. TURK. Anforderungsanalyse für Elektronische Produktkataloge. Technical Report, FR-1998-003, Bavarian Reserach Center for Knowledge-Based Systems, 1998.

Stochastic Models for Spontaneous Speech
(Akustische und linguistische Wahrscheinlichkeitsmodelle für spontan produzierte lautsprachliche Äußerungen)

Partner: Univ. Erlangen, Dep. f. Pattern Recogn.	**Supported by:** DFG
Active: 1994 – 1999	**Contact:** F. Gallwitz

Objective:

Automatic recognition of spontaneous speech is a task that proves to be much more difficult than the recognition of read speech. While read utterances are usually grammatically correct, spontaeneous utterances are often ungrammatical and filled with phenomena that are a great challenge for automatic speech recognition systems. For example, loughing, coughing and different hesitations like "em" and "hm" have to be handled by the recognizer. Furthermore, spontaneous speech often contain corrections, restarts, incomplete words etc. that human listeners are mostly unaware of, but which make automatic processing a tough problem. In this project, stocastic language models and acoustic models for spontaneous speech to be developed. This includes the tackling of nonverbal phenomena and out-of-vocabulary (OOV) words as well as the integration of prosodic information into the speech recognition process.

Results:

Our experiments are based on spontaneous speech utterances collected by a train timetable inquiry system and on utterances collected in face-to-face appointment scheduling dialogues in the Verbmobil project. We investigated several approaches of integrating nonverbal sounds into the speech recognizer using Hidden Markov Models as acoustic models and stochastic n-gram models. Furthermore, we developed an integrated approach to detect and to classify OOV words. This algorithm enables the recognizer to provide category information for OOV words, e.g. "unknown train station", which can be used by parser and dialog modules. For the two class problem 'OOV train station" vs. "other OOV word" we achieve a classification accuracy of 94%. Currently, we are developing an integrated model for words and prosodic boundaries. We achieve a significant reduction of word error rate and provide boundary information that can be used by the parser to drastically reduce its search space and to understand ambigous word sequences.

Selected publications:
References

1. F. GALLWITZ, E. NÖTH, H. NIEMANN. A Category Based Approach for Recognition of Out-of-Vocabulary Words. In Proceedings of ICSLP'96, 228-231, Philadelphia, 1996.
2. F. GALLWITZ, S. HARBECK, A. BATLINER, J. BUCKOW, E. NÖTH, H. NIEMANN. Word Recognition with Integrated Detection of Phrase Boundaries. In 3rd SQEL Workshop on Multi-Lingual Information Retrieval Dialogs, 407-414, High Tatras, Slovakia, 1998.
3. E.G. SCHUKAT-TALAMAZZINI, F. GALLWITZ, S. HARBECK, V. WARNKE. Rational Interpolation of Maximum Likelihood Predictors in Stochastic Language Modeling. In EUROSPEECH'97, Rhodos, 2731-2334, 1997.

An interactive system for the rehabilitation of patients with facial paralysis
(SFB 603)

Partner: Department of Otorhino–Larygology	Supported by: DFG
Active: 04/1998 – 12/2000	Contact: A. Gebhard

Objective:

Facial paralysis is the most frequent paralysis which occurs isolated. At the Department of Otorhino–Larygology of the University Erlangen–Nuremberg over 100 patients with new appearances of paralysis are observed per year. The aim of the project is the development of an expert system that on the one hand assists the attending physician with the diagnosis on the other hand observes and improves the patient's rehabilitation training for a better and faster cure. No such system is known and published, yet, neither for diagnosis assistance nor for the support of the rehabilitation. The technical organisation of the system consists of a computer with a frame grabber and an computer–controlled active camera (with pan/tilt-unit and controllable focus, zoom, and aperture). That allows the patient to act in a confortable way. During training the recorded face of the patient is processed online to classify the paralysis in different face regions and to analyze the degree of severity in model driven way. The success of the rehabilitation training is judged by means of the analysis results and further exercises are selected in dependence of the progress in the cure. In the clinical application the system can perform diagnosis assistance based on an unbiased judgement of the paralysis level calculated by means of measurements. On the medical side it enables a systematic and automatic evaluation and documentation of cases of paralysis and its rehabilitation. A head/face model has to be developed which takes especially possible asymme tries and functional disturbances into account. By means of this model a camera is controlled by the computer in a way that the classification decisions, the analysis performance, and as a result the judgement of the exercises will be optimized. The closed-loop active control uses – besides the image data – the camera position and the adjustment of the lens for the analysis. The project is influenced by works about an unbiased diagnosis of facial paralysis and their rehabilitation performed at the Department of Otorhino-Larygology.

Results:

First results were published in [1].

Selected publications:
References

1. U. AHLRICHS, D. PAULUS, S. WOLF. Objektivierung der Beurteilung von Gesichtsasymmetrien durch Bildanalyse. In T. Lehmann, I. Scholl, K. Spitzer (eds.): Workshop Bildverarbeitung für die Medizin, Aachen, 1996, 125–130.

GeoMed (Geographical Mediation) - Public Planning and Decision Making Support

http://www-fit-ki.gmd.de/projects/geomed.html

Partner: The GeoMed consortium consists of: Intecs Sistemi (IT) [Coordinator], GMD (D) [Technical Director], Intrasoft (GR), Vrije Universiteit Brussel (B), TNO-FEL (NL), TNO-Bouw (NL), City of Bonn (D), City of Tilburg (NL), Tuscany Region (IT), and the Technical Chamber of Greece (GR).	**Supported by:** EU
Active: 01/1997 – 07/1998	**Contact:** Dr. T. Gordon

Objective:

Using the World-Wide Web as basic infrastructure, the project implements a distributed system that provides open access to geographic information resources (GIS data) for public planning and political decision making procedures, which typically involve a large number of people with different interests, backgrounds and technical eqipment. Pilot applications in real life urban and regional planning processes, resource management and environmental assessment procedures guide the evolution of the required technological support.

Results:

The ZENO system, developed by GMD, provides the basis for the mediation services of GeoMed. ZENO allows an arbitrary large number of interested parties in various locations to take part in decision making processes extending over a long period of time. ZENO places issues, positions and arguments into a "picture" which is richer, more precise and focused than mechanisms typical of other electronic news groups. As part of a feasibility study for GeoMed, a model was created in cooperation with the City of Bonn to demonstrate ZENO's potential benefits as a mediator's assistant.

Untersuchungen zur Kompetenzeinschätzung intelligenter Systeme
am Beispiel von Lernverfahren
(Graduiertenkolleg)

Partner: TU Darmstadt, GK ISIA	**Supported by:** DFG
Active: 5/1998 – 12/2000	**Contact:** G. Grieser

Objective:

This project receives its motivation from the field of Artificial Intelligence. Besides a large amount of theoretical work, the development of methods and tools, AI mainly produces special purpose systems. As impressive some results may be as problematic are and will be the question of how much confidence man can have in those systems. If any of them crosses the borderline of its competence then it may produce counter-productive results in a way that the user may not notice the problem. Unfortunately, the boundaries of an AI system can hardly be described. This motivates the question whether and how one can enrich inference mechanisms with the ability to know about its competence and limitations. This problem seems to become more and more

Reflexives Lernen aus Beispielen (REFLEX)

Partner: FIT Leipzig e.V.	Supported by: DFG
Active: 05/1996 – 04/1998	Contact: G. Grieser

Objective:

The project motivation stems from the field of Artificial Intelligence (AI). AI as a knowledge engineering discipline comes up with a wide variety of special purpose systems. Though many AI systems do a rather impressive job either in autonomous problem solving or in assistance to humans, there arises the crucial question of those systems' competence. How much confidence man can have in complex AI systems?

The borderline of a system's competence area is usually non-rigid and, even worse, mostly unknown. If a complex system is invoked on problems beyond its competence, it may produce counterproductive results in a way that the user might not become aware of the problem.

Unfortunately, the boundaries of problem domains to which particular AI system do appropriately apply can hardly be described. This motivates the question whether and how one can enrich inference mechanisms with the ability to know about its competence and limitations. This problem seems to become increasingly more relevant because with growing distribution of AI systems more and more naive users will be confronted with those systems and will face the question whether or not to trust in those AI system's results. Competence assessment lies beyond the capabilities of the normal user. In this project, the problem of competence assessment is investigated in the well–formalized area of Inductive Inference. Even more ambitious, the results are interpreted from the perspective of AI, in general.

Results:

Reflection is understood to be the ability of a system to draw conclusions about its own behaviour. Here, we confine it to the aspect of assessing whether or not a system can solve a certain problem. More precisely, when and how an inductive learner can be enriched with reflection abilities? First, reflective behaviour of inductive learners was formalized. Different approaches like an optimistic and a pessimistic one were developed and compared. For a class of learning criteria it was studied, how reflection abilities of the learner affect the learning behaviour. For learning in the limit, reflection remarkably restricts the learnable problems. On the other hand, the actual reflection behaviour (whether it works optimistically or pessimistically, e.g.) does not influence the learning power. In the opposite, learning machines which know about the final point of learning are very sensitive to the type of reflection. Lastly, there are learning criteria where a reflection component can be added without restraining the learner.

Selected publications:

1. K. P. JANTKE. Reflecting and self-confident inductive inference machines. In Jantke, Shinohara, and Zeugmann, editors, *Proceedings ALT'95*, 283–298. Springer-Verlag, LNAI 997, 1995.
2. G. GRIESER. Selbsteinschätzung im Lernen. In Jantke, Grieser, and Wittig, editors, *Impulse für Informatik-Innovationen*, 193–202. Infix, Sankt Augustin, 1997.

Language Generation within the scope of Action-Oriented Information Processing

http://coli.lili.uni-bielefeld.de/~goecke/road.html

(DFG Priority Programme Language Production)

Partner: University of Bielefeld	Supported by: DFG
Active: 10/1997 – 10/1999	Contact: K. U. Goecke

Objective:

The aim of the project is the development of a system that provides a testing environment for the sensoric conditions under which a *conceptualization process of linguistic structures* can take place. As an exemplifying case, we consider the generation of *situation/action descriptions (SADs)* from the perspective of a simulated, behavior-oriented assembly robot (see *CoRA*, Project D1 "Communicating Agents", SFB 360 "Situated Artificial Communicators", University of Bielefeld).

Additional to the insights about conceptualization that we hope to aquire, an application of our work in the area of service robotics is well imaginable.

Results:

The system *RoAD (Robot Action Description)* has been developed to validate our hypotheses about conceptualization processes. Its basic informational structure is a hierarchy of *interpretative schemata (ISM)*. Each schema maps sensor data accrueing in *CoRA* (visual, telemetric, tactile, internal activation data and joint parameters) onto a conceptual structure (CS, Jackendoff). Furthermore, some ISM can serve as additional selection criteria for other, "higher" ones. In case an ISM is activated, the corresponding CS is passed on to a parallel, incremental surface generation component which uses a blackboard model.

At present, about twenty ISM are realized integrating five sensoric modalities. Thus, subsymbolic, conceptual, and linguistic structures are correlated and form representational units which serve as basis for natural language generation. That way, SADs like *"I drive around the obstacle"* or *"I grasp the red cube"* can be generated. We plan to be able to generate descriptive utterances of the whole range of the robots' abilities by the end of the first project period. Additionally, the conceptualization of substantiations like *"I can't reach the object because it's too far away"* is scheduled until then.

We aspire to complete the implementation of *RoAD* (Java) and the interlinking with *CoRA*. Together, these systems add up to a situated, multimodal architecture of a linguistically competent, reactive system.

Selected publications:
References

1. J.-T. MILDE, K.U. GOECKE. Umsetzung von Sensordaten in Sprache. Accepted at KI-98, Workshop Cognitive Robotics, Bremen.
2. K.U. GOECKE, J.-T. MILDE. Situations- und Aktionsbeschreibungen durch einen teilautonomen Montageroboter. To appear in: Proceedings of Konvens 98, Bonn.

Formal Specification of Spatial Concepts and Structures with Definitions and Axiomatic Characterizations
(Axiomatics of Spatial Concepts)

Partner: none	Supported by: DFG
Active: 06/1996 – 05/2000	Contact: Prof. Dr. C. Habel

Objective:

The investigation of spatial concepts is a central topic in spatial cognition [5]. The main objective of the project is to built up an inventory of formal specifications for spatial concepts and evaluate different options. Definitions and axiomatic characterizations are used to specify individual concepts as well as families of concepts. The analysis of spatial expressions of natural language and the corresponding spatial concepts determine the requirements and functions as instance of evaluation.

Results:

In [3] we describe the specification of spatial concepts that are the basis of projective terms as 'right' and 'left' or 'in front of' and 'behind' in the framework of an ordering geometry. Furthermore, this can be used as the basis for interpreting complex spatial relations as German 'links vor' ('left in front of') [4]. Ordering geometry is also the framework for an axiomatic characterization of curves, which can be seen as geometric correlates of the contours of objects [2]. These characterizations including curves do not need methods or concepts from differential geometry; we propose such a "modest" axiomatization for spatial concepts used by natural language, since structures containing more information are not justified by cognitive requirements of language processing. This planar shape geometry allows to distinguish concepts as 'vertex', 'turning point' and 'smooth point' which are the basis of the specification of shape concepts and shape nouns, as 'corner' and 'kink'. Analogue to the differentiation of line and oriented line, which is introduced in [3], we define oriented curve in [1]. By representing trajectories as oriented curves it is possible to reason about motion in qualitative manner without commitment to measuring time and path of motion. The only temporal concept which is needed in this analysis is that of simultanity.

Selected publications:
References

1. C. ESCHENBACH, C. HABEL, L. KULIK. Representing simple trajectories as oriented curves. submitted to publication.
2. C. ESCHENBACH, C. HABEL, L. KULIK, A. LESSMÖLLMANN. Shape nouns and shape concepts: A geometry for 'corner'. In C. Freksa, C. Habel, K.F. Wender (eds.), Spatial Cognition, 177–201. Springer, 1998.
3. C. ESCHENBACH, L. KULIK. An axiomatic approach to the spatial relations underlying 'left'–'right' and 'in front of'–'behind'. In G. Brewka, C. Habel, B. Nebel (eds.), KI-97: Advances in Artificial Intelligence, 207–218. Springer, 1997.
4. C. ESCHENBACH, C. HABEL, A. LESSMÖLLMANN. The interpretation of complex spatial relations by integrating frames of reference. In P. Olivier (ed.) AAAI Workshop "Language and Space", AAAI-97, Providence, RI., 45–56.
5. C. HABEL, C. ESCHENBACH. Abstract structures in spatial cognition. In C. Freksa, M. Jantzen, R. Valk (eds.), Foundations of Computer Science – Potential – Theory – Cognition, 369–378. Berlin, 1997.

Processes of Conceptualization in Language Production: A Computational Model Based on the Empirical Investigation of Event Descriptions
http://www.informatik.uni-hamburg.de/WSV/sprachproduktion/index.html
(DFG Schwerpunkt Sprachproduktion)

Partner: none	Supported by: DFG
Active: 06/1997 – 06/1999	Contact: Prof. C. Habel

Objective:

For a cognitively plausible computational model of language production based on Levelt's psycholinguistic model subprocesses of conceptualisation have to be considered: Beyond the well investigated process of linearization we assume segmentation, structuring, and selection as fundamental for building up conceptual structures. The focus of our research lies on the conceptualization of events in contrast to generating descriptions of objects or static constellations. In order to restrict the influential parameters of event conceptualization, we currently investigate verbal descriptions of dynamic sketch maps, which have been elicited experimentaly. The subjects see the genesis of the drawings on a computer screen, so that distinct events do not take place simultaneously. In producing a description verbalizers have segment the unstructured stream of impressions into meaningful units by reconstructing graphical objects and subevents.

Results:

The starting point of our work is the analysis the graphical entities, which led to the conception of a sketch grammar, reflecting a persons competence underlying sketch map production and interpretation. It is based on principles of visual perception as well as on motor processes of hand writing and drawing [1]. Within the framework of referentiel nets [2], we build up a system to represent the objects and events used in conceptualizing the drawing of sketch maps. This knowledge base reflects the systematic relations between various representational layers (RL) that interact during the conceptualization of sketch maps, namely RL of the graphical objects (e.g. lines, squares,...), RL of the real world objects (e.g. the campus, the bus stop...), RL of the drawing events (e.g. a line appears, a square is being drawn, ...), and RL of the real world events (e.g. an arrival at the subway station, ...). The analyses of the verbal protocols gives evidence that the above mentioned representational levels are not only simultanously available but can moreover be refered to within a single utterance [3]. Our examination of the discourse structures underlying the spoken texts reveals that major principles like the right frontier principle are not violated by explicit mentioning of planning or vocabulary search processes and led to the introduction of new rhetorical relations [4].

Selected publications:

References

1. M. ERICHSEN. Wissensbasierte Analyse des graphischen Inventars von Freihandzeichnungen. Exam paper. University of Hamburg.
2. CH. HABEL. Prinzipien der Referentialität. Untersuchungen zur propositionalen Repräsentation von Wissen. Berlin: Springer.
3. H. TAPPE, CH. HABEL. Verbalization of Dynamic Sketch Maps: Layers of Representation and their Interaction. http://www.informatik.uni-hamburg.de/WSV/sprachproduktion/CogSci98.ps
4. H. TAPPE, F. SCHILDER. Coherence in Spoken Discourse. In the Proceedings of the Coling/ACL. Montreal, Canada. To appear.

DBR-MAT

http://nats-www.informatik.uni-hamburg.de/~dbrmat/

Partner: Bulgarian Academy of Sciences, Linguistic Modelling Laboratory; University of Bucharest, Faculty of Mathematics, Computer Science Department; Universität Hamburg, AB Natürlichsprachliche Systeme	Supported by: Volkswagen Foundation
Active: 05/1993 - 01/1999	Contact: Prof. Dr. W. von Hahn

Objective:

The project investigates a new MAT-paradigm where the human user is supported by linguistic as well as by subject information. The basic hypotheses of the approach are:

- domain knowledge is not encoded in the lexicon entries, i.e. we distinguish clearly between the language layer and the conceptual layer;
- the representation of domain knowledge is language independent and can encode most of the semantic entries in traditional terminological lexicons;
- the user accesses domain information by highlighting a text string and formulating a request for clarification using a menu-based interface;
- factual explanations to the user are clear and transparent although the underlying formalism for knowledge representation is rather complex;
- Conceptual Graphs (CGs) are adopted as the knowledge representation formalism due to their strong expressive power and well-defined operations. CGs seem rather suitable for representing and processing terminological knowledge with different granularity.

Results:

The results of the project is a demonstrator of the translation tool for German, Bulgarian, and Romanian with a syntactic component and test lexicons in three languages. The progress of the project is documented in the Technical Reports.

Selected publications:

References

1. W. v.HAHN. Handling Multilingual Technical Terms in a Knowledge Based System. In Gyde Hansen (ed.): LSP Texts and the Process of Translation, 31 - 57. Kopenhagen 1998.
2. W. v.HAHN, G. ANGELOVA, O. KALADIJEV. The Gain of Failures: Using Side-Effects of Anaphora Resolution for Term Consistency Checks. In: Proceedings of the AIMSA Conference. Sofia 1998.
3. W. v.HAHN. Die Verbindung lexikalischer und terminologischer Definition. Lösungen in einem Übersetzungs-Unterstützungssystem. In: C. Knobloch, B. Schaeder (eds.), Nomination - fachsprachlich und gemeinsprachlich, 187 - 214. Opladen 1996.
4. W. v.HAHN, G. ANGELOVA. Combining Terminology, Lexical Semantics and Knowledge Representation in Machine Aided Translation. In: C. Galinski, K.-D. Schmitz (eds.) TKE'96, Terminology and Knowledge Engineering, 304 - 314. Frankfurt 1996.

SoLaR - Study for Structures of Speech

Partner: University of Erlangen	**Supported by:** MEDAV
Active: 11/1994 –	**Contact:** S. Harbeck

Objective:
In this project automatic processing of speech signals with various kinds of distortions as cracks changing signal/noise ratios, fading and so on is investigated. For this type of signals a cascade of pattern classifiers are to be developed. On the top level there is the classifier of speech and non-speech signals. In a very short period of time it has to be decided if there is speech on the active channel or not. The second level of the cascade consists of a language classifier. To distinguish language prosodic or acoustic effects and phonotactic or lexical information can be useful.

On the next level of the classification cascade the type of information is of interest. This classification called "topic spotting" tries to categorize all utterance of a specific language into several different classes. A possible classification scheme might be to

Analysis, Coding and Processing of Light Fields

http://sfb-603.uni-erlangen.de/HTML/German/Zusammenfassung/z-C1/z-C1.html

Partner: none	Supported by: DFG
Active: 1998 – 2000	Contact: B. Heigl

Objective:

The goal of this project is the image based modelling and visualization of objects without explicit reconstruction of the exact geometry. The basis of this approach is the so called light field [4, 2]. To get such a model, views are recorded by a camera mounted on a robot's arm. In future, the light field will be recorded using a hand-held camera without a fixed recording system. Therefore the camera positions have to be determined from a given image stream, assuming an internally calibrated camera. For a realistic scene model many views have to be taken, so the data volume becomes huge. To reduce the size, approaches for compression are developed using hierarchical methods. Other goals of the project are to create efficient visualization tools and to represent the reflection properties of objects by modeling the relationship between incoming and outcoming light field. For a better visualization and compression, knowledge about the approximative geometry is advantageous. So another goal is to reconstruct it out from an existing light field.

Results:

At the moment the light field is recorded using a calibrated robot moving around the object and taking 289 color images with the total size of 54 MBytes per light field. To reduce this data volume, existing motion compensation methods are adapted to that representation, and compressions rates of 400:1 are achieved. For visualization an efficient method is implemented using texture mapping hardware and achieving frame rates of 10 to 20 frames per second. By applying a shape–from–contour method, an approximative model for the geometry can be built [1].

The light field already has been used in the field of pattern recognition for creating training sets for statistical object models [3] and in the field of computer graphics for simulating real light sources.

Selected publications:

References

1. J. DENZLER, B. HEIGL, H. NIEMANN. An efficient combination of 2d and 3d shape descriptions for contour based tracking of moving objects. In Computer Vision - ECCV 98, LNCS. Springer, LNCS, 1998. To appear.
2. S. J. GORTLER, R. GRZESZCZUK, R. SZELINSKI, M. F. COHEN. The lumigraph. *Computer Graphics (SIGGRAPH '96 Proceedings)*, 43–54, August 1996.
3. B. HEIGL, J. DENZLER, H. NIEMANN. On the application of light field reconstruction for statistical object recognition. In EUSIPCO 98 Proceedings. To appear.
4. M. LEVOY, P. HANRAHAN. Light field rendering. Computer Graphics (SIGGRAPH '96 Proceedings), 31–45, August 1996.

SFB 527 – Integration of Symbolic and Subsymbolic Information Processing in Adaptive Sensormotoric Systems Subproject D1: Symbolic knowledge processing for autonomous sensomotoric systems Subproject D2: Task planning for sensomotoric systems

http://www.informatik.uni-ulm.de/ki/sfb-d{1,2}.html

Partner: other departments at the Univ. of Ulm	**Supported by:** DFG
Active: 01/1997 – 01/2000	**Contact:** Prof. F. von Henke

Objective:

The purpose of SFB 527 is to investigate the combination of symbolic and subsymbolic techniques for controlling autonomous sensomotoric systems. The subprojects D1 and D2 address problems arising at the symbolic level of such systems, including planning the actions the system has to take to fulfill its tasks, and the interfaces to the subsymbolic levels that use, for example, techniques based on neural networks or control theory.

Results:

The research concentrates on developing planning techniques that make it possible to control autonomous vehicles in complicated environments where quick response to unpredictable events is required. First results concern the basic case of finding a sequence of actions that reach the current goal; here, techniques for improving the efficiency of existing planning algorithms have been developed. Future research will address different forms of uncertainty present in complicated domains, and the rationality and utility of the actions performed.

Selected publications:

References

1. J. RINTANEN. A planning algorithm not based on directional search. In A. G. Cohn, L. K. Schubert, S. C. Shapiro, Principles of Knowledge Representation and Reasoning: Proceedings of the Sixth International Conference (KR '98), 617–624, San Francisco, California, 1998.

TYPELAB – A verification environment based on type theory

http://www.informatik.uni-ulm.de/ki/typelab.html

(DFG-Schwerpunktprogramm "Deduktion")

Partner: none	**Supported by:** DFG
Active: 09/1995 - 09/1998	**Contact:** F.W. von Henke

Objective:

The aim of the TYPELAB project is to develop a specification and verification environment based on an expressive logic which permits to manipulate the objects arising in software and hardware verification in a homogeneous framework.

The core logic of TYPELAB is a variant of the Calculus of Constructions, extended with constructs that facilitate the stepwise development process of software and hardware. The following are distinctive features of the resulting language:

- The language has an executable subset. Consequently, programs can be defined in TYPELAB itself and can be executed or symbolically evaluated.
- The language is polymorphic, types are first-class values. Specifications can be represented as dependent record types. In particular, operations such as refinement of specifications or parameterization of specifications are internal functions of the language.
- An intuitionistic higher-order logic is embedded in the language via the *propositions-as-types*-principle.

Results:

The efforts so far have been concentrated on creating a sound infrastructure for the TYPELAB system in general and for support of deductive processes in particular. TYPELAB has a graphical user interface which facilitates moving between goals, displaying proof trees, resetting the proof state and applying tactics.

Furthermore, the theoretical foundations for deductive support in the system have been elaborated. The deductive machinery is based on a calculus with existential variables and explicit substitutions. For this calculus, a sequent-style proof method has been developed and implemented, equational reasoning has been incorporated.

The TYPELAB system is operational and can be demonstrated.

Selected publications:

References

1. F.W. VON HENKE, M. LUTHER, M. STRECKER. TYPELAB: An environment for modular program development. In M. Dauchet, M. Bidoit, editors, Proceedings TAPSOFT'97, 851–854. Springer LNCS 1214, 1997.
2. M. STRECKER, M. SOREA. Integrating an equality prover into a software development system based on type theory. In G. Brewka, Ch. Habel, B. Nebel, editors, Proceedings KI'97, 147–158. Springer LNAI 1303, 1997.
3. M. STRECKER, M. LUTHER, F.W. VON HENKE. Interactive and automated proof construction in type theory. In Bibel, Schmitt: Automated Deduction — A Basis for Applications. Kluwer Academic Publishers, 1998.

Functional Brain Analysis with AI Tools
http://aida.intellektik.informatik.tu-darmstadt.de/~chris/bmbf.html
(Max-Planck-Institute of Cognitive Neuroscience)

Partner: Clinic for Neurology, Mainz University Clinic; Supported by: BMBF
Walter Graphtek GmbH, Bad Oldesloe
Active: 04/1998 - 03/2001   Contact: Dr. C. Herrmann

Objective:
The project is subdivided into three parts:

- methodology (MPI Leipzig),
- rule-generation and -evaluation (Mainz University Clinic), and
- implementation (Walter Graphtek).

The project is intended to further develop the approach introduced in [1] for rule-based analysis of electroencephalograms (EEGs) into a clinically applicable tool for neurologists and brain researchers. The cooperation between a clinic which is specialized in neurology, a research institute working in the field of analyzing electrophysiological data and a company that produces digital EEG recording devices represents a tripartite round of development. In the first stage of development neurologists formulate the rules needed to detect certain phenomena in the EEG. In the second stage methodologists develop the necessary approaches to extract and manipulate appropriate parameters from the EEG signal which allows symbolical reasoning. In the final stage computer scientists implement the software and integrate it into their EEG recording devices. After one round of development the applicability of the system is evaluated by the neurologist. Rules that do not function properly on their target phenomena are revised and the round is renewed.

Approaches from signal analysis (e.g. frequency domain representation) are used for pre-processing. The artificially intelligent reasoning is subsequently carried out by a fuzzy rule-based system. In addition to the rules of the neurologist, a neural network automatically generates further rules.

Selected publications:

1. C.S. HERRMANN. Ein hybrides KI–System zur medizinischen Befundung: am Beispiel der Elektroenzephalographie. Dissertation, TH Darmstadt, FG Intellektik, Infix–Verlag, 1996.

AVAnTA - Automatical Video Analysis for Textual Annotation

(Strategic research initiative Distributed Processing and Exchange of Digital Documents)

Partner: The Bremen Radio and TV Station	**Supported by:** DFG
Active: 01/1998 – 01/2000	**Contact:** Prof. Dr. O. Herzog

Objective:

In this project research is performed in the areas of subsymbolic and symbolic analysis of video sequences including some audio features. The goal is to establish content analysis algorithms by combining the results of the analysis of the different input streams at a knowledge-based level. For each input stream, structured textual annotations are generated. These annotations will serve as input data for the content-based retrieval that integrates text, images, and video in distributed electronic libraries. We build upon the results of the IRIS project that has been carried through from 1994-1997. The algorithms that were developed there allow for a syntactical and semantical analysis of still images.

Selected publications:

References

1. P. ALSHUTH, TH. HERMES, J. KREYSS, M. RÖPER. Gesucht – gefunden!?: Wissensbasiertes Bildretrieval. KI(1), 1997.
2. O. HERZOG. Bild- und Videoretrieval für Digitale Bibliotheken. Proceedings of the 6. Heidelberger Bildverarbeitungsforum, July 1997, Kaiserslautern, Germany, 1997.

cosap: Ecological Impact Analysis

http://www.tzi.uni-bremen.de/grp/cosap

Partner: Institute for Environmental Process Engineering, University of Bremen	Supported by: Stadtwerke Bremen AG
Active: – 10/1997	Contact: Prof. Dr. O. Herzog

Results:

Main focus of work between 08/97 and 07/98: We have developed a software system which offers technical support for an ecological impact analysis. The system allows the user to model production processes in a stream-oriented way, to balance the contained materials and streams, and to identify ecological weak points automatically. Based upon this model, the Elwira-subsystem has been developed. Elwira supports the application of production-oriented environmental protection. The production processes modelled with cosap are screened for their environmental impact assessment (EIA) involving ecological criteria. A first prototype models the recycling of materials from sewage water within a particular production process.

Selected publications:

References

1. H. STUCKENSCHMIDT, I. TIMM, J. SCHRÖDER, D. HARTMANN. Elwira: wissensbasierte Methoden für den produktionsintegrierten Umweltschutz Umweltinformatik '97, 11. Symposium Informatik für den Umweltschutz, W. Geiger and A. Jaeschke, O. Rentz, E. Simon, Th. Spengler, L. Zilliox, T. Zundel, Reihe Umweltinformatik Aktuell. MetropolisVerlag, Marburg September 1997.
2. H. STUCKENSCHMIDT, I. TIMM, J. SCHRÖDER, D. HARTMANN. Elwira - Elemente eines wissensbasierten Systems zur Reduzierung umweltrelevanter Auswirkungen. In: Wissensbasierte Systeme in Umweltanwendungen, H. Keller, K.C. Ranze, Forschungsberichte FZKA, Karlsruhe 1997.

exupro/DECIDE

http://www.tzi.org/is/exupro/

Partner: Bremen Institute of Industrial Technology and Applied Work Science at Bremen University (BIBA), Heinrich Bühnen KG Ltd., Bremen, Junge & Warncken Ltd., Bremen	**Supported by:** State of Bremen
Active: 10/1995 – 06/1999	**Contact:** Prof. Dr. O. Herzog

Topics:

Knowledge based System, Multiagent System

Results:

Main focus of work between 08/97 and 07/98: exupro is a C/S system designed for the modeling and processing of assessment tasks. Assessment models are represented as compiled knowledge bases in relational databases. DECIDE (DECision support In Distributed Environments) is an agent-based extension of exupro to support a group of experts in order to find a common evaluation for several assessment goals. The experts within the DECIDE framework might be human or computer, with different types of assessment criteria. Different types of conflicts between the experts may be resolved through mediated negotiation. Different problem-solving methods are defined within task/method-slots with clear interfaces.

Selected publications:
References

1. K. C. RANZE, H. J. MÜLLER, O. HOLLMANN, O. HERZOG. Handling Conflicts in Distributed Assessment Situations. Accepted for Workshop Conflicts among agents: avoid or use them?, held during ECAI'98, Brighton.
2. M. ESSER, A. HOLSTEN, K. C. RANZE. exupro – Umweltbewertung von Produktionsdaten zur Umsetzung einer ökologischen Produktionsplanung und –steuerung. In H.-J. Bullinger, L.M. Hilty, C. Rautenstrauch (eds.): Betriebliche Umweltinformationssysteme in Produktion und Logistik. Metropolis, Marburg 1998.
3. H. J. MÜLLER, K. C. RANZE. Über den Einsatz von Multi-Agenten Systemen in Umweltanwendungen. In W. Geiger, A. Jaeschke, O. Rentz, E. Simon, T. Spengler, L. Zilliox, T. Zundel (eds.), Proceedings zum 11. Internationalen Symposium Informatik für den Umweltschutz. Metropolis, Marburg, 1997.

FlowTEC: IT support for Virtual Enterprises

http://www.informatik.uni-bremen.de/grp/flowtec/

Partner: none	Supported by: University of Bremen
Active: 10/1997 – 10/1999	Contact: Prof. Dr. O. Herzog

Topics:

KADS, AI-Technologies

Results:

Main focus of work between 08/97 and 07/98: Development of an information management system, that supports a Virtual Enterprise (VE). It will provide access to the Internet for Small and Medium sized Enterprizes (SME's). Within the project the functional specification for an IT system has been created to support a number of companies in respect to the IT structure of a Virtual Enterprise. The requirements for such a system are models of the organisation structure, models of the workflows, integration of existing CSCW systems and other applications, and the management of the creation and changes of documents. Another important aspect is the security management. It should be possible to generate the common tasks and the organisation structure of the VE. The parts of the individual organisation models and workflow definitions which coincide with VE must be mapped onto the FlowTEC system. The sys tem must be flexible, that means it has to allow changes of the organisation and workflow models at run time. KADS models are used in order to record the requirements.

Selected publications:

References

1. G. JOERIS. Cooperative and Integrated Workflow and Document Management for Engineering Applications. Proceedings of the 8th Int. Workshop on Database and Expert Systems Applications, Workshop on Workflow Management in Scientific and Engineering Applications, 68 – 73, Sept. '97, Toulouse, France, 1997.

Determination of Organism-Specific Oligonucleotide Sequences for Genetic Sensors
(BioRegio)

Partner: R & D Consortium 'Genetic Sensoring' of Bremen (BIAS, IMSAS, IOMC, TZI, UFT, ZHG)	Supported by: BMBF, State of Bremen
Active: 06/1998 – 03/2000	Contact: Prof. Dr. O. Herzog

Objective:

Genetic sensors can be used to analyze arbitrary probes containing nucleic acid material. Main application fields are the food industry, medicine and environmental protection. The analytical quality of such sensors depends on the selectivity and specifity of the used oligonucleotide sequences, which have to be extracted from international nucleic acid databases. This is a complex task requiring several intermediate steps. Each step produces results which have to be interpreted biologically and prepared for the next step. The goal of this project is to build a knowledge-based assistance system to support this process as much as possible.

Selected publications:
References

1. U. BOHNEBECK, W.SÄLTER, O. HERZOG, M. WISCHNEWSKY, D. BLOHM. An Approach to mRNA Signalstructure Detection through Knowledge Discovery. In D. Frishman, H.W. Mewes (eds.), Computer Science and Biology, Proceedings of the German Conference on Bioinformatics GCB'97, 1997.
2. U. BOHNEBECK, T. HORVATH, S. WROBEL. Term Comparisions in First-Order Similarity Measures. To appear in, Proceedings of the Eighth International Conference on Inductive Logic Programming (ILP'98), 1998.

Multi-Agent Systems Supporting Transport Logistics

Partner: none	**Supported by:** State of Bremen
Active: 01/1998 – 01/2001	**Contact:** Prof. Dr. O. Herzog

Topics:
Multi-Agent Systems, Dynamic Conflict Management, Machine Learning

Results:
Main focus of work between 01/98 and 07/98: This project is based on a scenario for the transportation domain. Within this scenario manufacturer and haulage companies are working in an alliance with the aim to reduce environmental pollution through planning and optimizing their transports. Negotiations and planning of this alliance are modelled with the help of a multi-agent system. Agents represent the companies associated with the alliance and follow economical business goals. This behaviour can lead to decision conflicts between the global goal of reducing environmental pollution and the individual goal of achieving maximal profit. Two different levels of conflicts can be identified, the conflict within negotiations and the conflict within the individual planning process of transport. The project is focused on conflict management in combination with behavior adaption. In this area we transfer results from decision and game theory to this domain and expand it by machine learning methods. Another research goal is to find an adequate communication protocol supporting the conflict management adequately. We will design new concepts of open protocols, where agents negotiate with agents to define common communication protocols on the base of elementary market-mechanism protocols.

Selected publications:
References

1. I. J. TIMM. Multi-Agentensysteme zur Unterstützung ökologischer Transportlogistik. Proceedings der Umweltinformatik Tagung 1998, Bremen. To appear.

Coordination of Material Flows in International Production Networks

Partner: Business Administration Department, University of Bremen, LEAR Corporation Ltd., Bremen	**Supported by:** State of Bremen
Active: 06/1998 – 06/2001	**Contact:** Prof. Dr. O. Herzog

Topics:

Multi-Agent Systems, Knowledge Representation.

Results:

Main focus of work between 08/97 and 07/98: In this project we investigate the coordination of material flow in international production networks. We use multi-agent systems on the basis of negotiation-oriented methods to model an inter-enterprise material flow management. For this, the material flow management between the collaborator LEAR Corporation Ltd. and its international sub-contractors will be exemplarily investigated. In particular, the objective is an efficient coordination of the individual production units with regards to environment, costs, and quality. One of the projects goals is the improvement of the order-related cooperation between LEAR Corporation and its sub-contractors in order to ensure just-in-time-production. Thus, the enterprise shall be supported in its endeavours to reorganize the processes in connection with the exchange of information and material with its subcontractors. At the same time this project represents a contribution to the optimization of the logistics management as well as to the support of the local automobile industry on regional and nationwide markets.

Selected publications:

References

1. G. JOERIS, CH. KLAUCK, O. HERZOG. Dynamical and Distributed Process Management based on Agent Technology. 6th Scandinavian Conference on Artificial Intelligence (SCAI'97), August '97, Helsinki, Finland, 187–198.
2. G. JOERIS. Change Management Needs Integrated Process and Configuration Management. European Software Engineering Conference (ESEC/FSE'97), Sept. '97, Zurich, Swiss, 125–141.
3. CH. KLAUCK, H.J. MÜLLER. Formal Business Process Engineering Based on Graph Grammars. International Journal on Production Economics 50, Special Issue on Business Process Reengineering (1997) 129–140.

ModE-U: Modeling Expertise under Uncertainty

Partner: none	**Supported by:** State of Bremen
Active: 01/1996 – 01/2001	**Contact:** Prof. Dr. O. Herzog

Objective:

Main focus of work between 08/97 and 07/98: The first stage of the project elaborates an approach to the explicit integration of uncertain reasoning mechanisms into conventional KADS-based models of expertise. We assume that uncertainty is present in the model of expertise in the sense that terminological knowledge is available but some assertions cannot be determined due to uncertainty. Therefore we have introduced an approach enabling the specification of uncertain knowledge in a logic-based setting. For this purpose we enhanced existing specification languages based on the well-known KADS model of expertise with a causal model of uncertainty which is based on the framework of valuation-based systems and Pearl's model of uncertainty.

Selected publications:

References

1. K.C. RANZE, H. STUCKENSCHMIDT. Modeling Uncertainty in Expertise. Accepted for IT&Knows, held during 15th IFIP World Computer Congress, Vienna, Budapest, August 30th - September 5th.
2. H. STUCKENSCHMIDT, K.C. RANZE. Extending KBS Specification Languages with a Causal Model of Uncertainty. Submitted to FroCoS'98,"Frontiers of Combining Systems", October 2-4, 1998, ILLC, University of Amsterdam.
3. K.C. RANZE, H. STUCKENSCHMIDT. Bridging Gaps in Models of Expertise. Submitted to Workshop Inference-Mechanisms in Knowledge-Based-Systems: Theory and Applications, held at KI-98, Bremen, 15–17. September 1998.

MOKASSIN: Innovative Approaches for Modelling and Integrating complex Processes and Systems

http://www.tzi.uni-bremen.de/grp/mokassin

(Initiative zur Förderung der Software-Technologie in Wirtschaft, Wissenschaft und Technik)

Partner: VSS GmbH, Bremen; Bremen Institute of Industrial Technology and Applied Work Science, University of Bremen	**Supported by:** BMBF
Active: 03/1996 – 03/1999	**Contact:** Prof. Dr. O. Herzog

Topics:

AI software engineering, knowledge representation, multi agent systems

Results:

Main focus of work between 08/97 and 07/98: In the MOKASSIN project we are developing a software tool - the MOKASSIN system - which actively supports the modelling and enactment of business processes. In MOKASSIN we extend workflow techniques with the ability of dynamic model changes in order to allow modifications of processes at any time. Furthermore, we support cooperated work within a workflow. Finally, in order to allow an uniform view of heterogeneous information systems we use enterprise ontologies for their integration. The framework of the MOKASSIN system is a multi-agent system. A first prototyp of the MOKASSIN system was presented ot CeBIT'98.

Selected publications:

References

1. G. JOERIS, CH. KLAUCK, O. HERZOG. Dynamical and Distributed Process Management based on Agent Technology. 6th Scandinavian Conference on Artificial Intelligence (SCAI'97), August '97, Helsinki, Finland, (1997) 187–198.
2. G. JOERIS. Change Management Needs Integrated Process and Configuration Management. European Software Engineering Conference (ESEC/FSE'97), Sept. '97, Zurich, Swiss, 125–141.
3. CH. KLAUCK, H.J. MÜLLER. Formal Business Process Engineering Based on Graph Grammars. International Journal on Production Economics 50, Special Issue on Business Process Reengineering 1997, 129–140.

Intelligent Measurement Interpretation of a Physical System as part of the PIUS-project

http://www.tzi.uni-bremen.de

Partner: Institute for Environmental Process Engineering, University of Bremen, Institute for Microsensors, –actuators and –systems, University of Bremen	Supported by: University of Bremen
Active: 09/1995 – 02/1999	Contact: Prof. Dr. O. Herzog

Topics:

Knowledge Based Systems, Learning

Results:

Main focus of work between 08/97 and 07/98: The automatic interpretation of measurement data is a problem with great practical importance. Due to the need of process control, a physical system is generally equipped with a lot of sensors. This project examines possibilities to use the acquired data to improve the insights into the system dynamics. Methods from machine learning and knowledge discovery are used to extract knowledge out of multiple time series of a physical system. The project is focused on rule extraction out of measurement data. For this task, we have developed a special pre–processing method for time series, and a new inductive learning algorithm was specified to handle continuous attributes in decision tree induction.

Selected publications:

References

1. M. BORONOWSKY. Automatisches Erstellen qualitativer Modelle von Abwasserbehandlungsanlagen. In: Elftes internationales Symposium der Gesellschaft für Informatik (GI), volum 15 -f IIm lti f   ·i' l· ll ^^· ^ ^

mRNA Signal Structure Detection Through Knowledge Discovery

Partner: University of Bremen, Department of Molecular Genetics and Biotechnology, and German National Research Center for Information Technology, SET.KI	Supported by: State of Bremen and ILP II end user club 1 [a]
	[a] associated with ESPRIT IV Long Term Research Project ILP II (No. 20237)
Active: 09/1995 – 02/1999	Contact: Prof. Dr. O. Herzog

Topics:

Inductive Logic Programming, Knowledge Discovery, Computational Molecular Biology

Results:

Main focus of work between 08/97 and 07/98: mRNA signal structure detection requires new approaches in computational molecular biology, especially classification and clustering methods for screening large data sets of mRNA secondary structures. Until now work was focused on classification of known mRNA signal structures, to develop a biologically founded similarity measure. Similarity measures used in firstorder IBL have been limited so far to the function-free case, but a lot of predictive power can be gained by allowing lists and other terms in the input representation. Therefore an appropriate similarity measure was developed, that works directly on these structures.

Selected publications:

References

1. U. BOHNEBECK, T. HORVATH, S. WROBEL. Term Comparisons in First-Order Similarity Measures. In D. Page, editor, Proceedings of the 8th International Workshop on Inductive Logic Programming. Springer 1998. To appear.
2. U. BOHNEBECK, T. HORVATH, W. SÄLTER, S. WROBEL. Klassifikation von mRNA-Signalstrukturen durch Relationales Lernen aus Beispielen. Workshop KI'98, 1998.
3. U. BOHNEBECK, W. SÄLTER, O. HERZOG, M. WISCHNEWSKY, D. BLOHM. An Approach to mRNA Signal Structure Detection through Knowledge Discovery. In Proceedings of GCB'97, 125–126, 1997.

3-dimensional Scene Interpretation
(ISP - Technology Investment Program)

Partner: BWM Bremen, DASA - RI, Bremen	**Supported by:** University of Bremen
Active: 02/1997 - 02/2000	**Contact:** Prof. Dr. O. Herzog

Objective:

Main focus of work between 08/97 and 07/98:

Development of a system aiming at a 3-dimensional scene interpretation as an intelligent navigation support for a mobile robot. A novel laser-camera, which has been developed by Dasa-RI, is integrated as an acquisition device in our system. This laser camera is an active visual system and provides both grey-level and distance images. A distance image is a 2-dimensional matrix, where each element of the matrix represents the distance value between the camera and a corresponding point of an object surface. Both images are processed by low-level image processing functions, like noise reduction, segmentation and thinning. The process of 3D-interpretation is based on the syntactic description of images. The first scenario is aimed at detecting special landmarks as spatial orientation objects and to estimate the self-localization of the camera in a room using a triangulation method. The geometry models of these landmarks are known a-priori. The 3-dimensional method comparing 2-dimensional with textured marks is well suited for an arbitrary textured background. The goal of another scenario is the model-based identification of different objects, estimation of their geometrical form, and their spatial position.

Results:

Our first highlight was presented during the Hannover Messe'98. The demonstrated system controls an industrial robot for the exact localization of an object in a box filled with objects of the same kind.

LOCAS: Situations, Actions, and Causality in Logic

http://pikas.inf.tu-dresden.de/projekte/lokas.html

(DFG Schwerpunktprogramm Deduktion)

Partner: TU Dresden	**Supported by:** DFG
Active: 01/1995–01/2001 (projected)	**Contact:** Prof. Dr. S. Hölldobler

Objective:

The goal of LOCAS is the combination of different approaches for deductive planning, like e.g. the linear connection method, fragments of linear/affine logic, and situation calculus, within one deductive system.

In LOCAS planning is considered as constructing a witness for the reachability of a set of *goal-states* from a given set of *initial-state* within a transition system. In order to perform planning deductively, one represents states and transitions in a fragment of a well-chosen logic, that allows to establish a simple correspondence between proofs and plans.

Based on the fluent-calculus [1] and the result of [2], where it was shown that the linear connection method, a fragment of linear logic, and the fluent calculus are similar expressive, concerning conjunctive resource-oriented planning problems, the fluent calculus is extended as a general technique for formalizing provability of various fragments of logics within equational logic. This extension allows to treat (specialized inference methods for) these fragments in a uniform way.

The results will be implemented in a distributed planning system.

Results:

The first part of the project was mainly theoretical oriented. We have focused on revealing the relations between resource sensitive logics, non-classical connection methods, and variants of the fluent calculus (e.g. [2,3]). In particular efficient methods for (disjunctive) resource-oriented planning were developed and implemented in a prototypical system.

Selected publications:

References

1. S. HÖLLDOBLER, J. SCHNEEBERGER. A New Deductive Approach to Planning. New Generation Computing, 8: 225-244, 1990.
2. G. GROSSE, S. HÖLLDOBLER, J. SCHNEEBERGER. Linear Deductive Planning. Journal of Logic and Computation, 6(2): 233-262, 1996.
3. E. SANDNER. From Linear Proofs to Direct Logic with Exponentials. KI-97: Advances in Artificial Intelligence, 135–146. Springer, LNAI 1303, 1997.

Foundations of Data Warehouse Quality (DWQ)

http://www.dbnet.ece.ntua.gr/~dwq/

(ESPRIT Long Term Research Project)

Partner: NTUA (Greece), RWTH Aachen, DFKI (Germany), INRIA (France), IRST, Uniroma (Italy)	Supported by: EU
Active: 10/1996 – 10/1999	Contact: Prof. Dr. M. Jarke

Objective:

Data warehouses (DW) are large scale information systems designed for decision support based upon information from various heterogeneous sources. DWQ is targeted at the development of techniques and tools to support the design, operation, and evolution of a DW based on a quality-oriented, semantically rich representation of meta-data. To achieve this goal, DWQ combines techniques from database research such as query optimisation and update propagation with methods developed in knowledge representation and reasoning. The latter methods play an important rôle for the conceptual modeling and provide sophisticated reasoning services used in DW design and evolution. A project overview is given in [4].

Results:

A novel DW architecture model represents explicitly the three different perspectives (conceptual, logical, and physical) of a DW. The model is linked to a quality model generalizing the goal-question-metric approach from software engineering. This meta information is stored in a repository and can be queried to analyse the structure and the quality of a DW [3]. Specialized reasoners can be attached to the repository for the evaluation of quantitative (e.g., performance, reliability, freshness) and qualitative (e.g., accessibility, completeness, consistency, view reusability) quality factors. As a basis for reasoners suited for the specific problems in DWs, the complexity of inference problems for Description Logics with specific aggregation functions was studied [1] and a new Description Logic for representing knowledge about abstract aggregation was developed [2].

Selected publications:

References

1. F. BAADER, U. SATTLER. Description logics with concrete domains and aggregation. In Proc. ECAI-98, 1998.
2. I. HORROCKS, U. SATTLER. A description logic with transitive and converse roles and role hierarchies. In Proc. Int. Workshop on Description Logics, Trento, 1998.
3. M. JARKE, M.A. JEUSFELD, C. QUIX, P. VASSILIADIS. Architecture and quality in data warehouses. In Proc. 10th Conf. Advanced Information Systems Eng., Pisa, 1998.
4. M. JARKE, Y. VASSILIOU. Data warehouse quality: A review of the DWQ project. In Proc. 2nd Conf. on Information Quality, MIT, Cambridge, MA, 1997.

MEMO
Mediating and Monitoring Electronic Commerce
http://infolab.kub.nl/prj/esprit/memo/
(ESPRIT)

Partner: ABN/AMRO Netherlands, Origin Spain, FEND Spain; RWTH Aachen, IHK Aachen, IMK Netherlands; Tilburg University, Sarenet Spain	**Supported by:** EU
Active: 06/1998 – 12/2000	**Contact:** Prof. Dr. M. Jarke

Objective:

The project MEMO aims to investigate the principles of an agent-like electronic broker system for the full life cycle of business-to-business commerce, i.e. from partner identification to bank-guaranteed international business transaction execution. Specifically, the broker system will assist partner campanies to manage business data (product and partner profiles), to search for business-related information, to negotiate about contract terms (using predefined chunks of a formal business communication language), and to enact the contract by an EDIFACT-based workflow engine. The broker system encorporates the semantically rich meta database system ConceptBase for representing knowledge and facts about the commerce of partner companies. The search engine utilizes concept definitions for vertical markets (business branches). Furthermore, the formal business communication language is founded on deontic logics.

Results:
- architecture for the electronic commerce broker
- identification of key tools (ConceptBase, FLBC)

Selected publications:
References

1. M.P. PAPAZOGLOU, M.A. JEUSFELD, H. WEIGAND, M. JARKE. Distributed, interoperable workflow support for Electronic Commerce. In Proc. GI/IFIP Conf. Trends in Electronic Commerce (TREC'98), Hamburg, Germany, June 3-5, 1998.

MIDAS: Explorative Data Mining in Business Applications
(Aachener Graduiertenkolleg Informatik und Technik)

Partner: Informatik V, RWTH Aachen; Tengelmann Warenhandelsgesellschaft	Supported by: DFG
Active: 2/1995-2/1998	Contact: Prof. Dr. M. Jarke

Objective:

Knowledge discovery in business applications requires an explorative data mining approach that combines human intuition and goal-finding with efficient automated segmentation, reasoning, and learning techniques. The MIDAS project investigates two integration issues: (a) the linking of segmentation and classification based on neural networks, with the generation of symbolic pattern descriptions based on fuzzy logic; (b) the two-way link between formal and visually interactive representations of identified knowledge. Specific project goals include the development of an experimental explorative data mining environment, called MIDAS, and its experimental evaluation in different application domains.

Results:

MIDAS consists of a set of visually oriented interaction tools backed up by a combination of subsymbolic and symbolic algorithms on top of a database [1]. Bridging the gap between numerical data and symbolic descriptions, a technique called STS constructs fuzzy-variables separating the feature space of data stored in a Kohonen map [2]. These terms together with learned interrelations between automatically discovered patterns [3], serve as a vocabulary for a learning algorithm, named mcF-ID3, which learns pattern descriptions. To enable interactive exploration functionalities, patterns are visualized based on a data structure called P-matrix [2,3]. Effects of learned or manually designed descriptions and terms as well as users' manipulations can directly be visualized by color overlay techniques within this structure. This enables a user to switch easily between data mining and visual exploration.

MIDAS has been used successfully in two commercial projects concerning the analysis of retail and of city population descriptive data. Incorporating users' insights gained by visual exploration into automatic data mining, and vice versa, led in both studies to remarkable results, which the users had great confidence in.

Selected publications:
References

1. M. GEBHARDT, M. JARKE, M. A. JEUSFELD, C. QUIX, S. SKLORZ. Tools for data warehouse quality. In Proc. 10th SSDBM, IEEE CS Press. Capri, Italy, July 1998.
2. S. SKLORZ, M. MÜCKE. A hybrid approach for medical data analysis. In Proc. of the 5th European Congr. on Intelligent Techniques and Soft Computing (EUFIT), 2:1162–1166. Aachen, Germany, Sept. 1997.
3. S. SKLORZ. A method for data analysis based on self-organizing feature maps. In Proc. of WAC'96, Soft Computing with Industrial Applications, 5:611–616. TSI Press Series. Montpellier, France, May 1996.

Verbmobil (Subtasks: End-to-end evaluation of current systems, testing of scenario settings, Wizard-of-Oz recordings, dialogue and prosody)

http://nats-www.informatik.uni-hamburg.de/~vm/
(Verbmobil Verbundprojekt)

Partner: DFKI Saarbrücken; Phondat LMU München; University of Bielefeld; FAU Erlangen; CMU Pittsburgh; Prof. Kurematsu, Tokyo; Universität Hamburg, AB Natürlichsprachliche Systeme	**Supported by:** BMBF
Active: 01/1998 - 01/2001	**Contact:** Dr. S. Jekat

Objective:

Verbmobil is a long-term interdisciplinary Language Technology project. The Verbmobil System recognizes spoken input, analyzes and translates it, and utters the translation. This speaker-independent system processes spontaneous speech. Verbmobil offers assistance in multilingual dialog situations in certain domains (e.g. scheduling appointments, travel planning and making hotel reservations). The project is a joint initiative involving information-technology companies, universities, and research centers.

The part of the project at the University of Hamburg is currently engaged in the evaluation of spoken language systems, in Wizard-of-Oz recordings and the testing of scenario settings, and in investigating the interface between dialogue and prosody.

Results:

Development of a corpus of multilingual spontaneous spoken language dialogues, contributions to Verbmobil scenario design and dialogue modelling, end-to-end evaluation of the current demonstrators.

Selected publications:

References

1. S. J. JEKAT, H. TAPPE, H. GERLACH, T. SCHOELLHAMMER. Dialogue Interpreting: Data and Analysis. VM-Report 189, Universität Hamburg, April 1997.
2. S. J. JEKAT, C. SCHEER, T. SCHULTZ. VMII Szenario I: Instruktionen für alle Sprachstellungen - VMII Scenario I: Instructions. VM-Techdoc 62, Universität Hamburg, LMU München, Universität Karlsruhe, September 1997.
3. D. CAVAR, U. JOST. End-to-End Evaluation des Verbmobil Herbstdemonstrators 1997 Verbmobil Memo.

Technology of Information for Communication and Cooperation
(SFB 467: Transformable Business Structures for Multi-Variant Serial Production)

Partner: Prof. Dr. P. Levi, Prof. Dr. K. Rothermel	**Supported by:** DFG
Active: 01/1997 – 12/1999	**Contact:** Prof. Dr. P. Levi

Objective:

This subproject aims to provide a platform which is necessary for the communication and cooperation infrastructure between distributed and autonomous performance units. The infrastructure has to be well suited for the increased requirements of adaptable corporate structures. First a general model for communication and cooperation will be developed. This model will be taken as a starting point to develop more specialized models for cooperation between software agents and between humans interacting with telecooperation tools. Both approaches will be integrated by analyzing the interactions, the media, data objects and the definition of the human computer interface.

Selected publications:
References

1. M. BECHT, M. MUSCHOLL, P. LEVI. Transformable Multi-Agent Systems: A specification language for cooperation processes. In Proceedings of the World Automation Congress (WAC), Sixth International Symposium on Manufacturing with Applications (ISOMA), 1998.
2. M. BECHT, M. MUSCHOLL, P. LEVI. Ein Framework für Kooperationsverfahren zwischen Roboteragenten. In P. Levi, Th. Bräunl, N. Oswald, editors: Autonome Mobile Systeme, Informatik aktuell, 166 - 177. Berlin u. a., 1997. Universität Stuttgart, Institut für Parallele und Verteilte Höchstleistungsrechner, Springer.

Multiagent softwarearchitecture for a Measuring and Testing centre

(SFB 514: Active Exploration by Sensor-Actor-Feedback for Adaptive Measurement and Inspection Technology)

Partner: none	**Supported by:** DFG
Active: 01/1998 - 01/2001	**Contact:** Prof. Dr. P. Levi

Objective:

The Topic of the SFB is the development of new extensions for industrial measuring and inspection technology. Through a coordinated interaction of mechanical actors the measurement procedure can be adapted flexibly to the current situation. As a result, the area of application of optical sensors is expanded and the test of optically and visual features (shine, color) is enabled. The main tasks for this project in the context of this SFB are the conception of a multiagent system architecture, development of models for high level image processing and integration of learning techniques.

Selected publications:

References

1. G. HETZEL, P. LEVI. Sensor-Aktor-Kopplung zur explorativen Bildauswertung. 5. Syposium Bildverarbeitung 1997, Technische Akademie Esslingen.

OBIDICOTE: On Board Identification, Diagnosis and Control of Gas Turbine Engines
(Programme of Brite/Euram Projekt)

Partner: Institut für Parallele und Verteilte Höchstleistungsrechner, Universität Stuttgart	**Supported by:** EU-Projekt **Projektpartner:** Alfa Romeo Avio, Lufthansa Technik AG, MTU Muenchen GmbH, Rolls-Royce plc, Snecma, Techspace Aero, Volvo Aero Corp AB, Chalmers University of Technology AB, TU Muenchen, National Technik University of Athens, Universite Catholique de Louvain
Active: 02/1998 – 02/2002	**Contact:** Prof. Dr. P. Levi

Objective:

Prototyp eines On Board Diagnosesystems für Flugzeugtriebwerke.

Makro - DEsign and realisation of an autonomous multi-segment sewer robot platform

http://www.gmd.de/FIT/KI/CogRob/Projects/Makro/makro-engl/makro-e.html

Partner: rhenag Rheinische Energie Aktiengesellschaft, Kln (Koordinator), FZI, Karlsruhe, Inspector Systems Rainer Hitzel GmbH, Rödermark.	**Supported by:** BMBF
Active: 10/1997 – 10/2000	**Contact:** F. Kirchner

Objective:

The goal of the MAKRO project is to develop a prototype of a multi-segment robot platform which can operate autonomously in sewer pipes of nominal diameters ranging from 300 mm through 600 mm. By the end of the project term, a working prototype shall be employable for the video inspection of a real, roughly cleaned sewer that is not flooded by rain. Depending on the actually achievable quality of a radio link, a human operator must be able to take over the control of the platform, if necessary.

Results:

MAKRO is based on results of the also funded feasibility investigation LAOKOON, which we conducted with partners in 1995. One result of this preliminary work is a concept of a robot platform and design studies of numerous details. Meanwhile, a first prototype of the active drive and joint elements, and the hardware/software control architecture have been completed, first experimental platform studies have been performed.

Selected publications:
References

1. J. HERTZBERG, TH. CHRISTALLER, F. KIRCHNER, U. LICHT, E. ROME. Sewer Robotics. Submitted to the Tenth Innovative Applications of Artificial Intelligence Conference, Madison, Wisconsin, July 26-30, 1998.
2. J. HERTZBERG, TH. CHRISTALLER, F. KIRCHNER, U. LICHT UND E. ROME. MAKRO - Serviceroboter im Kanalbetrieb. In J. Lenz (ed) Globalisierung der Märkte und internationale Arbeitsteilung - auch im Rohrleitungsbau? 12. Oldenburger Rohrleitungsforum, 643-652. Vulkan-Verlag, Essen, 1998.
3. F. KIRCHNER, J. HERTZBERG. A Prototype Study of an Autonomous Robot Platform for Sewerage System Maintenance. Autonomous Robots 4(4), 1997, S. 319-331.

DAWAI
Ressourcenbeschränkte Analyse gesprochener Sprache
http://nats-www.informatik.uni-hamburg.de/~dawai/

Partner: Humboldt-Universität zu Berlin, Lehrstuhl für Computerlinguistik Universität Hamburg, AB Natürlichsprachliche Systeme	**Supported by:** DFG
Active: 01/1997 – 12/1998	**Contact:** Prof. Dr. W. Menzel

Objective:

Spoken language processing requires the abilities to cope with deviant input and to adapt to constantly changing temporal restrictions. The project attempts to achieve a similar *anytime* behaviour within the framework of structural disambiguation using graded constraints. Based on the eliminative nature of constraint satisfaction techniques, the degree of remaining ambiguity is continuously monitored and constraint reinforcement strategies are applied to influence the temporal behaviour of the parsing procedure.

Results:

An experimental parsing system has been set up and used with different constraint sets to investigate the robustness of the system against unexpected input. The approach has also been successfully applied to the problem of error diagnosis in language tutoring systems.

Selected publications:
References

1. W. MENZEL. Constraint Satisfaction for Robust Parsing of Spoken Language. Journal of Experimental and Theoretical Artificial Intelligence, 10(1): 77 – 89.
2. W. MENZEL, I. SCHRÖDER. Constraint-based Diagnosis for Intelligent Language Tutoring Systems. To appear in Proc. IT& KNOWS, XV. IFIP World Computer Congress, Vienna/Budapest 1998.
3. W. MENZEL, I. SCHRÖDER. Model-based Diagnosis under Structural Uncertainty. Proc. 13th European Conference on Artificial Intelligence, ECAI'98, Brighton UK, 284 – 288.
4. J. HEINECKE, J. KUNZE, W. MENZEL, I. SCHRÖDER. Eliminative Parsing with Graded Constraints. To appear in Proc. 17th Int. Conference on Computational Linguistics. Montreal, Canada.
5. W. MENZEL, I. SCHRÖDER. Decision Procedures for Dependency Parsing Using Graded Constraints. To appear in Proc. Coling-ACL Workshop on Processing of Dependency Grammars. Montreal, Canada.
6. J. HEINECKE, I. SCHRÖDER. Robust Analysis of (Spoken) Language. To appear in Proc. KONVENS-98.

ISLE, Interactive Spoken Language Education

http://nats-www.informatik.uni-hamburg.de/ isle/
(Telematics, Language Engineering)

Partner: Dida*El S.r.l, Milano, Italy; Klett-Verlag, Stuttgart, Germany; Entropic Cambridge Research Lab, Cambridge, UK; University Leeds, UK; Universita' degli Studi di Milano, Italy; Universität Hamburg, AB Natürlichsprachliche Systeme	**Supported by:** EU
Active: 03/1998 – 03/2000	**Contact:** Prof. Dr. W. Menzel

Objective:

The project aims at introducing speech recognition technology into future commercial courseware products for Computer-Aided Language Learning. One of the most prominent goals will be to provide an appropriate level of feedback to the student in order to directly point out possible directions for the improvement of pronunciation.

Results:

Currently a user requirements study is under way.

COMRIS – Co-Habited Mixed-Reality Information Spaces

www-ai.cs.uni-dortmund.de/FORSCHUNG/MLTXT/COMRIS/comris.eng.html

(ESPRIT – intelligent information interfaces (i³))

Partner: University of Dortmund, Artificial Intelligence Unit (D), Riverland Next Generation (B), Instituut voor Perceptie Onderzoek (NL), GMD (D), The University of Reading (GB), IIIA – CSIC (E), Vrije Universiteit Brussel (B)	Supported by: EU
Active: 10/1997 – 9/2000	Contact: Prof. Dr. K. Morik

Objective:

The COMRIS project aims to develop, demonstrate and experimentally evaluate a scalable approach to integrating the Inhabited Information Spaces schema with a concept of software agents.

The COMRIS project uses a conference center as the thematic space and concrete context of work. In the mixed-reality conference center real and virtual conference activities are going on in parallel. Each participant wears his personal assistant, an electronic badge and ear-phone device, wirelessly hooked into an Intranet. This personal assistant – the COMRIS parrot – realizes a link between the real and virtual spaces. It observes what is going on around its host and it informs its host about potentially useful encounters, ongoing demonstrations that may be worthwhile attending, and so on. This information is gathered by several personal representatives, software agents that participate on behalf of a real person in the virtual conference. Each of them has the purpose to represent, defend and further a particular interest or objective of the real participant. The project brings together ideas from different backgrounds (software agents, virtuality, networking, robotics, machine learning, social science) into a coherent concept and technical approach. COMRIS pursues a radical information push model, in which information is actively imposed upon the user in his concrete minute-to-minute context of activities. Techniques of "interest based navigation" bring together those virtual agents whose interests are likely to fit into a productive social process. Their interactions accumulate an information context, mined from a variety of structured and unstructured sources, and related to the different interests involved. At all times, techniques of "competition for attention" focus the interactions and in particular the stream of information towards the user.

Machine Learning and Statistics SFB 475/A4
(SFB 475 Komplexitätsreduktion in multivariaten Datenstrukturen
www-ai.cs.uni-dortmund.de/FORSCHUNG/KDD/MLSTATISTIK/mlstatistik.html)

Partner: FB Statistik, Uni Dortmund	Supported by: DFG
Active: 7/1997 – 6/2000	Contact: Prof. Dr. K. Morik

Objective:
Both statistics and machine learning share the goal of analysing data to find regularities and predict future events. This project explores three forms of synergy arising between machine learning and statistics. Their effectiveness is analysed on selected problems.

- **Knowledge bases and statistics.** Support users of statistical methods using a knowledge based approach. Machine learning techniques are used for a balanced, cooperative modeling of the knowlegdge base, i.e. activities like knowledge maintainance or revision can be done by the system or the user.
- **Complexity reduction.** Support users of machine learning methods using tools from statistics. This involves drawing appropriate samples from large datasets, clustering numerical data as preprocessing and data reduction based on sufficiency, invariances etc.
- **Knowledge discovery in databases** using both methods from statistics and machine learning. In particular this will involve new techniques from inductive logic programming, which have the ability to represent relational concepts. This high expressive power leads to high computational demands making a reduction of the raw data mandatory. Potential solutions are the incorporation of statistical tests for dimensionality reduction and sampling into the induction algorithm.

This project aims to combine methods and experience from statistics and machine learning to build systems for analysing large datasets. To integrate and combine different methods, their theoretical charaterization as well as practical experience with such multi-strategy systems is crucial. The goal is to cross the border between the two disciplines and develop new methods more powerful than those in each field alone.

Results:
Developed software: SVM-light, support vector learning package

Selected publications:
References

1. T. JOACHIMS. Text Categorization with Support Vector Machines: Learning with Many Relevant Features. Machine Learning: ECML–98. Springer, LNAI 1398, 1998.
2. K. MORIK, P. BROCKHAUSEN. A Multistrategy Approach to Relational Knowledge Discovery in Databases. Machine Learning Journal, 27:3, 287–312, Kluwer, 1997.
3. K. MORIK, I. PIGEOT, U. ROBERS. The Use of Inductive Logic Programming for the Development of the Statistical Software Tool CORA. Workshop Logische Programmierung, München, 1997.

Reflective Teams - Active Learning and Information Integration in Open Environments

http://set.gmd.de/AS/rteams/proj.html

Partner: The project is part of the Real World Computing (RWC) Programme (http://www.rwcp.or.jp)	**Supported by:** MITI, Japan
Active: 04/1997 – 04/1999	**Contact:** Dr. H. Mühlenbein

Objective:

Research in R-TEAMS aims at the analysis and development of systems that operate on large data spaces with unknown properties or interact with technical or natural processes with unknown behavior. R-TEAMS is designed for the following problems, which might exist individually or in combinations.

Search of large data spaces: The data spaces are given in mathematical representation or, in the case of real-world data, as sets of value pairs obtained from observation or from simulation of real-world processes. Interaction with real-world processes: The tasks and the behavior of the processes cannot be completely taken into account when the system is designed, since the tasks are not known in advance nor the situations which they will refer to. Simulation of real-world processes: In complex applications data often cannot be generated by mathematical models, but has to be numerically computed by simulating the physical process.

Results:

A framework based on parallel distributed problem solving. Many agents of varying functionality and granularity cooperate or compete in teams, referred to as reflective teams. Current Applications are: Control of an anthropomorphic hand-eye robot with two manipulators and 3D stereo vision Placement of antennas for mobile radio communication Predicting the risk of a credit Optimization of decomposable functions

Database Marketing

http://www.forwiss.de/fg-we/DatabaseMarketing.html

Partner: FORWISS	Supported by: Daimler-Benz AG
Active: 04/1997 – 01/1999	Contact: M. Mueller

Objective:

The discovery of association rules is a very efficient data mining technique, especially suitable for large amounts of categorical data. The goal of the project Database Marketing was to develop a new algorithm for the discovery of association rules and sequential patterns over ordinal data which uses taxonomies as a specific form of background knowledge. In addition, a new absolute measure for the interestingness of quantitative association rules should be built. With this measure, rule extraction should be speeded up and rule evaluation should become more intuitive and transparent for users, compared to implicit interestingness relations and the standard measures support and confidence. The technical goal was to extend the commercial data mining tool Clementine with this algorithm which enables the system to support basket analysis. The performance of the methods to be developed should be evaluated with real-world data from a domain which was provided by Daimler-Benz AG.

Results:

First, previously proposed approaches of applying association rule discovery to numerical data as well were selected, reviewed, and analyzed. Q2, a new and fast algorithm for the discovery of multi-dimensional association rules over ordinal data, was designed and implemented. Experiments in which the new algorithm was compared against the previous approaches on real-world data showed that performance improvements of more than an order of magnitude could be obtained. A new interestingness measure was defined which is based on the view that quantitative association rules have to be interpreted on the background of their Boolean generalizations. This measure has two major benefits: rule extraction and evaluation became much faster, and the interpretation of the measure is easier for users now, compared to previous measures and relative interestingness computation. A rule browser was developed which supports the new methodology for exploration of ordinal data with quantitative association rules. This browser enables to filter, sort, and structure the flood of discovered rules. The integration of this new data mining technique into the Clementine system is planned in the near future.

Selected publications:
References

1. O. BÜCHTER, R. WIRTH. Discovery of Association Rules over Ordinal Data: A New and Faster Algorithm and its Application to Basket Analysis. In Research and Development in Knowledge Discovery and Data Mining (Proceedings of the Second Pacific-Asia Conference on Knowledge Discovery and Data Mining PAKDD-98). Springer, LNAI 1394, 1998.

Intelligente Überwachung des Wirknetzes von Mobilkommunikationssystemen durch modellbasierte KI-Systeme

(DFG-Schwerpunktprogramm Mobilkommunikation)

Partner: Institut für Allgemeine Nachricht-entechnik, Universitt Hannover	**Supported by:** DFG
Active: 11/1996 - 11/2000	**Contact:** Prof. Dr. W. Nejdl

Objective:

To interpret and condense alarm message cascades in mobile telecommunication systems. Operators in the operation and maintenance centers of cellular phone networks are regularly flooded with alarm messages generated by local and remote equipment. These messages reflect certain conditions of the equipment as noticed by the equipment itself or its proxies, and are usually rather primitive (crossing of a threshold, device not responding, etc.). It is the task of the operator to identify, from the available messages, the possible causes entailing those messages, and to find a suitable remedy. This is basically a diagnostic process which we intend to reproduce in terms of model-based diagnosis. In a two-year continuation of our project we plan to apply market-related principles to control problems of cellular phone networks. These will rely on customized trend detection methods designed to detect temporal patterns in the network management message stream.

Results:

We have mapped the technical system descriptions of base station subsystems (consisting of network elements, their topology and their interactions) into logical system descriptions in FOL, implementing in effect a simulation model. This allows us to infer the causes of all incoming alarm messages declared in the system description with the standard techniques of model-based diagnosis. We have adapted our own diagnostic engine, DRUM-II (Dynamic Revision and Update Machine) and demonstrated its potential for real-time, online diagnosis in the operation and maintenance centers of mobile telephone systems.

Selected publications:

References

1. P. FRÖHLICH, W. NEJDL, K. JOBMANN, H. WIETGREFE. Model-Based Alarm Correlation in Cellular Phone Networks. Fifth International Symposium on Modeling, Analysis, and Simulation of Computer and Telecommunication Systems (MASCOTS), January 1997.
2. P. FRÖHLICH, W. NEJDL. A Static Model-Based Engine for Model-Based Reasoning. IJCAI-97, Nagoya, 1997.

BAND - Benutzeradaptiver Netz-Informationdienst
http://www.lavielle.com/band.html

Partner: Lavielle EDV-Systemberatung	Supported by: Wirtschaftsbehörde
Labor für Künstliche Intelligenz	Hamburg
University of Hamburg	
Active: 12/1996 – 12/1998	Contact: Prof. Dr. B. Neumann

Objective:
In the project BAND we develop advanced technologies for adaptive information presentation and content-based information retrieval on the Internet. Though today most World Wide Web sites present information already with static or dynamic outlook, most of them fail to adapt to user needs. Answering to questions is possible with database queries or full text retrieval. For creating next generation web sites which offer the user adaptive behavior a new adaptive approach seems to be necessary. New tools and abstractions are needed which integrate dynamic servers and rich knowledge representation for presentation generation and information retrieval. A framework for providing network information services with user adaptivity is developed. Access and presentation of information are dynamically adapted according to user demands by knowledge based techniques. The innovative software techniques developed in this project can be used in the context of many applications such as help desk systems, intranet services, medical applications, etc. As an example application we consider a user adaptive TV assistant. Thereby user adaptivity is performed by intelligent information presentation (e.g., a TV program table specifically adapted to a sports fan's demands) and by content-based information retrieval where, for instance, similarities between TV broadcasts are computed and then used for information queries.

Results:
So far our system is able to demonstrate the main objectives of the project in the context of the "TV-Assistant". We have modeled several user types, and the TV program table is automatically adapted based on user interactions with the system. In addition, we provide application independent solutions for collecting information items and use formal terminological logics for content-based information retrieval of TV broadcasts.

Selected publications:
References

1. R. MÖLLER, V. HAARSLEV, B. NEUMANN. Semantics-Based Information Retrieval. International Conference on Information Technology and Knowledge Systems, Vienna, Budapest, August–September, 1998.
2. T. MANTAY, R. MÖLLER. Content-Based Information Retrieval by Computation of Least Common Subsumers in a Probabilistic Description Logic. Proceedings of the ECAI'98 Workshop Intelligent Information Integration, Brighton, UK, August 1998.

INDIA - Intelligent Diagnosis in Industrial Applications

http://lki-www.informatik.uni-hamburg.de/~india

(Intelligente Systeme)

Partner: Robert Bosch GmbH, Stuttgart; Fraunhofer-Institut für Informations- und Datenverarbeitung (IITB), Karlsruhe; Labor für Künstliche Intelligenz (LKI), University of Hamburg; MAZ Mikroelektronik Anwendungszentrum Hamburg GmbH; R.O.S.E. Informatik GmbH (RIG), Heidenheim a. d. Brenz; Still GmbH, Hamburg; Technical University of Munich; THEN Maschinen- und Apparatebau GmbH, Schwäbisch-Hall	**Supported by:** BMBF
Active: 07/1995 – 07/1999	**Contact:** Prof. B. Neumann

Objective:

INDIA aims at substantial contributions to knowledge-based - in particular: model-based - diagnosis of technical devices in order to facilitate industrial applications. To this end we want to prepare solutions which meet the demands of concrete applications (e. g. with respect to safety, ecology, variety, integration into development and runtime environment). We approach these aims from two sides. On the one hand we transfer recent results of research into industrial applications. On the other hand we analyze application problems to drive further research. The consortium consists of research institutes, vendors of diagnostic systems and users of diagnosis systems.

Results:

Innovative methods and several prototypical systems for diagnosis tasks are developed, e.g. 1. automatic generation of a cost optimal fault tree starting with a qualitative model of the electrics of fork lifters, 2. model-based generation of failure-mode and effects analysis by automatic derivation of the effect of component failures on an automotive system, and 3. modeling and analyzing dye houses using state charts.

Selected publications:

References

1. A. BRINKOP. Integrating Function and Behavior for Model-Based Diagnosis. IJCAI-97 Workshop on Modeling and Reasoning about Function, Y. Umeda (ed.), Nagoya, Japan, August 25, 1997, 1-10, 1997.
2. J. KAHL, L. HOTZ, H. MILDE, S. WESSEL. Automatic Generation of Decision Trees for Diagnosis: The MAD-System. Int. Conf. on Information Technology and Knowledge Systems, Vienna, Budapest, August–September 1998.
3. P. STRUSS, A. MALIK. Automated Diagnosis of Car-Subsystems Based on Qualitative Models. In: Expertensysteme 97, Beiträge zur 4. Deutschen Tagung Wissensbasierter Systeme (XPS-97), 5.-7. März 1997, Bad Honnef am Rhein. PAI Proceedings in Artificial Intelligence, Vol. 6, infix-Verlag, 157-166, 1997.

Prosody, linguistic analysis, and dialogue act modeling
(VERBMOBIL II)

Partner: VERBMOBIL consortium	**Supported by:** BMBF
Active: 01/1997 – 01/2001	**Contact:** Dr. E. Nöth

Objective:

Recognition and modeling of prosodic information (e.g., boundaries, accents, sentence modality, emotion); combination of different knowledge bases; use of prosodic information for linguistic analysis and dialog act recognition; modeling of speakers.

Results:

In the first phase of the VERBMOBIL project, in 1992 – 1996, we successfully classified prosodic information in German that could be used by the higher linguistic modules in the VERBMOBIL system. For boundary recognition, using only a language model and a large training corpus annotated with syntactic–prosodic boundaries, boundary vs. no boundary could be recognized with a high accuracy (94% correct classified). In the first phase of the VERBMOBIL project such a very good segmentation accuracy decreased the parsing time of the syntactic parser to 6% of the time needed without segmentation. We now started to develop analogously prosodic classifiers for American English and for Japanese.

Up to now, the prosodic component used information obtained by word recognition. Recently, we developed a feature vector with only frame based features that can be used in an incremental analysis without word information.

Other topics investigated are the modeling and the recognition of emotions, of speech repairs, and of salient information in dialogue act classification for the three languages German, American English and Japanese.

Selected publications:
References

1. A. KIESSLING. Extraktion und Klassifikation prosodischer Merkmale in der automatischen Sprachverarbeitung. Berichte aus der Informatik. Shaker Verlag, Aachen. 1997.
2. R. KOMPE. Prosody in Speech Understanding Systems. Springer, LNAI, 1997.
3. H. NIEMANN, E. NÖTH, A. KIESSLING, R. KOMPE, A. BATLINER. Prosodic Processing and its use in Verbmobil. In Proceedings of the International Conference on Acoustics, Speech, and Signal Processing (ICASSP), volume 1, 75-78, Munich, April 1997. IEEE Computer Society Press.
4. E. NÖTH, A. BATLINER, A. KIESSLING, R. KOMPE, F. GALLWITZ, V. WARNKE, H. NIEMANN. Spracherkennung und Prosodie. KI, 4:14-19, 1997

Short: Localization and Navigation for Autonomous Robots

http://www-info1.informatik.uni-wuerzburg.de/projects/DFG/dfg.e.html

(DFG-SPP Efficient Algorithms for Discrete Problems and their Applications)

Partner: Siemens ZFE (Neuperlach); FAW Dept. Autonomous Systems/Mechatronics (Ulm); Nomadic Technologies (Mountain View, CA)	**Supported by:** DFG
Active: 12/1995 – 12/1999	**Contact:** Prof. Dr. H. Noltemeier

Objective:

In industrial and service environments the design of landmark-independent navigation algorithms is necessary for the development of autonomous robots. In our setting we assume that a robot is in an indoor-environment, for which it has a map, and has to do a complete relocalization using only the distance information of its laser radar.

The aim of our research is to find an adequate representation for the localization problem, to develop algorithms for solving it, and to test our solutions in real-world applications.

Results:

Our approach to solving the localization problem is to use pattern matching strategies for comparing the laser scans with preprocessed parts of the map. This is done in an efficient way, which prevents us from doing unnecessary comparisons. We have implemented our localization strategy in C++ with several pattern matching algorithms and added some useful functions (e.g., for coping with partial scans, limited sensing range etc.). Currently we are going to evaluate our software in typical real-world scenarios.

Selected publications:

References

1. O. KARCH, H. NOLTEMEIER. Robot Localization — Theory and Practice. In Proceedings of the 10th IEEE/RSJ International Conference on Intelligent Robots and Systems (IROS '97), 850–856, 1997.
2. O. KARCH, TH. WAHL. Relocalization — Theory and Practice. Discrete Applied Mathematics (Special Issue on Computational Geometry), 1998. To appear.
3. O. KARCH, H. NOLTEMEIER, TH. WAHL. Using Polygon Distances for Localization. Accepted for Annual Conference of the IEEE Industrial Electronics Society, Aachen, Germany, August 31st–September 4th 1998.

SMART: Integration of Symbolic and Subsymbolic Information Processing in Adaptive Sensorimotor Systems
http://www.uni-ulm.de/SMART/
(SFB Special Research Center)

Partner: University of Ulm, FAW, DaimlerBenz Research Ulm	**Supported by:** DFG
Active: 1997–2008	**Contact:** Prof. Dr. G. Palm

Objective:
The main goals of project SMART are

1. the study of principles and methods for neurosymbolic integration,
2. the development of hybrid control architectures for sensorimotor systems,
3. the study of adaptivity and learning,
4. biological modeling of neural systems,
5. the design of advanced architectures for sensor fusion, and
6. integration of planning and control.

Results:
About one year after project start we have preliminary results in most subprojects. Some examples are

1. fast algorithms for computing foveal and peripheral optical flow,
2. mechanisms for brightness and contrast processing based on biological principles,
3. a multi-layered, hybrid architecture for spatial representation and dynamic world modeling,
4. modules for multimodal sensor fusion, and
5. EpsiloNN, a language for specifying neural networks, and compilers generating efficient parallel implementations.

Selected publications:
References

1. St. Enderle, G. Kraetzschmar, G. Palm. Neural Networks for Mapping Sonar Data to Egocentric Maps for Mobile Robots. Proceedings of NN-98, Magdeburg, 1998.
2. Th. Kämpke, R. Kober. Nonparametric Optimal Binarization. Proceedings of ICPR-98, Brisbane, 1998.
3. G. Krone, B. Talle, A. Wichert, G. Palm. Neural Architectures for Sensor Fusion in Speech Recognition. Proceedings of WS AVSP-97, Rhodes, Greece, 1997.
4. A. Strey. EpsiloNN – A Specification Language for the Efficient Parallel Implementation of Neuural Networks. Proceedings of Biological and Artificial Computation: From Neuroscience to Technology, LNCS 1240, 714-722. Springer 1997.
5. Ch. Töpfer, M. Wende, G. Baratoff, H. Neumann. Robot Navigation by Combining Central and Peripheral Optical Flow Detection on a Space-Variant Map. Proceedings of ICPR-98, Brisbane, 1998.

Computer Aided Diagnostics in Computed Tomography of the Lung

Partner: Institute of Computer Science, Department of Radiology; Johannes-Gutenberg University of Mainz Active: 11/1995–11/1998	Supported by: DFG Contact: Prof. Dr. J. Perl

Objective:

The purpose of the project is to develop and use intelligent image analysis methods in the computer-aided classification of computed tomography (CT) images. Especially the use of hierarchical, self organizing neural nets in connection with different, mutually linked analysis modules (logical rules, fuzzy logic, expert knowledge, textural features, semantic nets) is examined.

Results:

First prototype of the multi-level model HYBRIKON (HYBRides KONfigurationsmodell) is finished. HYBRIKON achieve a flexible and effective implementation of medical expert knowledge (global (pathological, anatomical) and local (morphological, microstructural) knowledge) with both classical image analysis methods (semantic networks, voxelseeding, textural parameters) and methods of the AI (hierarchical neural nets, fuzzy logic). The developed methods are (going to be) used in clinical and experimental radiological applications, as the automatic detection, quantification and visualization of

- Ground glass opacities on lung CT
- Airtrapping in inspiration-/exspiration pairs on lung CT
- Volumetry of the spleen

Selected publications:

1. HEITMANN, KAUCZOR, UTHMANN, MILDENBERGER, PERL, THELEN. Hybrid neural networks in the automatic detection and quantification of pathologies on HRCT and helical CT of the lung. In: Proc. of the 11th Int. Symp. and Exhib. on Computer Assisted Radiology and Surgery (CAR' 97, Berlin) 331-336.
2. HEITMANN, UTHMANN, DIAZ. HYBRIKON: Ein hybrides Multi-Ebenen Modell für die radiologische Bildanalyse. In: Tagungsband zum Workshop Einsatz von Methoden und Konzepten der KI in der medizinischen Informationsverarbeitung, KI-97, Freiburg. Informatik-Bericht der Johannes Gutenberg-Universität Mainz, Institut für Informatik, Nr. 7/97, 19-26.
3. HEITMANN, KAUCZOR, MILDENBERGER, UTHMANN, PERL, THELEN. Automatic detection of ground glass opacities on lung HRCT using multiple neural networks. Eur. Radiol. 7 1463-1472 (1997). Akzeptiert für: 1998 IMIA Yearbook of Medical Informatics.

Communicating Agents
http://coli.lili.uni-bielefeld.de/D1
(SFB 360 - Situated Artificial Communicators)

Partner: none	Supported by: DFG
Active: 07/1996 – 12/1999	Contact: K. Peters

Objective:
The project 'Communicating Agents' tries to model situated communication in a co-operative construction task. The communicating agent CoRA is a simulated assembly robot, which can be directed by natural language instructions. The agent is situated in the sense that it is able to perceive its environment and to execute certain actions semi-autonomously. Because of the complex interplay between language, perception and action, a correct semantic interpretation of utterances found in instruction situations can only be achieved by considering extralinguistic information.

Results:
In order to cope with these kind of communication situations, we developed a hybrid control architecture which contains a behavior-oriented base system and a deliberative system. The behavior system is embedded in the real world by means of sensors and actuators, which enable it to detect changes in the world and react to them immediately. It has the necessary competence for the autonomous execution of basic actions. The deliberative system is responsible for the sequencing of complex actions into simple basic actions and schedules the execution of these actions. As a consequence of the hybrid architecture, two types of action directives are distinguished: Simple directives called *interventions* can manipulate the behavior system directly, complex directives called *instructions* influence the deliberative system and only in the second step the behavior system. The behavior system integrates linguistic information into the current action, treating it just like any other sensor data. It is through the coupling of a deliberative system and a behavior-oriented base system, that the interpretation and flexible execution of all kinds of directives can be realized by the interplay of goal-directed and reactive behavior.

Selected publications:
References

1. K. U. GOECKE, K. PETERS, H. LOBIN. Aufgabenorientierte Verarbeitung von Interventionen und Instruktionen. Report 96/7, SFB 360 - Situierte Künstliche Kommunikatoren, Universität Bielefeld, 1996.
2. J.-T. MILDE, S. STRIPPGEN, K. PETERS. Situated Communication with Robots. In: Y. Wilks (ed.), Machine Conversation, Kluwer Academics 1998. To appear.
3. K. PETERS, S. STRIPPGEN, J.-T. MILDE. CoRA - An Instructable Robot. In: T. Lueth, R. Dillmann, P. Dario, H. Wörn (eds.), Distributed Autonomous Robotic Systems 3, pp. 247-256. Springer 1998.

Communicating Agents

http://coli.lili.uni-bielefeld.de/D1

(SFB 360 - Situated Artificial Communicators)

Partner: University of Bielefeld	**Supported by:** DFG
Active: 07/1996 – 12/1999	**Contact:** K. Peters

Objective:

The project 'Communicating Agents' tries to model situated communication in a cooperative construction task. The communicating agent CORA is a simulated assembly robot, which can be directed by natural language instructions. The agent is situated in the sense that it is able to perceive its environment and to execute certain actions semi-autonomously. Because of the complex interplay between language, perception and action, a correct semantic interpretation of utterances found in instruction situations can only be achieved by considering extralinguistic information.

Results:

In order to cope with these kind of communication situations, we developed a hybrid control architecture which contains a behavior-oriented base system and a deliberative system. The behavior system is embedded in the real world by means of sensors and actuators, which enable it to detect changes in the world and react to them immediately. It has the necessary competence for the autonomous execution of basic actions. The deliberative system is responsible for the sequencing of complex actions into simple basic actions and schedules the execution of these actions. As a consequence of the hybrid architecture, two types of action directives are distinguished: Simple directives - called interventions - can manipulate the behavior system directly, complex directives - called instructions - influence the deliberative system and only in the second step the behavior system. The behavior system integrates linguistic information into the current action, treating it just like any other sensor data. It is through the coupling of a deliberative system and a behavior-oriented base system, that the interpretation and flexible execution of all kinds of directives can be realized by the interplay of goal-directed and reactive behavior.

Selected publications:

References

1. K. U. GOECKE, K. PETERS, H. LOBIN. Aufgabenorientierte Verarbeitung von Interventionen und Instruktionen. Report 96/7, SFB 360 - Situierte Künstliche Kommunikatoren, Universität Bielefeld, 1996.
2. J.-T. MILDE, S. STRIPPGEN, K. PETERS. Situated Communication with Robots. In: Y. Wilks (ed.), *Machine Conversation*, Kluwer Academics 1998. To appear.
3. K. PETERS, S. STRIPPGEN, J.-T. MILDE. CORA - An Instructable Robot. In: T. Lueth, R. Dillmann, P. Dario, H. Wörn (eds.), Distributed Autonomous Robotic Systems 3, 247-256. Springer 1998.

READ (Recognition and Document Analysis) - Off-line handwritten character recognition

http://set.gmd.de/EIA/read.html

Partner: Siemens EletroCom GmbH, Konstanz CGK Computer Gesellschaft, Konstanz Daimler-Benz AG, Ulm DFKI, Kaiserslautern GMD-SET GMD-IPSI Graphikon, Berlin Siemens, Mnchen TU Braunschweig Univ. Koblenz-Landau Univ. Magdeburg	**Supported by:** BMBF
Active: 08/1995 – 08/1998	**Contact:** Dr. L. Peters

Objective:

The project Read aims at increasing the efficiency of the current *Recognition and Document Analysis* technology. The main goal in Read is to combine and refine document analysis techniques, ranging from low level picture processing over document structure analysis to linguistic extraction, into a general framework.

Results:

The FOHDEL language, which was developed by GMD-SET for on-line character recognition, is extended and applied to represent the fuzzy rules for word recognition. Neural networks supplement the fuzzy set theoretic techniques to generate the expert information automatically and thus generate the rule-bases for the recognition process. This capability is developed also to adapt the recognition system on-the-fly to new document environments. Another major activity is the integration of the various object recognition approaches developed by GMD, Siemens EletroCom and Univ. Koblenz into a unique toolbox.

Selected publications:
References

1. L. PETERS, A. MALAVIYA, F. IVANCIC. Verfahren zur automatisierten Regelgenerierung für die Klassifizierung von Bilddaten. (Automatic rule generation for the classification of visual data). Europäische Patentanmeldung, April 1998.
2. F. IVANCIC, A. MALAVIYA, L. PETERS. An Automatic Rule Base Generation Method for Fuzzy Pattern Recognition with Multi-phased Clustering. IEEE Proceedings of KES'98, Adelaide, 1998.
3. L. PETERS, C. LEJA, A. MALAVIYA. A fuzzy Statistical Rule Generation Method for Handwriting Recognition. Expert Systems, February 1998, Vol. 15, No.1, 1998.
4. A. MALAVIYA, L. PETERS. A syntactic approach to Handwriting Recognition. Accepted for publication in Fuzzy Sets and Systems in 1998.
5. A. MALAVIYA, C. LEJA, L. PETERS. A Hybrid Approach of automatic fuzzy rule generation for handwriting recognition. Editor: Downtown und Impedevo Progress in Handwriting Recognition, World Scientific, Singapore, 1997.

Meta Knowledge for Medical Critiquing Systems

Partner: Universität Würzburg	**Supported by:** DFG
Lehrstuhl für Künstliche Intelligenz	
und Angewandte Informatik	
Active: 09/1996 – 09/1998	**Contact:** Prof. Dr. F. Puppe

Objective:

A critiquing system has been defined in a recent textbook on medical informatics as a *decision support system that allows the user to make the decision first; the system then gives its advice when the user requests it or when the user's decision is out of the system's permissible range.* However, despite its broad theoretical acceptance little work has been done on critiquing systems since the seminal work of Perry Miller in the eighties. A promising approach is similar to intelligent training systems: Comparing the solution derived by an expert system with the solution of the user and criticizing major differences. This approach assumes that the expert systems expertise is superior to the user. While this assumption might be fulfilled for students and preselected well-known cases, it is rarely true for experts and arbitrary cases. Therefore, in this project we investigate what kind of additional knowledge a diagnostic critiquing system needs if based on a conventional diagnostic expert system.

Results:

Additional knowledge types for critiquing systems include: 1.Knowledge for the analysis of the reliability of a diagnostic conclusion for a given case taking into account reliability and completeness of data, reliability of the diagnostic knowledge and the explanation of the diagnostic conclusion. 2. Knowledge about the importance of a diagnosis (e.g. treatibility, danger, urgency), and 3. Multiple diagnostic models including partial knowledge like explicit critiquing rules or guidelines. An implementation with the shell kit D3 is under way.

Selected publications:

References

1. U. RHEIN-DESEL, F. PUPPE. Concepts for a Diagnostic Critiquing System in Vague Domains. To appear in: Proc. of KI-98, Springer, 1998.

Cooperating Diagnostic Expert Systems for Complexity Reduction to build very large Knowledge Bases
(BMBF, Arbeit und Technik)

Partner: Universität Würzburg (Prof. Puppe); TU-HH Technologie GmbH (Prof. Malsch); Koenig & Bauer-Albert AG, Würzburg (Hr. Hessler) **Active:** 08/1995 – 04/1999	**Supported by:** BMBF, AuT **Contact:** Prof. Dr. F. Puppe

Objective:

The implementation, maintenance and fault finding in complex machines is an important and knowledge intensive task, which can be well supported by diagnostics and information systems. However, the conventional methodology of building monolithic knowledge bases has two major inherent drawbacks: How to control the resulting complexity of the knowledge base and how to encourage a broad participation of different domain experts.

Results:

These problems can be avoided to a large degree, if the domain experts develop lots of small specialized knowledge bases on their own. We call the resulting small diagnostic systems "agents". An agent needs to have additional knowledge for communication, e.g. to know, what other agents might be competent for a problem not lying in its core knowledge and how to exchange data and intermediate results with other agents using different terminologies. We accordingly extended our diagnostic shell kit D3 to enable cooperation of agents and implemented the approach with our project partner Koenig&Bauer Albert AG for building a diagnostic and information system for printing machines. The third project partner TuHH Technology GmbH with competence in the social sciences and in particular with technology transfer deals with the inevitable difficult organizational and qualificational issues arising in such a joint innovative project.

Selected publications:
References

1. S. BAMBERGER. Cooperating Diagnostic Expert Systems to Solve complex Diagnosis Tasks. In Proc. KI-97, 21st German Conference of Artificial Intelligence, 325-336, LNAI 1303. Springer, 1997.
2. S. LANDVOGT, S. BAMBERGER, J. HUPP, R. KESTLER, S. HESSLER. KBA-D3: ein Experten- und Informationssystem zur Fehlerdiagnose von Druckmaschinen. In Proc. XPS-97 (Expertensysteme-97), PAI 6. infix-Verlag, 61-78, 1997.
3. S. ZIEGLER, S. SCHWINGELER. Rekontextualisierung als Konzept einer Systemschulung: Ein Tutorial für die Selbstakquisition mit dem Expertensystem-Shell-Baukasten D3. In: J.-P. Pahl et al. (eds.): Lern- und Arbeitsumgebungen in der Instandhaltungsausbildung, 171-187. Kallmeyersche Verlagsbuchhandlung, Seelze-Velber, 1997.

Multimedial Knowledge- and Case-Based Training and Information Systems in Medicine
(BMBF)

Partner: Universität Würzburg (Prof. F. Puppe); **Supported by:** BMBF
Medizinische Universitätsklinik Würzburg
(Dr. B. Puppe); Universität München
(LMU), Poliklinik (Prof. S. Schewe)
Active: 01/1997 – 10/1999   **Contact:** Prof. Dr. F. Puppe

Objective:

Solving problems in simulated environments is a powerful training method in many domains. This project aims at building and evaluating an authoring tool for medical diagnostic training, with which experts can formulate their general knowledge and enter case descriptions, where symptoms might be illustrated by pictures. From this input, the system generates training scenarios. Cases are presented to the students incrementally, who have to interpret the pictures, to ask for additional information about the case and to find out the correct diagnoses and therapies. The system criticizes the students' actions by comparing them with its own actions based on the data known so far and its knowledge base.

Results:

A first prototype of the authoring tool is completed and has been used to build and evaluate large medical training systems in neurology, rheumatology and hepatology. It is based on the diagnostic shell kit D3 and reuses existing knowledge bases, so that the same knowledge can be used both for consulting and training. Only the knowledge about pictures and their interpretation has to be added specifically for the training system. The main focus of the current work lies in enhancing the system by offering various didactic strategies ranging from a quick but simplified presentation to a more realistic, but time-consuming work-up of a training case. A major concern is to minimize the amount of additional knowledge the expert has to enter, so that most of the options can be configured at run-time by predefined switches.

Selected publications:
References

1. F. PUPPE, S. SCHEWE. Mehrfachverwendung von diagnostischen Wissensbasen in der Medizin. Künstliche Intelligenz 97/3, 15-23, 1997.
2. F. PUPPE, B. PUPPE, B. REINHARDT, S. SCHEWE, H.P. BUSCHER. Evaluation medizinischer Diagnostik-Expertensysteme zur Wissensvermittlung. Informatik, Biometrie und Epidemiologie in Medizin und Biologie 29 (1), 48-59.
3. F. PUPPE, B. REINHARDT. Generating Case-Oriented Training from Diagnostic Expert Systems. Machine Mediated Learning, Vol 5, Nr. 3&4, 199-219, 1995.

MOVIS - Mobile Optoelectronic Visual-Interpretative System for the Blind and Visually Impaired
(Elektronisches Auge)

Partner: JURCA Optoelektronik GmbH, Rodgau CORRSYS GmbH, Wetzlar empirica De-lasasse GmbH, Köln Technical University of Hamburg-Harburg, Prof. H. Burkhardt (now: University of Freiburg) University of Hamburg, Prof. B. Neumann	**Supported by:** BMBF
Active: 06/1994 – 09/1997	**Contact:** Dr. A. Reuter

Objective:
MOVIS is the name of an opto-electronic seeing aid for the blind developed in a project which was also called MOVIS. The goal of the first three years (1994 - 1997) is a laboratory prototype of a spectacle-like device, involving two CCD-cameras, which lets blind navigators (1) recognize special objects like pedestrian crossings and telephone booths, (2) record and recognize "landmarks", i.e. views of places important for their navigational needs. The output of the device consists of acoustical signals and generated speech. Further development steps including additional functionality and miniaturization are planned for subsequent years. The ultimate goal of MOVIS is to improve the living quality of thousands of blind persons by means of advanced computer vision technology.

Results:
A laboratory prototype has been completed and its performance has been demonstrated in September 1997. During the demonstration, a person could navigate an indoors environment and test the algorithms on both a real telephone booth and a real post-box as well as a scaled down (80an-crossing. Using an 8-processor parallel computer, recognition and calculation of the distance could be shown in real time. MOVIS has been selected as a national project for Expo 2000 in Hanover.

Selected publications:
References

1. A. LUO, W. TAO, H. BURKHARDT. A new multilevel line-based stereo vision algorithm based on fuzzy techniques. Proc. 13th International Conf. on Pattern Recognition, pp. 383-387, Vienna, Austria, August 1996.
2. B. NEUMANN, H. KIRSCHKE. MOVIS - Anforderungen und Entwurf. Bericht des Labors für Künstliche Intelligenz, Universität Hamburg, Mai 1996.
3. S. UTCKE. Grouping based on projective geometry constraints and uncertainty. Proc. Sixth International Conf. on Computer Vision, Bombay, India, January 1998. Narosa Publishing House.

IMAGINE
IMage- and Atlas-Guided Interventions in NEurosurgery
http://kogs-www.informatik.uni-hamburg.de/PROJECTS/imagine/Imagine.html

Partner: Univ. Hamburg, Philips Hamburg	**Supported by:** Philips Hamburg
Active: 1994 – 2000	**Contact:** Dr. K. Rohr

Objective:
Development of algorithms and methods for computer-assisted analysis of 3D multi-modality medical images (e.g., CT and MR images). Applications are the planning and simulation of neurosurgical interventions as well as intraoperative navigation. There are three main work areas: (i) Elastic registration of images and digital atlasses of the human brain to enable the combination of complementary image information, (ii) localization of anatomical landmarks which serve as features for image registration, and (iii) biomechanical models to predict brain deformations.

Results:
We have generalized an existing approach to elastic registration based on thin-plate splines from an interpolation to an approximation scheme. This extension is important in clinical applications since it allows to take into account landmark localization errors. Also, we have proposed a new approach to incorporate additional knowledge in form of attributes (e.g., directions) at landmarks. To localize anatomical landmarks in 3D images of the human brain, we have developed new 3D differential operators. These operators are applied within a semi-automatic user-interaction procedure and yield voxel or even subvoxel positions of landmarks.

Selected publications:
References

1. M. FORNEFETT, R. SPRENGEL, K. ROHR, H.S. STIEHL. Elastic Medical Image Registration Using Orientation Attributes at Landmarks. Proc. Medical Image Understanding and Analysis (MIUA'98), Univ. of Leeds/UK, 6-7 July 1998.
2. S. FRANTZ, K. ROHR, H.S. STIEHL. Refined Localization of Three-Dimensional Anatomical Point Landmarks Using Multi-step Differential Approaches. Proc. SPIE Int. Symposium, Vol. 3338, Medical Imaging 1998 – Image Processing (MI'98), Febr. 21-27, 1998, San Diego/CA.
3. K. ROHR. On 3D Differential Operators for Detecting Point Landmarks. Image and Vision Computing 15:3 (1997) 219–233.
4. K. ROHR, H.S. STIEHL, R. SPRENGEL, W. BEIL, T.M. BUZUG, J. WEESE, M.H. KUHN. Point-Based Elastic Registration of Medical Image Data Using Approximating Thin-Plate Splines. In K.H. Höhne, R. Kikinis (eds.) Proc. 4th Int. Conf. Visualization in Biomedical Computing (VBC'96), Hamburg, Sept. 22-25, 1996, LNCS 1131, 297–306. Springer 1996.
5. K. ROHR, R. SPRENGEL, H.S. STIEHL. Incorporation of Landmark Error Ellipsoids for Image Registration based on Approximating Thin-Plate Splines. In H.U. Lemke, M.W. Vannier, K. Inamura (eds.) Proc. Computer Assisted Radiology and Surgery (CAR'97), 234-239. Elsevier 1997.

KIKon - Configuring customer-specific telecommunication systems

http://nathan.gmd.de/projects/kikon.html

Partner: Deutsche Telekom AG, Dialogis GmbH, GMD-TKT in Darmstadt, GMD-MMK, GMD-SET	**Supported by:** Deutsche Telekom AG
Active: 01/1998 - 01/1999	**Contact:** J. Schaaf

Objective:
Support of cooperative, interactive configuration of telecommunication systems

Results:
Software prototype of an interactive configuration tool which enables a user to set up configuations in a hierarchic-modular, axiomatic and functional dialogue and to compose them to new configurations.

Selected publications:
References

1. W. EMDE, J. RAHMER, A. VOSS, C. BEILKEN, J. BÖRDING, J. ORTH, U. PETERSEN, J.W. SCHAAF, M. SPENKE, S. WROBEL. Interactive Configuration in KIKon In: P. Mertens, Voss, Hans (eds.): Expertensysteme '97 – Beiträge zur 4. Deutschen Tagung Wissensbasierte Systeme. Sankt Augustin [infix] 1997, 79 - 92.

Wissensbasiertes System zur Entwöhnung von künstlicher Beatmung

Partner: Klinik für Anästhesiologie Institut für Informatik, Johannes Gutenberg-Universität Mainz **Active:** 03/1997 – 12/1999	**Supported by:** Drägerwerk AG, Lübeck **Contact:** T. Semmel – Griebeler

Objective:

Entwicklung eines wissensbasierten Systems (Evita Weaning System (EWS)) zur Steuerung eines Beatmungsgertes. Als Beatmungsgerät verwenden wir die "Evita" der Drägerwerk AG, Lübeck. Die für die Durchführung einer Beatmung eines Patienten mit der Evita wesentlichen Parameter werden von dem EWS so bestimmt, daß ein Patient automatisch ausreichend beatmet wird. Hierfür verwendet EWS einerseits Meßdaten, die das Beatmungsgerät liefert, andererseits können optional Informationen vom Pflegepersonal berücksichtigt werden. Da der Patient möglichst schnell und schonend von dem Beatmungsgerät entwöhnt werden soll, muß die Eigenatmung möglichst zu einem frühen Zeitpunkt angeregt werden. Die Spontanatmung kann durch Verringerung der maschinellen Unterstützung erreicht werden. Ein "standardisiertes" Vorgehen wird jedoch durch verschiedene Typen von Patienten erschwert. So kann ein Mensch nach einer einfachen Operation sicherlich anders als ein Langzeitbeatmungspatient entwöhnt werden. Besonders kritisch kann aber ein scheinbar "einfacher" Patient sein. Falls plötzlich doch eine nicht bekannte Komplikation eintritt, muß gewährleistet sein, daß der Patient immer noch ausreichend beatmet wird. Das Konzept für ein Weaningsystem (Entwöhnungssystem) muß sicherstellen, daß in jeder Situation eine ausreichende Sauerstoffversorgung gewährleistet ist.

Results:

Als erster Schritt wurde interdisziplinär (Klinik für Anästhesiologie und Institut für Informatik, Johannes Gutenberg-Universität Mainz) ein geeignetes Modell zur Entwöhnung ausgearbeitet. Auf dieser Basis wurde ein Entwurf für ein erstes, einfaches System mit sog. "sicherer Klassifikation" erstellt und mit Hilfe der Expertensystem-Shell D3 in einem ersten Prototyp implementiert (D3 wurde an der Universität Würzburg am Lehrstuhl für Künstliche Intelligenz (Prof. Puppe) entwickelt). D3 enthält verschiedene Problemlösungmodule. Für den ersten Prototyp wurde das Expertenwissen auf eine regelbasierte Datenstruktur abgebildet. Die Vorversion des EWS wurde an einer mechanischen Lunge und an einem Patientensimulator mit Erfolg getestet. Aufgrund der Ergebnisse und Erfahrungen dieser ersten Tests wird zur Zeit eine Revison und Erweiterung des Prototypen durchgeführt. Als nächster Schritt ist dann ein Einsatz am menschlichen Patienten unter ständiger Beobachtung eines Arztes geplant.

ForeignSGML
Quality Management of Multilingual Technical Documents
http://www.forwiss.de/fg-we/ForeignSGML.html

Partner: FORWISS, eidon GmbH	**Supported by:** BFS
Active: 10/1996 – 10/1998	**Contact:** H. Silberhorn

Objective:

The project ForeignSGML integrates the production of translations into document management based on SGML. The goal of ForeignSGML is to develop methods and tools to guarantee the consistency of multilingual technical documents. Using content-based structuring of documents, ForeignSGML incorporates and expands approaches of computer aided translation and analysis of document structure. Thereby it offers new possibilities to reuse existing translations of documents in part or as a whole. As it is based on the international standard SGML, the interoperability of documents is insured and they can be used within a wide range of hardware and software.

Results:

The heart of the project is a document management system based on SGML which facilitates a structured approach to working with multilingual documents. Components to support maintenance and production of versions and variants, as well as to detect changes in a document and transfer them to multilingual versions of the document, have been built on top of the SGML document environment. Besides, modules to detect automatically structurally or terminologically inconsistent document parts in translations and to reuse existing translations have been developed. In addition, the ForeignSGML system comprises interfaces to adapt to external translation supporting tools like terminology databases, translation memories, machine translation, spell checkers etc. Furthermore, ForeignSGML automates steps in the production of translations and simplifies and optimizes translation tasks.

The incorporation of the translation process into an SGML environment opens up new possibilities to link various language versions of documents to each other and to access them based on the content of their subsections. Time and resources needed to produce and manage multilingual documents can be reduced by working with ForeignSGML. At the same time the quality can be increased and new possibilities arise in particular for guaranteeing the consistency of multilingual documents and for keeping them up to date.

Selected publications:

References

1. H. SILBERHORN. ForeignSGML – A New Approach to Processing Complex Multilingual Technical Documentation. internal report, 1998.

KIT-MARKER
Development of a lexicon of discourse markers for automatic text generation

http://www.cs.tu-berlin.de/kit/markerD.html

(DFG-Schwerpunkt Sprachproduktion)

Partner: Technische Universität Berlin, FB Informatik, Forschungsgruppe KIT	**Supported by:** DFG
Active: 07/1997 – 07/1999	**Contact:** Dr. M. Stede

Objective:

Discourse markers ('cue words') are lexical items that signal the kind of coherence relation holding between adjacent text spans; for example, *because*, *since*, and *for this reason* are different markers for causal relations. Discourse markers are a syntactically quite heterogeneous group of words, many of which are traditionally treated as function words belonging to the realm of grammar rather than to the lexicon. But for a single discourse relation there is often a set of similar markers, allowing for a range of paraphrases for expressing the relation. To capture the similarities and differences between these, and to represent them adequately, we are developing DiMLex, a lexicon of discourse markers. With the help of this lexicon, an automatic text generator can choose the most suitable verbalization of a given discourse relation in a particular context. Thus, a central part of the lexicon entries concerns the constraints that the marker places on its syntactic and semantic environment.

Results:

In the first phase of the project we examined the discourse relations CONTRAST and CONCESSION and their German markers. Building on our analyses, we constructed sample lexicon entries for these markers. in parallel, we developed a language generation system on the basis of several pre-existing modules, which serves as a testbed for our prototypical marker lexicon. Our current application domain is the production of instructional text such as user manuals.

Selected publications:

References

1. M. STEDE, C. UMBACH. DiMLex: A lexicon of discourse markers for text generation and understanding. To appear in: Proceedings of Coling-ACL-98, Montreal, 1998.
2. B. GROTE, M. STEDE. Discourse marker choice in sentence planning. To appear in: Proceedings of the 9th International Workshop on Natural Language Generation, Niagara-on-the-Lake, 1998.

RELAX: Nonlinear Relaxation Networks for Multi–Dimensional Signal Processing and Segmentation

(German Research Foundation – Priority Programme: System– und Schaltungstechnik für hochgradige Parallelverarbeitung)

Partner: TU Hamburg–Harburg	**Supported by:** DFG
Active: 04/1996 – 04/1999	**Contact:** Prof. Stiehl

Objective:

Basis of the project is a class of well–understood variational approaches for nonlinear adaptive image smoothing and segmentation [1–3]. Goal of the project is the realization of analogue VLSI systems for the case of 2D images that work in real–time. A key issue is the interplay between theory, numerics, algorithmic complexity, VLSI design constraints, component perturbation models, and discrete simulation.

Results:

In 1998, a one–dimensional prototype with 32 cells has been fabricated using 0.8 μm technology, based on an analysis of how various approximations and perturbations of the underlying mathematical model affect both theoretically achievable results and the VLSI design. The chip is fully functional with an overall error less than 1% [4].

As a by–product, an efficient hardware architecture suitable for mixed–mode VLSI–implementation has been devised, where the connections of circularly arranged cells can by dynamically reconfigured. This results in a nonlinear adaptive filter kernel which can be virtually shifted over infinite–length signals [4].

Currently, we are exploiting these results further for the case of 2D intensity images.

Selected publications:

References

1. C. SCHNÖRR. Unique Reconstruction of Piecewise Smooth Images by Minimizing Strictly Convex Non-Quadratic Functionals. J. of Math. Imaging and Vision 4: 189–198, 1994.
2. C. SCHNÖRR. A Study of a Convex Variational Diffusion Approach for Image Segmentation and Feature Extraction. J. of Math. Imaging and Vision 8: 271–292, 1998.
3. C. SCHNÖRR, H.-S. STIEHL, R.-R. GRIGAT. On globally asymptotically stable continuous-time CNNs for adaptive smoothing of multidimensional signals. Proc. 4th IEEE Int. Workshop on Cellular Neural Networks and their Applications, Seville, Spain, June 24-26, 1996.
4. K. WIEHLER, R.-R. GRIGAT, J. HEERS, C. SCHNÖRR, H.S. STIEHL. Dynamic Circular Cellular Networks for Adaptive Smoothing of Multi-Dimensional Signals. Proc. 5th Int. Workshop on Cellular Neural Networks and Their Applications, London, April 14-17, 1998.

Work Oriented Design of Knowledge Systems (WORKS)
(Wissensbasierte Systeme, Wissensmanagement)

Partner: Institut AIFB (Universität Karlsruhe); **Supported by:** BMBF Hochschule für Kunst und Design (Halle); Werkstatt fî Design & Informatik GmbH (Chemnitz); Fachhochschule Schmalkalden **Active:** 10/1995 – 10/1998   **Contact:** Prof. Dr. R. Studer

Objective:

The objectives of the WORKS project are the development of methods and tools for supporting knowledge intensive work processes. As a test case for the new methods and tools, a knowledge-based system for ergonomic consulting in industrial design named ERBUS has to be developed.

Results:

At the AIFB the system Ontobroker has been developed, which realizes an ontology based access to informal, semiformal and formal knowledge. Ontobroker is based on deductive techniques and uses an inovative query interface. Based on Ontobroker and in close cooperation with the Werkstatt für Design & Informatik GmbH, the core of a Knowledge Management System supporting industrial designers has been realized.

Selected publications:
References

1. S. DECKER, M. DANIEL, M. ERDMANN, R. STUDER. An Enterprise Reference Scheme for Integrating Model Based Knowledge Engineering and Enterprise Modelling. In: Proceedings of the 10th European Workshop on Knowledge Acquisition, Modeling, and Management (EKAW'97), Sant Feliu de Guixols, Spain. Springer, LNAI 1319, 1997.
2. D. FENSEL, S. DECKER, M. ERDMANN, R. STUDER. Ontobroker: The Very High Idea. In: Proceedings of the 11th Florida Artificial Intelligence Research Symposium (FLAIRS-98), Sanibel Island, Florida, May 1998.

Stochastic Local Search
(Graduiertenkolleg ISIA)

Partner: TU Darmstadt, GK ISIA	Supported by: DFG
Active: 07/1995 – 07/1998	Contact: T. Stützle

Objective:

Many problems from Artificial Intelligence and Operations Research are of a combinatorial nature and very difficult to solve as they are typically $\mathcal{NP}$-hard. Stochastic Local Search (SLS) algorithms have been proved to be particularly suited for the solution of such problems. Such problems include important ones from AI applications, like constraint satisfaction problems and propositional satisfiability, as well as optimization problems like the traveling salesman problem. Within this field we concentrate on the empirical analysis and improvement of established SLS methods for propositional satisfiability and constraint satisfaction problems. Many algorithmic improvements in the ability to solve combinatorial optimization problems have been inspired by analogies to natural phenomena. Among those we work with ant colony optimization, a promising new algorithmic approach inspired by the foraging behaviour of real ant colonies.

Results:

The results of the project are twofold. For the application of SLS to constraint satisfaction problems and propositional satisfiability we have shown that the use of Tabu Search for the guidance of the local search algorithm significantly improves the performance. Additionally, the empirical methodology used for the evaluation of local search algorithms in this domain has been refined using run-time distributions to investigate the behaviour of SLS algorithms. Regarding ant colony optimization, previous algorithmic approaches could be improved significantly. In particular, for the traveling salesman problem and the quadratic assignment problem our approaches are among the best algorithms known for these problems.

Selected publications:
References

1. T. STÜTZLE, H. HOOS. The $\mathcal{MAX}$-$\mathcal{MIN}$ Ant System and Local Search for the Traveling Salesman Problem. In Proc. of ICEC'97, IEEE Press, 309–314, 1997.
2. T. STÜTZLE, H. HOOS. Improvements on the Ant System: Introducing $\mathcal{MAX}$-$\mathcal{MIN}$ Ant System. In Proc. of ICANNGA97, 245–249. Springer 1997.
3. O. STEINMANN, A. STROHMAIER, T. STÜTZLE. Tabu Search vs. Random Walk. In KI-97: Advances in Artificial Intelligence, LNCS 1303. Springer 1997.
4. H. HOOS, T. STÜTZLE. Evaluating Las Vegas Algorithms — Pitfalls and Remedies. To appear in Proc. of UAI98. Morgan Kaufmann 1998.

SpeeData
http://www.forwiss.uni-erlangen.de/~uebler/
(Language Engineering)

Partner: Informatica Trentina, IRST (Trento), Regione Autonoma di Trento–Alto Adige, Bundesjustizministerium Austria	**Supported by:** EU
Active: 11/1995 – 03/1998	**Contact:** U. Übler

Objective:

The goal of this project was to develop a bilingual system for efficient data-entry of historic master books by means of natural speech, keyboard, and mouse. The system is designed to be used in the land register offices in the bilingual (Italian/German) region of South Tyrol in Italy. Special aspects of this project were among other to deal with accent of non-native speakers and with the dialects of the speakers which vary a lot between the standard German and the respective local dialects. Another aspect was to deal with the high number of proper names of persons, villages that appear in both languages. With this project, a reduction of labour cost of up to 40% is expected.

Results:

In a first step, together with the users of the system the interface and the communication between the means of data-entry was designed in order to allow an efficient data-entry. With this specification and some first data, a prototype was designed which again was discussed with the users. With this, the final version of the prototype was developed. For this prototype, ways were found to deal with the composita of the German language and the proper names of both languages. Research on speaker adaptation was done on adaptation sentences of the users. The performance of the system finally yielded a recognition rate for the speaker adapted version of 96.7 (90.6) for Italian (German). At present, the system is being installed at the land register offices in South Tyrol and will be used by the employees.

Selected publications:

References

1. U. ACKERMANN, B. ANGELINI, F. BRUGNARA, M. FEDERICO, D. GIULIANI, R. GRETTER, G. LAZZARI, H. NIEMANN. SpeeData: Multilingual Spoken Data Entry. Proc. Int. Conf. on Spoken Language Processing, Philadelphia, 1996.
2. U. ACKERMANN, B. ANGELINI, F. BRUGNARA, M. FEDERICO, D. GIULIANI, R. GRETTER, H. NIEMANN. SpeeData – a Prototype for Multilingual Spoken Data-Entry. Proc. European Conf. on Speech Communication and Technology, Rhodes, Greece, 1997.

OASES - Our Approach to Simulate Experimental Studies
http://www.informatik.uni-ulm.de/ki/oases.html
(Landesschwerpunktprogramm Baden-Württemberg)

Partner: Department of Orthopaedic Research and Biomechanics, University of Ulm	Supported by: Land Baden-Wuerttemberg
Active: 04/1996 – 01/1998	Contact: Dr. A.M. Uhrmacher

Objective:
Simulation means experimenting with the model of a domain. General rules to describe the causal relations of a domain are often difficult to obtain. Rather than basing simulation on an explicit model, OASES utilizes intensively cases for simulation. Given a specific situation, similar cases are identified and their relevance weighted. Finally, the most suitable cases are adapted to predict the likely outcome.

To measure relevance and suitability and to guide the process of adaptation, case-based reasoning systems require a predefinition of relevant parameters, if they cannot determine them inductively. Depending on the given case, the relevance of single parameters might vary drastically, hampering this approach. To avoid the need to generalize the assessment of similarity and adaptation between cases, OASES applies cases to compute suitability and to process adaptation.

Results:
OASES has been put to test in the domain of bone healing. The case base entails 650 cases extracted from about 50 publications. The set of variables and their scaling niveau varies from study to study within which about 70 parameters were measured or comparatively assessed. OASES was evaluated by extracting single studies from the case-base and asking it to predict the likely outcome of the experimental setting. Although the case base showed no obvious redundance, OASES performed the 80 test runs persuasively. The evaluation was facilitated by a graphical user interface, which presents reasoning steps in a hierarchical and case-based manner.

Selected publications:
References

1. D. DAMM, F.W. VON HENKE, A. SEITZ, A.M. UHRMACHER, L. CLAES, S. WOLF. Ein fallbasiertes System für die Interpretation von Literatur zur Knochenheilung. Technical Report Nr. 98-01. Ulmer Informatik-Berichte, Ulm, 1998.
2. A.M. UHRMACHER, A. SEITZ. Fallbasierte Simulation ökologischer und biologischer Systeme. 8th Workshop, AK5, GI-Fachgruppe 4.5.9/4.6.3. To be published in: Metropolis Verlag, 1998.
3. A. SEITZ, A.M. UHRMACHER. The Treatment of Time in a Case-Based Analysis of Experimental Medical Studies. To appear in: Proceedings of the KI-98. Bremen, 1998.

DAISY: DAiry Improvement SYstem using NN & AI Techniques for Breeding Decisions

http://www.fit.qut.edu.au/NRC/projects/daisy/daisy.html

Partner: Neurocomputing Research Centre, Queensland University of Technology, Brisbane, Australia Queensland Department of Primary Industries (QDPI), Australia	**Supported by:** ARC, Canberra, Australia
Active: 01/1998 – 01/2001	**Contact:** Dr. U. Visser

Topics:
Neural Networks, Rule–Extraction, artificial intelligence techniques, advanced statistics

Results:
Main focus of work between 08/97 and 07/98: This project investigates computerized techniques for the support of dairy breeding decisions by farmers in Australia. In particular, statistical methods, neurocomputing and artificial intelligence techniques are evaluated. The comparison will be done by methods such as cross-validation and bootstrap, as well as by the use of "real world scenarios." The objective is an integrated information system which combines these techniques and aims at a performance which cannot be achieved by any of the above mentioned methods in isolation. The outcome is a PC–based standalone system which supports a farmer wrt. animal breeding decisions.

Selected publications:

References

1. R. ANDREWS, J. DIEDERICH, A.B. TICKLE. A survey and critique of techniques for extracting rules from trained artificial neural networks. Knowledge-Based Systems, 8:373 – 389, 1995.
2. G. FINN, R. LISTER, T. SZABO, D. SIMONETTA, H. MULDER, R. YOUNG. Neural Networks applied to a large biological database to analyse dairy breeding patterns. Neural Computing and Applications, 4:237 – 253, 1996.
3. U. VISSER, R. NAYAK, M. T. WONG. Rule extraction from trained neural networks & connectionist knowledge representation for the determination of pesticide mixtures. Proceedings of the Australian Conference of Neural Networks (ACNN 98), 138 – 142, Brisbane, Australia, February 1998.

The CODY Project: Dynamic Conceptualization
Integration of structural and imaginal representations for dynamic conceptualization of objects and aggregates in assembly tasks

http://www.TechFak.Uni-Bielefeld.DE/techfak/ags/wbski/cody/

(SFB 360 Situated Artificial Communicators)

Partner: University of Bielefeld	**Supported by:** DFG
Active: 1993 – 1996	**Contact:** Prof. Dr. I. Wachsmuth

Objective:

In an experimental setting of mechanical-object assembly, the CODY project is concerned with the development of knowledge representations and inference methods that are able to dynamically conceptualize the changing situation in the task environment. A central aim is to enable an artificial agent to understand and process natural-language instructions of a human partner. Instructions may build on the current perception of the assembly environment on the one hand, and on the other on the knowledge-based understanding of grouped structures in the developing construct. To this end, a dynamic conceptualization must integrate information not only describing the types of the objects involved, but also their functional roles in, and the spatial layout of, changing assembly structures.

Results:

One of the main results of the first funding period (1993-1996) is the development of an operational knowledge representation formalism, COAR ("Concepts for Objects, Assemblies, and Roles"). Inferences concern the assertion or retraction of aggregate representations in a dynamic knowledge base, as well as the computation of role changes for individual objects associated herewith. In the second funding period (1996-1999), our investigations focus on an additional, imaginal kind of representation besides the structural representations we developed so far. These imaginal prototypes are parametric spatial representations of objects and aggregates that capture the generic 3D shape of artifacts at different levels of abstraction. Our results are integrated in a 3D computergraphics simulation environment, the CODY Virtual Constructor, which enables the interactive assembly 3D visualized mechanical parts to complex aggregates by way of natural language instructions and direct manipulation and which furnishes high-level representations to cognitive robotic systems developed in SFB 360.

Selected publications:
References

1. I. WACHSMUTH, B. JUNG. Dynamic Conceptualization in a Mechanical-Object Assembly Environment. Artificial Intelligence Review, 10 (3-4): 345 – 368, 1996.
2. B. JUNG. Wissensverarbeitung für Montageaufgaben in virtuellen und realen Umgebungen. Dissertationen der Künstlichen Intelligenz, Bd. 157, Infix, 1997.
3. B. JUNG, M. HOFFHENKE, I. WACHSMUTH. Virtual Assembly with Construction Kits. In Proceedings of the 1998 ASME Design for Engineering Technical Conferences (DECT-DFM '98), 1998. To appear.

SGIM: Speech and Gesture Interfaces for Multimedia

http://www.TechFak.Uni-Bielefeld.DE/techfak/ags/wbski/sgim/

(Multimedia NRW: The Virtual Knowledge Factory)

Partner: University of Bielefeld	**Supported by:** MWF-NRW
Active: 1996 – 1999	**Contact:** Prof. I. Wachsmuth

Objective:

The working group "Multimedia NRW: The Virtual Knowledge Factory (Die virtuelle Wissensfabrik)", founded in 1996, is a collaborative effort to bundle research from different areas of human-machine interaction. The SGIM project contributes to this effort by developing techniques for communicating with multimedia systems through the detection and interpretation of a user's verbal (speech) and coarse gestural input. The aim is to overcome the physical limitations of common computer displays and input devices, to enable enhanced interaction methods when using large-screen displays (wall projections, workbenches, caves), and thus allowing the user to operate an application system in a more natural and convenient manner.

Results:

In an experimental application of virtual construction users' gestural communication is supported by simple speech input. Object types and locations can be referenced via verbal expressions, e.g. "...this wheel", to identify objects and locations in cases where sole gestural communication is unnatural or reaches technical limitations. Therefore, the gestural data gathered by electromagnetic 6DOF position- and orientation sensors (trackers) is integrated with output from a speech analyser to form multimodal inputs for the multimedia system. The construction of a mobile platform ("City-Mobile"), based on large-screen projected CAD-models, serves as a shared testbed application which integrates the results achieved by the different research groups.

Close project cooperations exist with research groups in the Collaborative Research Center 'Situated Artificial Communicators (SFB 360)' and the Graduate Study Program 'Task-oriented Communication', University of Bielefeld. Further project partners are the European Centre for Mechatronic in Aachen and the Institute for Media Communication in St. Augustin. The research project SGIM is sponsored by the Ministry of Science and Research of the Federal State North-Rhine-Westphalia under grant no IV A 3 - 107 032 96.

Selected publications:
References

1. M. LATOSCHIK, I. WACHSMUTH. Exploiting distant pointing gestures for object selection in a virtual environment. In I. Wachsmuth, M. Fröhlich (eds.): Gesture and Sign Language in Human-Computer Interaction, 185-196. Springer, LNAI 1371, 1998.
2. M. LATOSCHIK, M. FRÖHLICH, B. JUNG, I. WACHSMUTH. Utilize speech and gestures to realize natural interaction in a virtual environment. In Proc. IECON'98, Special Session Advanced Man-Machine Interaction. To appear.

Verbmobil: Multilingual Processing of Spontaneous Speech

http://www.dfki.de/verbmobil

Partner: ATR International, Kyoto, Japan (Sub-contractor) Carnegie Mellon University, Pittsburgh, USA (Subcontractor) Center for the Study of Language and Information, Stanford, USA DFKI GmbH LMU München RWTH Aachen TU Berlin TU Dresden TU München Univ Bielefeld Univ Bochum Univ Bonn Univ Braunschweig Univ d. Saarlandes Univ Erlangen Univ Hamburg Univ Karlsruhe Univ Stuttgart Univ Tübingen Daimler-Benz AG DASA Philips Siemens AG	**Supported by:** BMBF
Active: 1993 – 2000	**Contact:** Prof. Dr. W. Wahlster

Objective:

Verbmobil is a long-term interdisciplinary Language Technology project. The Verbmobil System recognizes spoken input, analyzes and translates it, and utters the translation. This speaker-independent system processes spontaneous speech. Verbmobil offers assistance in multilingual dialog situations in certain domains (e.g. scheduling appointments, travel planning and making hotel reservations). The project is a joint initiative involving information-technology companies, universities, and research centers. The project is controlled by the German Aerospace Research Establishment (DLR). The Verbmobil milestones are reviewed twice a year by an international advisory board.

Results:

Distinguishing features of the Verbmobil Research Prototype (1996):

- Recognition of continuous and spontaneous German and Japanese using a close-speaking microphone.
- Vocabulary of around 2,500 words for translation from German to English.
- Speaker-independent speech recognition.
- Use of prosodic information for disambiguation.
- Linguistically motivated grammar for spontaneous German, including deep and shallow analysis.
- Spoken clarification dialogs between the Verbmobil System and the user.
- Semantic transfer for German/English and Japanese/English dialogs.
- Context-sensitive dialog processing.
- Completely software-based solutions for all modules on standard hardware.
- Processing time that is less than six times the length of the input signal.

Selected publications:

http://www.dfki.de/verbmobil

Automated Theorem Proving by Induction
(DFG Project)

Partner: none	**Supported by:** DFG
Active: 1992 – 1999	**Contact:** Prof. Dr. C. Walther

Objective:

Induction is the essential proof method for the verification of programs. Several techniques have been developed to perform induction proofs automatically. However, for an application of induction theorem proving in practice, the degree of automation still has to be increased. As there are two research paradigms for the automation of induction proofs, viz. explicit and implicit induction, our aim is to analyze the connections and benefits of these two approaches in order to refine the existing techniques for automated induction proofs.

Results:

In [7,9] methods are investigated which compute suitable induction relations automatically and techniques for the combination of induction relations are presented in [8]. The methods are refined further by a new approach which postpones the formulation of induction hypotheses until they are needed during the proof [4,5]. To detect false conjectures, methods are developed to generate counterexamples [3] and to transform flawed conjectures into valid ones [6]. Since the existing approaches for automated induction proofs are only sound for total functions, in [2] it is investigated under which prerequisites they may be extended to partial functions. Finally, to benefit from the results from both explicit and implicit induction theorem proving, a detailed comparison between these two approaches is worked out in [1].

Selected publications:
References

1. S. GERBERDING. Implizite und explizite Induktionsbeweisverfahren. Doctoral Dissertation, Infix-Verlag, St. Augustin, 1997.
2. J. GIESL. Induction Proofs With Partial Functions. Technical Report IBN 98/48, Darmstadt University of Technology, Germany, 1998.
3. M. PROTZEN. Disproving Conjectures. In Proceedings of CADE-92, LNAI 607, Saratoga Springs, NY, 340-354, 1992.
4. M. PROTZEN. Lazy Generation of Induction Hypotheses. In Proceedings of CADE-94, LNAI 814, Nancy, France, pages 42-56, 1994.
5. M. PROTZEN. Lazy Generation of Induction Hypotheses. Doctoral Dissertation, Infix-Verlag, St. Augustin, 1995.
6. M. PROTZEN. Patching Faulty Conjectures. In Proceedings of CADE-96, LNAI 1104, New Brunswick, NJ, pages 77-91, 1996.
7. C. WALTHER. Computing Induction Axioms. In Proceedings of LPAR-92, LNAI 624, St. Petersburg, Russia, 1992.
8. C. WALTHER. Combining Induction Axioms by Machine. In Proceedings of IJCAI-93, Morgan Kaufmann, Chambery, France, 95-101, 1993.
9. C. WALTHER. Mathematical Induction. *Handbook of Logic in Artificial Intelligence and Logic Programming*, Vol. 2, Gabbay, Hogger & Robinson (eds.), Oxford Univ. Pr., 1994.

Termination of Algorithms
(DFG Schwerpunkt Deduktion)

Partner: none	**Supported by:** DFG
Active: 1995 – 1999	**Contact:** Prof. Dr. C. Walther

Objective:

Proving termination is a central problem in software development. Our aim is to investigate the automation of termination proofs for functional programs as well as for (imperative) loop programs.

Results:

To prove termination of a functional algorithm, one has to find a well-founded relation such that the arguments in recursive calls are smaller than the corresponding inputs. In previous approaches the relations used were either fixed or had to be provided by the user. To increase their power, we developed a new technique for automated termination proofs which allows an automatic synthesis of suitable well-founded relations. Our approach proved successful on a large collection of examples (including algorithms with nested and mutual recursion), cf. [4-10].

The methods developed have been proved useful for termination analysis of term rewriting systems, too [1]. We also investigate the termination behaviour of partial functions by synthesizing termination predicates which approximate the domains of such functions. In particular, these problems arise during the analysis of loops in imperative programs [2,3,8].

Selected publications:
References

1. T. ARTS, J. GIESL. Termination of Term Rewriting Using Dependency Pairs. Theoretical Computer Science. To appear.
2. J. BRAUBURGER, J. GIESL. Termination Analysis for Partial Functions. In Proceedings of SAS '96, LNCS 1145, Aachen, Germany, pages 113-127, 1996.
3. J. BRAUBURGER, J. GIESL. Termination Analysis by Inductive Evaluation. In Proceedings of CADE '98, LNAI, Lindau, Germany, 1998.
4. J. GIESL. Generating Polynomial Orderings for Termination Proofs. In Proceedings of RTA-95, LNCS 914, Kaiserslautern, Germany, pages 426-431, 1995.
5. J. GIESL. Automated Termination Proofs with Measure Functions. In Proceedings of KI '95, LNAI 981, Bielefeld, Germany, 1995.
6. J. GIESL. Termination Analysis for Functional Programs using Term Orderings. In Proceedings of SAS '95, LNCS 983, Glasgow, Scotland, 1995.
7. J. GIESL. Termination of Nested and Mutually Recursive Algorithms. Journal of Automated Reasoning 19:1-29, 1997.
8. J. GIESL, C. WALTHER, J. BRAUBURGER. Termination Analysis for Functional Programs. In Automated Deduction – A Basis for Applications, Vol. 3 (Applications), W. Bibel, P. Schmitt (eds.), 135-164, Kluwer Academic Publishers, 1998.
9. C. WALTHER. On Proving the Termination of Algorithms by Machine. Artificial Intelligence 71:101-157, 1994.
10. C. WALTHER. Criteria for Termination. Research Report, Darmstadt University of Technology, 1998.

An Optimization Approach on the Integration of Multiple Images for Classification

http://sfb-603.uni-erlangen.de

Partner: none	Supported by: DFG
Active: 1998 – 2000	Contact: M. Zobel

Objective:

Until this day, the integration of different images based on optimization techniques to solve classification tasks in computer vision is still an open problem. Therefore the aim of this project is the development and the verification of approaches based on optimization techniques for sensor data fusion of multiple cameras for detection, tracking, and classification of objects in a natural environment. Unlike the available methods, detection and tracking are performed by the use of different resolutions (multi–resolution–hierarchies). These are technically realized by cameras with different focal lengths. The images of a camera with relative small focal length are used for the motion detection based on active contours or active rays. The images of a camera with a large focal length are used for classification and if necessary for the exact localization of objects (sensor data fusion). For object recognition a global overview and a local detail inspection are combined in such a way that the results from the classification and localization are as reliable as possible. Appropriate models are used for the identification of the objects (model–based object recognition). The models are not only represented geometrically, but also as parametric probability density functions. The models are created automatically from sample views of the object. The innovation on the whole approach is the optimized and data driven employment of images of multiple cameras for the classification of objects (optimization approach).

Results:

The base of the research in this project is build on the results of current research in the fields of active contours, active rays, and probabilistic object modelling and recognition.

Selected publications:

References

1. J. DENZLER, H. NIEMANN. Real-time pedestrian tracking in natural scenes. In G. Sommer, K. Daniliidis, J. Pauli (editors), Computer Analysis of Images and Patterns, CAIP'97, 42–49, 1997.
2. J. DENZLER, H. NIEMANN. Active rays: Polar-transformed active contours for real-time contour tracking. Journal on Real-Time Imaging, 1998. To appear.
3. J. HORNEGGER, H. NIEMANN. Statistical Learning, Localization, and Identification of Objects. ICCV 95, 914–919, 1996.
4. J. PÖSL, H. NIEMANN. Wavelet Features for Statistical Object Localization without Segmentation. ICIP 97, 170–173, 1997.

2 List of Project Contacts

U. Ahlrichs Spracherkennung ; Fachbereich Informatik; Universität Erlangen ; Martensstraße 3, 91058 Erlangen ; Germany
phone: +49 (0)9131 / 85 7874 ; fax: +49 (0)9131 / 303811
email: ahlrichs@informatik.uni-erlangen.de
www: http://faui56s2.informatik.uni-erlangen.de/HTML/English/Persons/MA/ah/index.html

Dr. M. Aretoulaki Spracherkennung ; Fachbereich Informatik; Universität Erlangen ; Martensstrae 3, 91058 Erlangen ; Germany
email: aretoula@informatik.uni-erlangen.de

Prof. Dr. F. Baader Lehr- und Forschungsgebiet Theoretische Informatik ; RWTH Aachen ; Ahornstr. 55 ; 52074 Aachen ; Germany
phone: +49 (0)241 / 8021 130 ; fax: +49 (0)241 / 8888 360
email: baader@informatik.rwth-aachen.de
www: http://cantor.informatik.rwth-aachen.de/ti/baader-uk.html

D. Bartmann Institut für Informatik ; Technische Universität München ; 80290 München ; Germany
phone: +49 (0)89 / 289 28419 ; fax: +49 (0)89 / 289 28483
email: bartmann@informatik.tu-muenchen.de
www: http://wwwbrauer.informatik.tu-muenchen.de/~bartmann/

Prof. Dr. C. Beierle Lehrgebiet Praktische Informatik VIII ; Fernuniversität Hagen ; Feithstr. 140 ; Informatikzentrum ; 58084 Hagen; Germany
phone: +49 (0)2331 / 987 4293 ; fax: +49 (0)2331 / 987 4288
email: christoph.beierle@fernuni-hagen.de

Prof. Dr. G. Brewka Intelligent Systems Department ; Computer Science Institute ; University of Leipzig ; Augustusplatz 10-11 ; 04109 Leipzig ; Germany
phone: +49 (0)341 / 973 2235
email: brewka@informatik.uni-leipzig.de
www: http://www.informatik.uni-leipzig.de/~brewka/

Prof. Dr. H.-D. Burkhard Lehr- und Forschungsgebiet Künstliche Intelligenz ; Institut für Informatik ; Humboldt-Universität zu Berlin ; Germany
phone: +49 (0)30 / 20181 213 ; fax: +49 (0)30 / 20181 216
email: hdb@informatik.hu-berlin.de
www: http://www.informatik.hu-berlin.de/~hdb

Prof. Dr. A. B. Cremers Institut für Informatik III ; Universität Bonn ; Römerstr. 164 ; 53117 Bonn ; Germany
phone: +49 (0)228 / 7345 00 (-01) ; fax: +49 (0)228 / 73 4382
email: abc@uni-bonn.de
www: http://www.informatik.uni-bonn.de/~abc

Prof. Dr. R. Dillmann Fakultät Informatik ; Univerität Karlsruhe ; Germany
phone: +49 (0)721 / 608 3846 ; fax: +49 (0)721 / 608 7141
email: dillmann@ira.uka.de

Dr. J. Dix Fachbereich Informatik ; Universität Koblenz ; Rheinau 1 ; 56075 Koblenz ; Germany
phone: +49 (0)261 / 9119 420 ; fax: +49 (0)261 / 9119 496
email: dix@informatik.uni-koblenz.de www: http://www.uni-koblenz.de/~dix/

C. Drexler

Prof. C. Freksa, PhD. Fachbereich Informatik ; Universität Hamburg ; Vogt-Kölln-Strasse 30 ; 22527 Hamburg ; Germany
phone: +49 (0)40 / 5994 2418 (-2416); fax: +49 (0)40 / 5994 2572
email: freksa@informatik.uni-hamburg.de
www: http://www.informatik.uni-hamburg.de/WSV/hp/freksa.html

Prof. Dr. U. Furbach Künstliche Intelligenz ; Fakultät Informatik ; Universität Koblenz ; Rheinau 1 ; 56075 Koblenz ; Germany
phone: +49 (0)261 / 9119 433 ; fax: +49 (0)261 / 9119 496
email: uli@informatik.uni-koblenz.de
www: http://www.uni-koblenz.de/~uli/

B. Gaede FORWISS - Bayerisches Forschungszentrum für Wissensbasierte Systeme ; Am Weichselgarten 7 ; 91058 Erlangen-Tennenlohe
phone: +49 (0)9131 / 691 198 ; fax: +49 (0)9131 / 691 185
email: bernd.gaede@forwiss.uni-erlangen.de

F. Gallwitz

A. Gebhard

K. U. Goecke Fakultät für Linguistik und Literaturwissenschaft ; Universität Bielefeld ; Germany
phone: +49 (0)521 / 106 3716
email: goecke@lili.uni-bielefeld.de
www: http://coli.lili.uni-bielefeld.de/~goecke/

Dr. T. Gordon GMD FI/KI ; Schloss Birlinghoven ; 53754 Sankt Augustin ; Germany
phone: +49 (0)2241 / 142 665 ; fax: +49 (0)2241 / 142 072
email: thomas.gordon@gmd.de
www: http://nathan.gmd.de/persons/thomas.gordon.html

G. Grieser Fachgebiet Intellektik ; Fachbereich Informatik ; Technische Universität Darmstadt; Alexanderstr. 10 ; 64283 Darmstadt ; Germany
email: gunter@intellektik.informatik.tu-darmstadt.de
www: http://www.intellektik.informatik.th-darmstadt.de/~gunter/

Prof. Dr. C. Habel Arbeitsbereich WSV ; Fachbereich Informatik; Universität Hamburg ; Vogt-Kölln-Straße 30; 22527 Hamburg; Germany
phone: +49 (0)40 / 5494 2417 (-2416)
email: habel@informatik.uni-hamburg.de
www: http://www.informatik.uni-hamburg.de/WSV/hp/christopher-english.html

Prof. Dr. W. von Hahn Natural Language Systems ; Computer Science Department ; University of Hamburg ; Vogt-Köhlln-Str. 30 ; 22527 Hamburg ; Germany.
phone: +49 (0)40 / 5494 2433 ; fax: +49 (0)40 / 5494 2515
email: vhahn@informatik.uni-hamburg.de
www: http://nats-www.informatik.uni-hamburg.de/~vhahn/

S. Harbeck

B. Heigl Spracherkennung ; Fachbereich Informatik; Universität Erlangen ; Martensstrae 3, 91058 Erlangen ; Germany
phone: +49 (0)9131 / 857891 ; fax: +49 (0)9131 / 303811
email: heigl@informatik.uni-erlangen.de
www: http://faui56s2.informatik.uni-erlangen.de/HTML/English/Persons/MA/he/he.html

Prof. F. von Henke Abtl. Künstliche Intelligenz ; Universität Ulm ; 89069 Ulm ; Germany
phone: +49 (0)731 / 50 24120 ; fax: +49 (0)731 / 50 24120
email: vhenke@ki.informatik.uni-ulm.de
www: http://www.informatik.uni-ulm.de/ki/vhenke.html

Dr. C. Herrmann Max-Planck-Institute of Cognitive Neuroscience ; Inselstr. 22-26 ; 04103 Leipzig ; Germany
phone: +49 (0)341 / 9940 250 ; fax: +49 (0)341 / 9940 113
email: herrmann@cns.mpg.de
www: http://www.intellektik.informatik.th-darmstadt.de/ chris/

Prof. Dr. O. Herzog TZI - Center for Computing Technologies - FB 3 ; University of Bremen ; P.O. Box 33 0440 ; D-28334 Bremen, Germany
phone: +49 (0)421 / 218 7089 (-7090); fax: +49 (0)421 / 218 7196
email: herzog@informatik.uni-bremen.de
www: http://www.informatik.uni-bremen.de/~herzog/

Prof. Dr. S. Hölldobler Institut für Künstliche Intelligenz ; Fakultät Informatik ; Technische Universität Dresden ; Hans-Grundig Str. 25 ; 01307 Dresden ; Germany
phone: +49 (0)351 / 463 8340 ; fax: +49 (0)351 / 463 8342
email: sh@inf.tu-dresden.de
www: http://wv.inf.tu-dresden.de/steffen/sh.html

Prof. Dr. M. Jarke Lehrstuhl für Informatik V ; RWTH Aachen ; Ahornstr. 55 ; 52056 Aachen ; Germany
phone: +49 (0)241 / 8021 501 ; fax : +49 (0)241 / 8888 321
email: jarke@informatik.rwth-aachen.de

Dr. S. Jekat Natural Language Systems ; Computer Science Department ; University of Hamburg ; Vogt-Köhlln-Str. 30 ; 22527 Hamburg ; Germany.
phone: +49 (0)40 / 5494 2520 ; fax: +49 (0)40 / 5494 2515
email: jekat@informatik.uni-hamburg.de
www: http://nats-www.informatik.uni-hamburg.de/~jekat/

Prof. Dr. P. Levi Bildverstehen ; Institut für Parallele und Verteilte Höchstleistungsrechner ; Universität Stuttgart ; Breitwiesenstr. 20-22; 70565 Stuttgart ; Germany
phone: +49 (0)711 / 7816 387 ; fax: +49 (0)711 / 7816 250
email: paul.levi@informatik.uni-stuttgart.de
www: http://www.informatik.uni-stuttgart.de/ipvr/bv/personen/levi.html

F. Kirchner GMD ; Schloss Birlinghoven ; 53754 Sankt Augustin ; Germany
phone: +49 (0)2241 / 142 402
email: frank.kirchner@gmd.de
www: http://www.gmd.de/People/Frank.Kirchner/

Prof. Dr. W. Menzel Natural Language Systems ; Computer Science Department ; University of Hamburg ; Vogt-Köhlln-Str. 30 ; 22527 Hamburg ; Germany.
phone: +49 (0)40 / 5494 2435 ; fax: +49 (0)40 / 5494 2515
email: menzel@informatik.uni-hamburg.de
www: http://nats-www.informatik.uni-hamburg.de/~wolfgang/

Prof. Dr. K. Morik Lehrstuhl für Künstliche Intelligenz ; Fachbereich Informatik ; Universität Dortmund ; Germany
phone: +49 (0)231 / 755 5101 ; fax: +49 (0)231 / 755 5105
email: morik@ls8.cs.uni-dortmund.de
www: http://www-ai.cs.uni-dortmund.de/PERSONAL/morik.html

Dr. H. Mühlenbein GMD SET; Schloss Birlinghoven ; 53754 Sankt Augustin ; Germany
phone: +49 (0)2241 / 14 2405 ; fax: +49 (0)2241 / 14 2342
email: heinz.muehlenbein@gmd.de
www: http://set.gmd.de/SET/mitarbeiter/Heinz.Muehlenbein.htm

M. Müller FORWISS - Bayerisches Forschungszentrum für Wissensbasierte Systeme ; Am Weichselgarten 7 ; 91058 Erlangen-Tennenlohe
phone: +49 (0)9131 / 691 198 ; fax: +49 (0)9131 / 691 185
email: mlmuelle@forwiss.uni-erlangen.de
www: http://www.forwiss.uni-erlangen.de/~mlmuelle/

Prof. Dr. W. Nejdl

Prof. Dr. B. Neumann Fachbereich Informatik ; Universität Hamburg ; Vogt-Kölln-Strasse 30 ; 22527 Hamburg ; Germany
phone: +49 (0)40 / 5994 2450 ; fax: +49 (0)40 / 5994 2572
email: neumann@informatik.uni-hamburg.de
www: http://lki-www.informatik.uni-hamburg.de/~neumann/home.html

Dr. B. Nöth

Prof. Dr. H. Noltemeier Lehrstuhl für Informatik I ; Universität Wrzburg ; Am Hubland ; 97074 Wrzburg ; Germany
phone: +49 (0)931 / 888 5055 ; fax: +49 (0)931 / 888 4600
email: noltemei@informatik.uni-wuerzburg.de
www: http://www-info1.informatik.uni-wuerzburg.de/staff/noltemeier.html

Prof. Dr. G. Palm Abteilung Neuroinformatik ; Fakultät für Informatik ; Universität Ulm 89069 Ulm ; Germany
phone: +49 (0)731 / 502 4151 ; fax: +49 (0)731 / 502 4156
email: gpalm@neuro.informatik.uni-ulm.de
www: http://www.informatik.uni-ulm.de/abt/ni/mitarbeiter/GPalm.html

Prof. Dr. J. Perl

K. Peters Teilprojekt D1 SFB 360 Kommunizierende Agenten ; Universität Bielefeld ;
Germany
phone: +49 (0)521 / 106 3514
email: conny@coli.uni-bielefeld.de
www: http://coli.lili.uni-bielefeld.de/~conny/

Dr. L. Peters GMD SET; Schloss Birlinghoven ; 53754 Sankt Augustin ; Germany
phone: +49 (0)2241 / 14 2855 ; fax: +49 (0)2241 / 14 2072
email: liliane.peters@gmd.de
www: http://set.gmd.de/SET/mitarbeiter/Liliane.Peters.htm

Prof. Dr. F. Puppe Lehrstuhl für Künstliche Intelligenz und angewandte Informatik ;
Institut für Informatik ; Universität Wrzburg ; Allesgrundweg 12 ; 97218 Gerbrunn ;
Germany
phone: +49 (0)931 / 70561 10 ; fax: +49 (0)931 / 70561 20
email: puppe@informatik.uni-wuerzburg.de
www: http://ki-server.informatik.uni-wuerzburg.de/~puppe/

Dr. A. Reuter JURCA Optoelektronik GmbH ; Rodgau ; Germany
phone: +49 (0)6106 / 8290 32

Dr. K. Rohr Universitt Hamburg ; Vogt-Kölln-Straße 30 ; D-22527 Hamburg ; Germany
phone: +49 (0)40 / 5494 2575 ; fax: +49 (0)40 / 5494 2572
email: rohr@informatik.uni-hamburg.de
www: http://kogs-www.informatik.uni-hamburg.de/~rohr/home.html

J. Schaaf GMD FIT/KI; Schloss Birlinghoven ; 53754 Sankt Augustin ; Germany
phone: +49 (0)2241 / 142 855 ; fax: +49 (0)2241 / 142 072
email: joerg.schaaf@gmd.de
www: http://nathan.gmd.de/persons/joerg.schaaf/joerg.schaaf.html

T. Semmel-Griebeler FB 17 ; Institut für Informatik ; Universität Mainz ; 55099 Mainz
; Germany
phone: +49 (0)6131 / 39 3616 (-3378) ; fax: +49 (0)6131 / 39 3534
email: semmel@informatik.uni-mainz.de
www: http://www.informatik.uni-mainz.de/PERSONEN/SemmelG.html

H. Silberhorn FORWISS - Bayerisches Forschungszentrum für Wissensbasierte Systeme
; Am Weichselgarten 7 ; 91058 Erlangen-Tennenlohe
email: horst.silberhorn@forwiss.de

Dr. M. Stede Projektgruppe KIT ; Fachbereich Informatik ; Technische Universität
Berlin ; Franklinstraße 28/29 ; 10587 Berlin ; Germany
phone: +49 (0)30 / 314 24944 ; fax: +49 (0)30 / 314 24929
email: stede@cs.tu-berlin.de
www: http://www.cs.tu-berlin.de/~stede/

Prof. Dr. S. Stiehl

T. Stützle Fachgebiet Intellektik ; Fachbereich Informatik ; Technische Universität Darmstadt; Alexanderstr. 10 ; 64283 Darmstadt ; Germany
email: tom@intellektik.informatik.tu-darmstadt.de
www: http://www.intellektik.informatik.th-darmstadt.de/~tom/

Prof. Dr. R. Studer Institut fr Angewandte Informatik und Formale Beschreibungsver-
fahren ; Universität Karlsruhe ; 76128 Karlsruhe ; Germany
phone: +49 (0)721 / 608 3923 (-4750) ; fax: +49 (0)721 / 693 3717
email: studer@aifb.uni-karlsruhe.de
www: http://www.aifb.uni-karlsruhe.de/Staff/studer.html

U. Übler FORWISS - Bayerisches Forschungszentrum für Wissensbasierte Systeme ; Am
Weichselgarten 7 ; 91058 Erlangen-Tennenlohe
phone: +49 (0)9131 / 691 258 ; fax: +49 (0)9131 / 691 185
email: uebler@forwiss.de
www: http://www.forwiss.uni-erlangen.de/~uebler/

Dr. A. Uhrmacher Abtl. Künstliche Intelligenz ; Universität Ulm ; 89069 Ulm ; Germany
phone: +49 (0)731 / 50 24123 ; fax: +49 (0)731 / 50 24119
email: lin@ki.informatik.uni-ulm.de
www: http://www.informatik.uni-ulm.de/ki/uhrmacher.html

Dr. U. Visser TZI - Center for Computing Technologies - FB 3; University of Bremen
PO Box 330 440 ; D-28334 Bremen ; Germany.
phone: +49 (0)421 / 218 7840 (-7090); fax: +49 (0)421 / 218 7196
email: visser@tzi.de
www: http://www.tzi.de/~visser/

Prof. Dr. I. Wachsmuth Arbeitsgruppe Wissensbasierte Systeme ; Technische Fakultät
; Universität Bielefeld
phone: +49 (0)521 / 106 2924 (-6999)
email: ipke@techfak.uni-bielefeld.de
www: http://www.TechFak.Uni-Bielefeld.DE/techfak/persons/ipke/

Author Index

Springer
and the
environment

At Springer we firmly believe that an international science publisher has a special obligation to the environment, and our corporate policies consistently reflect this conviction.
We also expect our business partners – paper mills, printers, packaging manufacturers, etc. – to commit themselves to using materials and production processes that do not harm the environment. The paper in this book is made from low- or no-chlorine pulp and is acid free, in conformance with international standards for paper permanency.

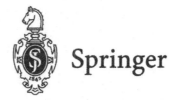 Springer

Lecture Notes in Artificial Intelligence (LNAI)

Lecture Notes in Computer Science